MASTER THE BOARDS
USMLE™ Step 2 CK

RELATED TITLES

Other products by Conrad Fischer, MD

USMLE Medical Ethics*

Master the Boards USMLE Step 3*

USMLE Diagnostic Test Flashcards*

USMLE Examination Flashcards*
The 200 "Most Likely Diagnosis" Questions You will See on the Exam for Steps 2 and 3

USMLE Pharmacology and Treatment Flashcards*

USMLE Physical Findings Flashcards*

Master the Boards: Internal Medicine

Internal Medicine Question Book

Applications for iPhone

Dr. Conrad Fischer's USMLE Disease Deck

*Also available in eBook format

MASTER THE BOARDS
USMLE™ Step 2 CK

Conrad Fischer, MD

—Kaplan's award-winning medical educator, teaching and mentoring tomorrow's leaders in medicine

© 2011 by Conrad Fischer, Inc.

The authors of the following sections have granted Conrad Fischer, MD, and Kaplan Publishing exclusive use of their work:
Elizabeth V. August, MD: Section 6, Obstetrics and Gynecology
Alina Gonzalez-Mayo, MD: Section 9, Psychiatry
Niket Sonpal, MD: Section 4, Surgery and Section 5, Pediatrics

Published by Kaplan Publishing, a division of Kaplan, Inc.
395 Hudson Street
New York, NY 10014

Printed in the United States of America

10 9 8 7 6 5

ISBN-13: 978-1-60714-653-7

Kaplan Publishing books are available at special quantity discounts to use for sales promotions, employee premiums, or educational purposes. For more information or to purchase books, please call the Simon & Schuster special sales department at 866-506-1949.

DEDICATION

This book is dedicated to:

Maureen McMahon,

President, Kaplan Publishing

Maureen is a consummate professional for whom I have the highest possible respect.

Maureen, you are the GREATEST ever! I can't tell you how much I appreciate your personal caretaking of all of my creative work and how lucky I feel to have the chance to collaborate with you.

ACKNOWLEDGMENTS

The author wishes to acknowledge, with gratitude, the support of his chief of service, **Dr. Thomas Santucci, MD**, Chairman, Department of Medicine, Jamaica Hospital Medical Center, whose constant warmth, devotion to patients, and decency have sustained this corner of Queens, New York, the hub of the world, these many years; and **Mr. Howard Rosen**, Administrator, Department of Medicine, who always keeps what really matters in sight.

Elizabeth August wishes to acknowledge Professor Edward C. August, Mrs. Donna M. August, and Eric D. August for their love, generosity, and unwavering support. Without them, my dreams would not be a reality. Dr. August also wishes to acknowledge Robert D. Biagiotti, who is my inspiration.

Niket Sonpal wishes to acknowledge Mr. Navin Sonpal, Mahendra Patel, Raj Patel, and Dr. Mukul Arya for their unwavering support, hope, and stance by me through thick and thin. Without them my path to becoming a physician would not have been possible.

The authors wish to acknowledge the expert attention to detail of Dr. Ana Franceschi.

About the Author

Conrad Fischer, MD, is Director of Educational Development for the Department of Medicine at Jamaica Hospital Medical Center in New York City. Dr. Fischer is also Chairman of Medicine for Kaplan Medical, teaching USMLE Step 2 and 3, Internal Medicine Board Review and Attending Recertification, and USMLE Step 1 Physiology. Jamaica Hospital is a robust window on the world of medicine. Dr. Fischer is responsible for advancing the scholarly environment at the hospital, expanding research and publications, and launching subspecialty fellowships.

Section Authors

Elizabeth V. August, MD, author of Obstetrics and Gynecology sections, is a resident of family medicine at the University of Medicine and Dentistry of New Jersey, Hoboken University Medical Center, in Hoboken, New Jersey.

Alina Gonzalez-Mayo, MD, author of Psychiatry sections, is a psychiatrist at Bay Pines VA Medical Center in Bay Pines, Florida.

Niket Sonpal, MD, author of Surgery and Pediatrics sections, is a house staff member of the department of internal medicine at Lenox Hill Hospital in New York, New York.

SECTION EDITORS

The author expresses his appreciation to the:

Faculty of the Department of Medicine at Jamaica Hospital Medical Center for assuring the accuracy of each of the following sections:

Cardiology: Rajpal Manchandani, MD; Mohammed Uddin, MD

Endocrinology: Richard Pinsker, MD

Ethics: Sudheer Chauhan, MD

Gastroenterology: Asit Mehta, MD; Avani Patel, MD

Hematology: Kaushik Doshi, MD; Alireza Eghtedar, MD

Infectious Diseases: Farshad Bagheri, MD

Nephrology: Parenkumar Patel, MD; Dhaval Satani, MD

Neurology: Mohammed Maruf, MD

Oncology: Kaushik Doshi, MD

Preventive Medicine: Ayaz Alwani, MD; Naveen Pathak, MD

Pulmonary: Craig Thurm, MD; Mohammad Babury, MD; Mahendra C. Patel, MD; Artur Shalonov, MD; Samir Sarkar, MD

Radiology: Sabiha Raouf, MD

Rheumatology: Jebun Nahar, MD; Prakashkumar Patel, MD

KAPLAN MEDICAL EXPERT REVIEW PANEL

TABLE OF CONTENTS

AUTHOR'S NOTE

Master the Boards: Step 2 CK is a complete book for your preparation for USMLE Step 2 CK. You do not need to use other books. As an educator, I get asked a lot of questions on the best way to prep. Here's the question I hear most: "Is this enough?" The answer to that question is a definite "yes!" Additional materials will still help you to reinforce what you have learned, but this is a smart first step to Step 2 CK success. Another question I get is about how to maximize medical knowledge. The best preparation for Step 2 CK is to learn more medicine.

YOUR GUIDE TO THE USMLE

Frequently, medical students wonder when they should take Step 2 CK. Well, the answer to this question depends on your background and level of knowledge. There is no requirement to have to take Step 1 before you take Step 2 CK, although for U.S. graduates, this is almost certainly what happens. Remember, U.S. graduates do not have to take Step 2 CK in order to participate in the annual residency match. International graduates must take Step 2 CK to be ECFMG certified. ECFMG certification is required for international graduates in order to be in the match.

For the vast majority of U.S. medical students, USMLE Step 1 is generally taken at the end of the second year of medical school. Some schools will, in fact, require passage of Step 1 in order to be allowed promotion into the third year of school and to participate in clinical rotations. For some international schools, particularly those in the Caribbean in which virtually the entirety of the class is headed for residency in the United States, they will follow this pattern as well.

Timing can be a factor for some U.S. graduates, too. For example, if you have a great grade on USMLE Step 1 and you are applying to a moderately competitive specialty, you may want to consider delaying your Step 2 CK examination until after you have applied and interviewed for residency. For instance, if you have a 250 or 260 on Step 1 and you get a 240 on Step 2 CK, it makes you look bad. If you are applying in Internal Medicine, or Psychiatry or Pediatrics, I do not think this helped you. If, however, you got a 220 on Step 1 then the same grade of 240 makes you look better. However, if you are applying to Ophthalmology, Dermatology, Orthopedics or a very competitive specialty, you will need to establish high grades on both Step 1 and Step 2 CK to gain credibility. The bottom line is, if you are a U.S. student with a high score on

Step 1 and do not absolutely need a great grade on Step 2 CK to get in, then why chance it? Wait until February or March or April of your fourth year when you are past the application process.

RESIDENCY AND USMLE

Here's another frequently asked question: How late can I take Step 2 CK and still be competitive in the Match? The Electronic Residency Application Service (ERAS) opens for applications at the beginning of September. To be competitive, you should plan on having your application complete by the end of September. You may think that the program directors are sitting in their offices over Labor Day weekend waiting for applications to come in over ERAS so they can give out interviews. This is not true. Remember that many programs will not consider an application "complete" until they have received the "Dean's letter." Often, the Dean's letter does not go out from the U.S. schools until October and in some cases, November. However, if you are an international graduate, they will not be waiting for the Dean's letters to arrive since the majority of international schools do not have this concept.

▶ TIP

Do not take the exam before you are ready. You cannot retake Step 2 CK if you pass with a poor grade. It is better to delay to prepare more than to take the exam ill-prepared.

If you think it is better to fail than to pass with a low grade, you are wrong. **You cannot hide the grade on previous attempts at Step 2 CK.** It is better to delay your test than to risk a lower grade. Unfortunately, it is true that if you wait to take Step 2 CK until November or December, you will lose interview spots. However, if you take the test prematurely and fail or pass with a minimal score, that grade will follow you around through your entire application process. I would go so far as to say that **it would be better to sit out a year and fully prepare than take a chance on a failing or low grade**.

Students often wonder, "Is Step 1 or Step 2 CK more important to my future? Again, the answer to this question may depend on your background. For U.S. graduates, Step 1 is often the more important examination because that is the only test result that is submitted with your ERAS application for residency. There is no intrinsic superiority of either examination. Program directors will be split in their opinion on this question. Step 1 may be perceived as a "harder" examination, however, the pass rate for first-time U.S. graduate test takers is about 93%. On the other hand, for many clinically oriented specialties, the perception may be that your performance on a clinically oriented examination such as Step 2 CK is more important than an examination more oriented to basic sciences. **For international graduates, Step 1 and Step 2 CK are generally of equal importance since the program directors will see both grades.**

WHAT DO PROGRAM DIRECTORS LOOK FOR?

Program directors all agree on a few important criteria:

- **Where did you go to school?**
- USMLE scores
- **Transcript** and Dean's letter for U.S. graduates
- **Visa status** for international graduates

Other criteria such as research, publications, letters of recommendation, extra-curricular activities, and the personal statement are much harder to define and are not universally valued. Some programs may highly prize research, some may not even look at your publications until after you arrive for an interview. The personal statement often has no value because it says nothing personal or original about you at all. Letters of recommendation often all sound the same.

> USMLE is the only worldwide, uniform measure across schools.

The reason that **USMLE carries such importance is because it is the only worldwide uniform measure across schools**. If you are a U.S. medical student, how do you prove to a program director that you have greater value than a student applying from a school with a very highly prized and famous name? Your USMLE score may be the only thing that gives you an edge. If you are indeed from a school with a highly prized and famous name, **how do you prove that you are a better applicant than another candidate from a similarly highly prized and famous name school?** The answer is your transcript and your USMLE score. If you are an international graduate, how do you overcome the fact that you need a visa or perhaps you are applying as an older graduate? The answer is the same: USMLE.

Is this fair? Is it right? The system is generally fair. **The test taken by U.S. and international graduates is the same.** The test is **not** graded on a curve. That means that theoretically, everyone taking the test on a particular day could get a 99. Whether or not you think it's right, one thing we know for sure is that the USMLE is of colossal importance to your professional future.

Nothing makes a student more anxious than the programmatic requirement for "United States Clinical Experience." The truth is, unless you are at an international school that is specifically geared to return you to the United States, **you are often simply not going to be able to get this U.S. experience. Do not worry!**

Many, many future doctors obtain residency each year as international graduates without U.S. clinical experience. A high score on Step 2 CK is also far more valuable than some "fake" experience where you "hang around" an office. How is "observing" measurable? What did you do there? I know you will get anxious about this. If you can get meaningful U.S. experience, that's great, however, **a higher score on Step 2 CK is always valuable.** An "observership" or "externship" is of extremely inconclusive value.

HOW DOES AN APPLICANT LOOK TO A PROGRAM DIRECTOR?

After separating applicants into groups based on where they went to school and for international graduates their visa status, the program director often has no readily quantifiable way to assess the applicant. There is enormous pressure to make sure that the pool he or she selects into the residency is highly qualified. Research, **observerships, and clinical grades are hard to measure.** Is one school a harder grader than another? Does one school practice grade inflation so that all the transcripts show high grades? Does another school fail many students to prove they are serious? These are all factors that may be considered. Take time to understand how your credentials stack up.

WHAT IF I FAILED?

The best way to show that your failure on Step 2 CK is not an accurate measure of your ability, knowledge, or intelligence is to **pass with a very high score when you DO pass.** If you failed Step 1, there is a lot riding on your Step 2 CK grade. This book is constructed to help you pass. Take your time. **Study day and night.** If you need more practice, use question banks to prepare and assess your knowledge base. If necessary, delay the exam until you are ready. Several years ago, the size of incoming classes in United States medical schools started to increase after more than 30 years with the same class size. In addition, **many new schools are opening.** This has enormous impact on both U.S. and international graduates. In many specialties, simply being a U.S. graduate automatically put you in the top half of the applicant pool. That is no longer true. **The incoming class size for U.S. schools will be increasing by several hundred every year for the next several years.** This will increase the competition for everyone trying to get a good residency position.

United States medical students pass Step 2 CK at a rate of approximately 93%, doctors of osteopathy (DO) pass at a rate of about 87%, and international graduates pass at a rate of approximately 80%.

YOUR FINAL STEP

You have worked very hard to get into medical school and to do well there. This is your last step. A great score on Step 2 CK will mean that all of your professional dreams in medicine are about to come true. Success on Step 2 CK will enormously influence what specialty and at what kind of training program you match into. Your best bet is to invest the time and energy required to ensure you get a high score.

Now is not the time to spare yourself. **You can rest later.** Now is the time to learn everything in this book. Practice hard and remember that everything you are learning here is medicine. It will help people. A high grade on Step 2 CK is not a phony numerical statistic. What you are learning here will, with 100% certainty, help someone. You will save lives. You will relieve suffering. You will do good for humanity. It is with this emotional power that you should go forth to work hard and to test the limits of your endurance. **Do not spare yourself.** Through your work, someone will be saved and protected through what you learn here. These are not superfluous facts.

What you learn here, through your heart and mind and the power of your hands will protect those who suffer in their hour of need.

I wish you well in your quest. If you see what you are learning here as "as bunch of stuff to cram in that you will forget," you will not get as good a grade and the information will quickly fade. If you can study knowing that a sick person that you have not yet met is depending on you, their very life is depending on you, then you will absorb this energy and make the studying you must do a sense of devotion.

We, you and I, commit ourselves at this moment to our sacred calling. To offer humanity the best of our art, and to **put the needs of others above our own needs**, now and always.

Dr. Conrad Fischer

August 2010

HOW TO USE THIS BOOK

Congratulations! By studying for your Step 2 CK exam, you are well on your way to becoming a doctor. This book contains information to help you perform well on the test and target areas of study. *Master the Boards USMLE Step 2 CK* offers a complete outline for Step 2 CK preparation in a convenient, colorful format. For many medical students, this book may be all the review you need, since your concurrent medical training offers hands-on learning opportunities to reinforce the medical principles and best practices tested on the USMLE.

Depending on how well you recall the topics in any given section of this book, you will be able to customize your study appropriately. For example, if you find yourself not recalling some major topics in the cardiology section, go back and review your primary texts, and consider supplementing with question banks and practice questions. Some students like to use a Master the Boards book before taking an in-depth live course, or to recap the content after the course concludes. The content in this book is not identical to the Kaplan Medical live classroom course books, but they work well to complement each other.

This book contains exam-style questions and it offers the opportunity to test your knowledge as you review. The answer explanations are another way to reinforce knowledge. Therefore, this book can be used in tandem with Kaplan Medical's USMLE qBooks and question banks or any other case studies program.

The Master the Boards series is arranged by medical specialty. Each section contains:

- Tips for recognizing incorrect answers
- Mini cases with detailed answer explanations to reinforce learning
- Full-color images of relevant items from the text

ABOUT THE USMLE STEP 2 CK

The USMLE Step 2 CK (Clinical Knowledge) is typically taken as the second test in a series of three national certifying examinations that are necessary to obtain a license to practice medicine in the United States. **Step 2 CK is usually taken between the end of the third year of medical school and the end of the fourth year.** How is Step 2 CK different than Step 1? Generally speaking, Step 2 CK is more clinically based than Step 1. Although there is no requirement to take Step 1 before Step 2 CK, this is the typical sequence for U.S. graduates. According to the test maker, the questions on Step 2 CK measure the ability to apply medical knowledge, skills, and understanding of clinical science as they pertain to patient care (under supervision), with emphasis on health promotion and disease prevention. Clinical Knowledge is one of two components of Step 2; the other, Clinical Skills (CS), uses model patients to test the ability to perform in a real clinical setting. Step 2 CK provides the foundation for the safe and effective practice of medicine by future medical doctors.

Results of the USMLE are reported to medical licensing authorities in the United States and its territories for use in granting the initial license to practice medicine. The sponsors of the USMLE are the Federation of State Medical Boards (FSMB) and the National Board of Medical Examiners (NBME).

ABOUT THE USMLE STEP 2 CK: EXAM BLUEPRINT

USMLE Step 2 CK is a computer-based test that consists of 352 questions taken over a 9-hour period. The test is divided into 8 blocks, each of which lasts 60 minutes. Once you have completed a block or your 60 minutes has run out, you will not be able to go back and review or change any of your work on that block. You will have 45 minutes of break time, which is used to transition between blocks and for longer breaks that require you to leave your seat (i.e., authorized breaks). The computer keeps track of your break time. You must be sure not to exceed the 45 minutes or you will be penalized by having any overage break time taken from the 60 minutes allotted for the last block of the test.

Structure of Step 2 CK Questions

The majority of Step 2 CK questions are single best answer (multiple-choice) questions with a clinical vignette followed by a question. The basic structure is:

- History of present illness
- Physical examination
- Possibly laboratory and radiologic tests

Here are the basic Step 2 CK question types, and consequently, the very structure around which this book is created.

1. What is the **most likely diagnosis**?
2. What is the **best initial diagnostic test**?
3. What is the **most accurate diagnostic test**?
4. Which physical finding is most likely to be associated with this patient?
5. What is the **best initial therapy**?

When the question reads: "What is the most appropriate **next step** in the management of this patient?" this can refer to **either a test or a treatment**. The phrase, *most appropriate next step* can also be referred to as *action,* *management,* or simply *what should you do next*? In all of these cases, the words *step, action, do*, or *management* can mean **either a test or a treatment**.

The most frequently asked question on Step 2 CK is "**What is the most likely diagnosis?**" As a result, many of the chapters in this book have a specific section labeled "What is the most likely diagnosis?" One of the many unique attributes of the Master the Boards format is that the diseases are presented with the specific goal of answering these questions.

Sequential Questions and Matching

A smaller number of Step 2 CK questions are sequential. This means you can have multiple questions following a single clinical story or vignette. Once you answer the first question, you will not be able to go back to the original question. This is because the second and third questions may give a clue to the answer to the first question. Some of the questions in the sequence are essentially matching questions. This means there are between 4 and 26 separate answers, and several cases may use the same answers. The answers can be used once, more than once, or not at all.

> The best preparation for Step 2 CK is to learn more medicine.

USMLE REGISTRATION

Depending on your situation, the registration process will differ. For the most accurate and up-to-date information about registration and test day procedures, go to http://www.usmle.org. At the time of publication, the registration fee is $740.

ON THE DAY OF THE EXAM

1. Arrive at the test center at least 30 minutes before your scheduled testing time to allow for check-in. If you arrive late, you may not be permitted to take the exam. If you arrive more than 30 minutes after your scheduled test time, you will not be permitted to take the exam.

2. You **must** bring your scheduling permit and an acceptable, **unexpired** form of identification with a recent (within the last 10 years) photograph. Acceptable forms of identification include a passport, a driver's license with photograph, a national identity card, another type of government-issued identification with a recent photograph, or an identification card issued by the *Educational Commission for Foreign Medical Graduates* (ECFMG). Identification without a signature must be supported by a separate unexpired form of identification such as a credit card with a signature.

> U.S. medical graduates do not have to take Step 2 CK in order to participate in the annual residency match. However, international medical graduates **must** take Step 2 CK to be certified by the *Educational Commission for Foreign Medical Graduates*. ECFMG certification is required for international graduates in order to participate in the match.

SCORING

Score Reporting

When you finish taking Step 2 CK, your answers are recorded for scoring. Your correct answers are converted to a 3-digit score (as of publication, typically between 140 and 260) and a 2-digit score. The 2-digit score is calculated based on your 3-digit score. The 2-digit score is always calculated so that 75 is the minimum passing score; this is because some licensing boards mention a "passing score of 75." Score reports and transcripts will show your 2-digit score, your 3-digit score, and either "Pass" or "Fail." Score reports, not transcripts, also show how you did on certain topics on the exam. This will help you assess your strengths and weaknesses as you move forward with your studies.

A Passing Score

At the time of publication, the 3-digit passing score was 184. **The 3-digit passing score does and will increase over time.** This is for a very simple reason: Current medical students continue to improve their knowledge. The average score is currently 220. This will also rise as students improve their knowledge. The 2-digit passing score is always 75 and will not change, although the 3-digit score corresponding to a 75 rises. As aforementioned, this is because several states have written into their laws that the requirement for a license is a "passing score of 75."

You must answer between 60% and 70% of questions correctly in order to get a passing score. There are always a number of new or experimental questions on each exam to test new questions for future exams. Every attempt is made to keep the exam fair and to allow the test to serve as an accurate measure of your knowledge level.

Good Luck!

SECTION 1
INTERNAL MEDICINE

INFECTIOUS DISEASES   1

INTRODUCTION TO ANTIBIOTICS

The organisms associated with particular diseases do not change over time, but the antibiotics that treat the infections can change. The single most important thing for you to learn in infectious diseases is the antibiotics that are associated with each group of organisms.

Principles of Answering Infectious Diseases Questions

1. The radiologic test is never "the most accurate test."
2. Risk factors for an infection are not as important as the individual presentation.
3. Beta-lactam antibiotics have greater efficacy than other classes.

Beta-lactam Antibiotics: Penicillins, Cephalosporins, Carbapenems, Aztreonam

Penicillins

Penicillin (G, VK, benzathine): viridans group streptococci, *Streptococcus pyogenes*, oral anaerobes, syphilis, *Leptospira*

Ampicillin and amoxicillin: cover the same organisms as penicillin, as well as *E. coli*, Lyme disease, and a few other gram-negative bacilli.

Gram-negative bacteria covered by amoxicillin:

(HELPS)

***H. influenzae*, *E. coli*, *Listeria*, *Proteus*, and *Salmonella*.**

→ *Ampicillin | Amoxicillin*

They are the "best initial therapy" for:

- Otitis media
- Dental infection and endocarditis prophylaxis
- Lyme disease limited to rash, joint, or seventh cranial nerve involvement
- Urinary tract infection (UTI) in pregnant women
- *Listeria monocytogenes*
- Enterococcal infections

→ Penicillinase-resistant penicillins (PRPs): oxacillin, cloxacillin, dicloxacillin, and nafcillin.

These drugs are used to treat:

- Skin infections: cellulitis, impetigo, erysipelas
- Endocarditis, meningitis, and bacteremia from staphylococci
- Osteomyelitis and septic arthritis only when the organism is proven sensitive

They are not active against methicillin-resistant *Staphylococcus aureus* (MRSA) or *Enterococcus*.

> **Methicillin sensitive or resistant really means oxacillin sensitive or resistant.**

▶ **TIP**

Methicillin is never the right answer. It causes renal failure from allergic interstitial nephritis.

Piperacillin, ticarcillin, azlocillin, mezlocillin: These agents cover gram-negative bacilli (eg, *E. coli*, *Proteus*) from the large enterobacteriaciae group as well as pseudomonads. They are the "best initial therapy" for:

- Cholecystitis and ascending cholangitis
- Pyelonephritis
- Bacteremia
- Hospital-acquired and ventilator-associated pneumonia
- Neutropenia and fever

Although these agents cover streptococci and anaerobes, they are not the answer when the infection is exclusively from these single organisms. You would use a narrower agent. They are nearly always used in combination with a beta-lactamase inhibitor such as tazobactam or clavulanic acid.

Cephalosporins

> *Listeria*, MRSA, and *Enterococcus* are resistant to all forms of cephalosporins.

The amount of cross-reaction between penicillin and cephalosporins is very small (3% to 5%). All cephalosporins, in every class, will cover group A, B, and C streptococci, viridans group streptococci, *E. coli*, *Klebsiella*, and *Proteus mirabilis*.

▶ **TIP**

If the case describes a <u>rash</u> to penicillin: Answer **cephalosporins**.

If the case describes **anaphylaxis**, you must use a **non-beta-lactam antibiotic.**

RASH TO PEN = CEPHALOSPORINS

ANAPHYLAXIS = NON-BETA-LACTAM

First Generation: Cefazolin, Cephalexin, Cephradrine, Cefadroxyl

First-generation cephalosporins are used to treat:

- Staphylococci: **methicillin sensitive = oxacillin sensitive = cephalosporin sensitive**
- Streptococci (except *Enterococcus*)
- Some gram-negative bacilli such as *E. coli*, but not *Pseudomonas*
- Osteomyelitis, septic arthritis, endocarditis, cellulitis

Second Generation: Cefotetan, Cefoxitin, Cefaclor, Cefprozil, Cefuroxime, Loracarbef

These agents cover all the same organisms as first-generation cephalosporins and add coverage for anaerobes and more gram-negative bacilli.

- Cefotetan or cefoxitin: Best initial therapy for pelvic inflammatory disease (PID) combined with doxycycline. Warning: Cefotetan and cefoxitin increase the risk of bleeding and give a disulfiramlike reaction with alcohol.
- Cefuroxime, loracarbef, cefprozil, cefaclor: Respiratory infections such as bronchitis, otitis media, and sinusitis.

Third Generation: Ceftriaxone, Cefotaxime, Ceftazidime

- Ceftriaxone: First-line for pneumococcus, including partially insensitive organisms
  - Meningitis
  - Community-acquired pneumonia (in combination with macrolides)
  - Gonorrhea
  - Lyme involving the heart or brain
- **Avoid ceftriaxone in neonates** because of impaired biliary metabolism.
- Cefotaxime
  - Superior to ceftriaxone in neonates
  - Spontaneous bacterial peritonitis
- **Ceftazidime has pseudomonal coverage**.

Fourth Generation: Cefepime

Cefepime has better staphylococcal coverage compared with the third-generation cephalosporins. It is used to treat:

- Neutropenia and fever
- Ventilator-associated pneumonia

Adverse Effects of Cephalosporins

Cefoxitin and cefotetan deplete prothrombin and increase risk of bleeding.

With ceftriaxone, there is inadequate biliary metabolism.

Carbapenems (Imipenem, Meropenem, Ertapenem, Doripenem)

Carbapenems cover gram-negative bacilli, including many that are resistant, anaerobes, streptococci, and staphylococci. They are used to treat neutropenia and fever.

> Ertapenem differs from the other carbapenems. Ertapenem does not cover *Pseudomonas*.

Aztreonam

This is the only drug in the class of monobactams.

- Exclusively for **gram-negative** bacilli including *Pseudomonas*
- **No cross-reaction with penicillin**

Fluoroquinolones (Ciprofloxacin, Gemifloxacin, Levofloxacin, Moxifloxacin)

- Best therapy for **community-acquired pneumonia**, including penicillin-resistant pneumococcus
- Gram-negative bacilli including most pseudomonads
- **Ciprofloxacin for cystitis** and pyelonephritis. Moxifloxacin will not enter the urine in high enough concentrations to treat cystitis.
- Diverticulitis and GI infections, but ciprofloxacin, gemifloxacin, and levofloxacin must be combined with metronidazole because they don't cover anaerobes except for moxifloxacin. **Moxifloxacin can be used as a single agent for diverticulitis** and does not need metronidazole.

Quinolones cause:

- **Bone growth abnormalities** in children and pregnant women
- **Tendonitis** and Achilles tendon rupture
- Gatifloxacin removed because of glucose abnormalities

Aminoglycosides (Gentamicin, Tobramycin, Amikacin)

- Gram-negative bacilli (bowel, urine, bacteremia)
- Synergistic with beta-lactam antibiotics for enterococci and staphylococci

- **No effect against anaerobes**, since they need oxygen to work
- **Nephrotoxic** and **ototoxic**

Doxycycline

- *Chlamydia*
- Lyme disease limited to rash, joint, or seventh cranial nerve palsy
- *Rickettsia*
- Primary and secondary syphilis in those allergic to penicillin
- *Borrelia, Ehrlichia*, and *Mycoplasma*
- Adverse effects: tooth discoloration (children), Fanconi syndrome (Type II RTA proximal), photosensitivity, esophagitis/ulcer

> Nitrofurantoin has one indication: cystitis, especially in pregnant women.

Trimethoprim/Sulfamethoxazole

- Cystitis
- Pneumocystis pneumonia treatment and prophylaxis
- MRSA of skin and soft tissue (cellulitis)
- Besides **rash**, it causes **hemolysis** with G6 PD deficiency and **bone marrow suppression** because it is a **folate antagonist**.

Beta-lactam/Beta-lactamase Combinations

- Amoxicillin/clavulanate
- Ticarcillin/clavulanate
- Ampicillin/sulbactam
- Piperacillin/tazobactam

Beta-lactamase adds coverage against sensitive staphylococci to these agents.

Specific Organism Groups and Their Treatments

Gram-positive Cocci: Staphylococci and Streptococci

The best initial therapy for gram-positive organisms are:

- Oxacillin, cloxacillin, dicloxacillin, nafcillin
- First-generation cephalosporins: cefazolin, cephalexin
- Fluoroquinolones
- Macrolides (azithromycin, clarithromycin, erythromycin) are third-line agents because they have less efficacy than oxacillin or cephalosporins. Erythromycin is also more toxic.

Oxacillin (Methicillin)-Resistant *Staphylococcus*

These are best treated with:

- Vancomycin
- Linezolid: reversible bone marrow toxicity

- Daptomycin: elevated CPK
- Tigecycline

Minor MRSA infections of the skin are treated with:

- TMP/SMX
- Clindamycin
- Doxycycline

Anaerobes

Oral (above the diaphragm)

- Penicillin (G, VK, ampicillin, amoxicillin)
- Clindamycin

Abdominal/gastrointestinal

- Metronidazole

Piperacillin, carbapenems, and second-generation cephalosporins also cover anaerobes.

Gram-Negative Bacilli *(E. coli, Klebsiella, Proteus, Pseudomonas, Enterobacter, Citrobacter)*

These organisms cause infections of the bowel (peritonitis, diverticulitis); urinary tract (pyelonephritis); and liver (cholecystitis, cholangitis).

All of these agents cover gram-negative bacilli:

- Quinolones
- Aminoglycosides
- Carbapenems
- Piperacillin, ticarcillin
- Aztreonam
- Cephalosporins

A man is admitted with E. coli bacteremia.

Which of the following is the most appropriate therapy?

a. Vancomycin
b. Linezolid
c. Quinolones, aminoglycosides, carbapenems, piperacillin, ticarcillin, or aztreonam
d. Doxycycline
e. Clindamycin
f. Oxacillin

*Answer: The correct answer is **(C)**. **All of the agents** listed under "Gram-Negative Bacilli" could be the right answer. It is like an IQ test: "Which of these is different from the other choices?" Choice **(C)** would be the only one covering gram-negative bacilli.*

CENTRAL NERVOUS SYSTEM INFECTIONS

All central nervous system (CNS) infections **may** present with fever, headache, nausea, and vomiting. All of them can lead to seizures.

[Handwritten margin note: FEVER / HA / NAUSEA / VOMITING]

Clues to Answering the "Most Likely Diagnosis" Question	
Symptom	**Diagnosis**
Stiff neck, photophobia, meningismus	Meningitis
Confusion	Encephalitis
Focal neurological findings	Abscess

Meningitis

DEFINITION/ETIOLOGY

Meningitis is an infection or inflammation of the covering or **meninges** of the central nervous system. Virtually any infection could cause this, but *Streptococcus pneumonia* (60%), group B streptococci (14%), *Haemophilus influenzae* (7%), *Neisseria meningitidis* (15%), and *Listeria* (2%) account for over 95% of cases. *Staphylococcus* occurs in those with recent neurosurgery.

[Handwritten margin note: IN NEONATE / -E. coli / -GROUP B STREP / -LISTERIA / -HERPES → AMP & GENT (+ CEFOTAXIME + VANC) / CEFTRI + VANC / + DEXAMETHASONE]

PRESENTATION

Look for a **fever, headache, neck stiffness** (nuchal rigidity), and **photophobia**. Acute bacterial meningitis presents over several hours. Focal neurological abnormalities occur in up to 30% of patients. If confusion occurs, you will not be able to answer "What is the most likely diagnosis?" without a CT and lumbar puncture (LP). Cryptococcal meningitis may be present for several weeks.

Organism Specific Presentations/"What is the Most Likely Diagnosis?"	
Presentation	**The most likely diagnosis is...**
AIDS with <100 CD4 cells/μl	*Cryptococcus*
Camper/hiker, **rash shaped like a target**, joint pain, facial palsy, tick remembered in **20%**	Lyme disease
Camper/hiker, rash **moves from arms/legs to trunk**, tick remembered in **60%**	Rocky Mountain spotted fever (*Rickettsia*)
Pulmonary TB in 85%	Tuberculosis
None	Viral
Adolescent, petechial rash	*Neisseria*

[Handwritten margin note: → ENTEROVIRUSES COXSACKIE]

DIAGNOSTIC TESTS

The best initial test and most accurate test is an LP.

CAN SEE HYPONATREMIA IS A SIGN

Cerebrospinal Fluid Evaluation				
	Bacterial meningitis	Cryptococcus, Lyme, Rickettsia	Tuberculosis	Viral
Cell count	1000s, neutrophils	10s–100s lymphocytes	10s–100s lymphocytes	10s–100s lymphocytes
Protein level	Elevated	Possibly elevated	Markedly elevated	Usually normal
Glucose level	Decreased	Possibly decreased	May be low	Usually normal
Stain and culture	Stain: 50–70%; culture: 90%	Negative	Negative	Negative

NML
<5
20-45
40-70
Pressure 50-180

When Is a Head CT the Best Initial Test?

Head CT is necessary prior to an LP only if there is the possibility that a space-occupying lesion may cause herniation. Answer **head CT first** when any of the following is present:

- **Papilledema**
- **Seizures**
- **Focal** neurological abnormalities
- **Confusion** interfering with the neurological examination

Blurred disc margin

Figure 1.1: Papilledema is a blurred, fuzzy disc margin from increased intracranial pressure. *Source: Conrad Fischer, MD*

In order to be accurate, a neurological examination needs a cooperative patient who can understand and follow instructions and answer questions.

> You cannot do an accurate neurological examination if the patient is severely confused.

> Better to treat and decrease the accuracy of a test than to risk permanent brain damage.

▶ **TIP**

If there is a contraindication to **immediate** LP, giving antibiotics is the best initial step in management.

Bacterial Antigen Detection (Latex Agglutination Tests)

These tests are similar to a Gram stain. If antigen detection methods are positive, they are extremely specific. If they are negative, the person could still have the infection. These tests by themselves are not sufficiently sensitive to exclude bacterial meningitis.

When is a bacterial antigen test indicated? When the patient has received antibiotics prior to the LP and the culture may be falsely negative.

Organism Specific Diagnostic Tests/"What is the Most Accurate Diagnostic Test?"

Tuberculosis: Acid fast stain and culture on 3 high-volume lumbar punctures. Centrifuge the specimen to concentrate the organisms. TB has the highest cerebrospinal fluid (CSF) protein level. An acid fast stain of a single, uncentrifuged sample of CSF has only 10% sensitivity.

Lyme and *Rickettsia*: Specific serologic testing, ELISA, western blot, PCR.

Cryptococcus: India ink is 60% to 70% sensitive. Cryptococcal antigen is more than 95% sensitive and specific.

Viral: Generally a diagnosis of exclusion.

TREATMENT

The best initial treatment for bacterial meningitis is ceftriaxone, vancomycin, and steroids. **You will base your treatment answer on the cell count**. Culture takes 2 to 3 days and is never available at the time that a treatment decision is made. **Gram stain is good if it is positive**; however, the false negative rate is 30% to 50%. **Protein and glucose levels are too nonspecific to allow for a treatment decision**.

Although steroids (dexamethasone) have been proven to lower mortality only in *S. pneumoniae* infection, you must give them when you see thousands of neutrophils because you will not know the culture results for several days.

> Thousands of neutrophils on CSF = ceftriaxone, vancomycin, and steroids. Add ampicillin if immunocompromised for *Listeria*.

Listeria Monocytogenes

Listeria is **resistant to all cephalosporins but** sensitive to penicillins. You must add ampicillin to ceftriaxone and vancomycin if the case describes risk factors for *Listeria*. These risk factors are:

- Elderly
- Neonates
- Steroid use
- AIDS or HIV
- Immunocompromised, including alcoholism
- Pregnant

ACETOMENOPHEN / IVF / Abx UNTIL BACTERIAL RULED OUT FOR VIRAL

INTRATHECAL AMPHOTERICIN B FOR FUNGAL

R.I.P.E. FOR TB

Neisseria meningitidis: Additional Management

- Respiratory isolation
- Rifampin or ciprofloxacin to the close contacts to decrease nasopharyngeal carriage
  - "**Close contacts**" means those who have major respiratory fluid contact, such as **household contacts**, **kissing**, or **sharing cigarettes** or **eating** utensils.
  - Routine school and work contacts are not close contacts. Sitting in class with someone with *Neisseria* infection does not make them a close contact.
  - Healthcare workers qualify only if they intubate the patient, perform suctioning, or have contact with respiratory secretions.

A man comes to the emergency department with fever, severe headache, neck stiffness, and photophobia. On physical examination he is found to have weakness of his left arm and leg. What is the most appropriate next step in the management of this patient?

a. Ceftriaxone, vancomycin, and steroids
b. Head CT
c. Ceftriaxone
d. Neurology consultation
e. Steroids

Answer: The correct answer is (A). When there is a contraindication to an immediate LP, the most important step is to initiate treatment. Ceftriaxone or steroids alone would not be sufficient. This patient's presentation is clear for meningitis. Although antibiotics may decrease the sensitivity of the CSF culture, it is more important to prevent neurological damage from untreated meningitis than it is to have a specific microbiological diagnosis. You can also still use the Gram stain and bacterial antigen detection methods to establish a diagnosis after the start of antibiotics, although they cannot tell sensitivity patterns. A head CT is important for this patient because of focal neurological deficits, but it is more important to initiate therapy. In addition, if the head CT shows a mass lesion, you may never be able to perform an LP.

▶ **TIP**

Consultation is almost always a wrong answer on USMLE Step 2 CK.

Encephalitis

Look for the **acute** onset of **fever** and **confusion**. Although there are many causes of encephalitis, **herpes simplex is by far the most common cause**. You must do a **head CT first** because of the presence of confusion. ↳ TEMPORAL LOBE

> What is the most common neurological deficit of untreated bacterial meningitis? Eighth cranial nerve deficit or deafness.

[handwritten notes:]
SEIZURES
MR
SPASTIC PARALYSIS
↓
DEXMETHASONE HELPS
AVOID THESE

[handwritten notes:]
WEST NILE VIRUS
LOOKS LIKE FLU IN THE SUMMER
1/150 CASES GET ENCEPHALITIS W/ MUSCLE WEAKNESS & FLACCID PARALYSIS

What is the most accurate test of herpes encephalitis?

a. *Brain biopsy*
b. *PCR of CSF*
c. *MRI*
d. *Viral culture of CSF*
e. *Tzanck prep*
f. *Serology for herpes (IgG, IgM)*

*Answer: The correct answer is **(B)**. **PCR is more accurate than a brain biopsy**. Serology for herpes is useless; 95% of the population will be positive, since blood serology cannot distinguish oral herpes from a routine cold sore, genital herpes, or encephalitis. Tzanck prep can be done as the initial test on a genital ulcerative lesion. Viral culture is the most accurate test of genital or skin lesions, but not of CSF or the brain.*

TREATMENT

Acyclovir is the best initial therapy for herpes encephalitis. Famciclovir and valacyclovir are not available as intravenous formulations. **Foscarnet is used for acyclovir-resistant herpes**.

A woman is admitted for herpes encephalitis confirmed by PCR. After 4 days of acyclovir her creatinine level begins to rise.

What is the most appropriate next step in management?

a. *Stop acyclovir.*
b. *Reduce the dose of acyclovir and hydrate.*
c. *Switch to oral famciclovir or valacyclovir.*
d. *Switch to foscarnet.*

*Answer: The correct answer is **(B)**. Oral medications such as famciclovir and valacyclovir are insufficient for herpes encephalitis. Although acyclovir may occasionally be renal toxic because the medication precipitates in the renal tubules, foscarnet has far more renal toxicity.*

HEAD AND NECK INFECTIONS

Otitis Media

Otitis media presents with redness, immobility, bulging, and a decreased light reflex of the tympanic membrane. Pain is common. Decreased hearing and fever also occur.

Which of the following is the most sensitive physical finding for otitis media?

a. *Redness*
b. *Immobility*
c. *Bulging*
d. *Decreased light reflex*
e. *Decreased hearing*

[Handwritten note:]
REYES SYNDROME (HEPATOENCEPHALITIS)
VOMITING | IRRITABILITY | AGGRESSION | CONFUSION | LETHARGY | COMA
DISCONTINUE SALICYLATES
EUGLYCEMIA
ISOVOLEMIA
IF SEIZURES → PHENYTOIN

*Answer: The correct answer is (B). Immobility is so sensitive a physical finding that a fully mobile tympanic membrane essentially excludes **otitis** media.*

▶ **TIP**

Radiologic tests for otitis are always the wrong answer.

DIAGNOSTIC TESTS/TREATMENT

Tympanocentesis for a sample of fluid for culture is the most accurate diagnostic test. Choose **tympanocentesis** if there are **multiple recurrences** or if there is no response to multiple antibiotics. Amoxicillin is the best initial therapy. If there is no response, or the patient is described as having been recently treated with amoxicillin, the answer is:

- Amoxicillin/clavulanate
- Azithromycin, clarithromycin
- Cefuroxime, loracarbef
- Levofloxacin, gemifloxacin, moxifloxacin

> Quinolones are relatively contraindicated in children.

Handwritten note (left margin): DON'T NECESSARILY MEAN NEED Abx IF GETTING BETTER IN 48 Hours

Sinusitis

A 34-year-old woman presents with facial pain, discolored nasal discharge, bad taste in her mouth, and fever. On physical examination she has facial tenderness.

Which of the following is the most accurate diagnostic test?

a. Sinus biopsy or aspirate
b. CT scan
c. X-ray
d. Culture of the discharge
e. Transillumination

*Answer: The correct answer is (A). Remember that in infectious diseases, the radiologic test is never "the most accurate test." Only a biopsy or aspirate can give you a precise microbiological diagnosis. There is a difference between a question that says "What is the **most accurate** test?" and one that asks "What will you **do**?" CT scan is the most common wrong answer to this question. You cannot stain or culture a CT scan.*

▶ **TIP**

Culture of nasal discharge is always the wrong answer for sinusitis.

Use of Sinus Biopsy or Aspirate

A **biopsy** in sinusitis is needed only if:

- Infection frequently **recurs**.
- There is **no response** to different empiric therapies.

Handwritten note (left margin): SINUSITIS — Sx OF 7 OR MORE DAYS — PURULENT NASAL D/c — MAXILLARY FACIAL PAIN UNILATERAL — WORSENING AFTER INITIAL IMPROVEMENT

Handwritten note (left margin): TREATMENT — TEMP < 101 = No Tx IN HEALTHY PT's — NASAL SALINE IRIGATION — TOPICAL DECONGESTANTS — PSEUDOEPHEDRINE/PHENYLEPHRINE — Abx AMOX 10-14 DAYS CEPH FLOROS MACROLIDES — NASAL STEROIDS IF ALLERGIC CAUSE

Handwritten note (right): IF CHRONIC ORAL STEROIDS Abx - 3-6 WEEKS

A 34-year-old woman presents with facial pain, a discolored nasal discharge, bad taste in her mouth, and fever. On physical examination she has facial tenderness.

What is the most appropriate next step OR action OR management?

a. *Linezolid*
b. *CT scan*
c. *X-ray*
d. *Amoxicillin and a decongestant*
e. *Erythromycin and a decongestant*

Answer: The correct answer is (D). When the diagnosis is as clear as in this case, radiologic testing is unnecessary. Amoxicillin, doxycycline, and trimethoprim/sulfamethoxazole remain first-line therapy for both otitis and sinusitis. The efficacy of these agents is the same as newer or more "broad spectrum" agents such as amoxicillin-clavulanate or quinolones. Imaging is done if the diagnosis is equivocal. A decongestant is used in all cases to promote sinus drainage.

Erythromycin is inadequate because of poorer coverage for Streptococcus pneumoniae. *Linezolid, although excellent for resistant gram-positive organisms, would not cover Haemophilus.*

Pharyngitis

Presents with:

- **Pain** on swallowing
- Enlarged lymph **node** in the neck
- **Exudate** in the pharynx
- Fever
- No cough and no hoarseness

When these features are present, the likelihood of streptococcal pharyngitis exceeds 90%.

DIAGNOSTIC TESTS

The best initial test is the "**rapid strep test**." This is an office/clinic-based test that determines within minutes whether a patient has group A beta hemolytic streptococci. A negative test is considered sufficiently sensitive to exclude disease and no antibiotics are needed.

Positive rapid strep test = positive pharyngeal culture.

- Small vesicles or ulcers: HSV or herpangina
- Membranous exudates: diphtheria, Vincent angina, or EBV

TREATMENT

1. Penicillin or **amoxicillin** is the best initial therapy.
2. Penicillin allergic patients are treated with **cephalexin if the reaction is only a rash**. If the allergy is anaphylaxis, use clindamycin or a macrolide.

> Streptococcal pharyngitis is treated to prevent rheumatic fever.

Influenza (The "Flu")

Influenza presents with:

- Arthralgias/myalgias
- Cough
- Fever
- Headache and sore throat
- Nausea, vomiting, or diarrhea, especially in children

The "most appropriate next step in management" depends on the time course from presentation. If within 48 hours since the onset of symptoms, perform a nasopharyngeal swab or wash in order to rapidly detect the antigen associated with influenza.

TREATMENT

Less than 48 hours of symptoms: oseltamivir, zanamivir. Neuraminidase inhibitors shorten the duration of symptoms. These drugs treat both influenza A and B.

More than 48 hours of symptoms: Symptomatic treatment only. Analgesics, rest, antipyretics, hydration.

> Oseltamivir and zanamivir do not successfully treat complications of influenza, such as pneumonia.

INFECTIOUS DIARRHEA

Blood and WBCs in Stool

- *Salmonella*: poultry
- *Campylobacter*: most common cause, associated with GBS
- *E. coli* 0157:H7—hemolytic uremic syndrome (HUS)
- *Shigella*: second most common association with HUS
- *Vibrio parahaemolyticus*: shellfish and cruise ships
- *Vibrio vulnificus*: shellfish, history of liver disease, skin lesions
- **Yersinia**: high affinity for **iron**, hemochromatosis, blood transfusions
- Clostridium difficile: white and red cells in stool

The **best initial test is for blood and/or fecal leukocytes**, but this will not determine a specific organism. Stool lactoferrin has greater sensitivity and specificity compared with stool leukocytes. Lactoferrin is a better answer than fecal leukocytes if it is one of the choices. The most accurate test is stool culture.

No Blood or WBCs in Stool

- Viral
- *Giardia*: camping/hiking and unfiltered fresh water
- Cryptosporidiosis: AIDS with less than 100 CD4 cells; detect with modified acid fast stain

- *Bacillus cereus*: vomiting
- *Staphylococcus*: vomiting

Scombroid

- Most rapid onset
- Wheezing, flushing, rash
- Found in fish
- Treat with antihistamines

TREATMENT

Mild disease: Oral fluid replacement

Severe disease: Fluid replacement and oral antibiotics such as ciprofloxacin

---

"Severe" infectious diarrhea means:

- Hypotension
- Tachycardia
- Fever
- Abdominal pain
- Bloody diarrhea
- Metabolic acidosis

Disease-Specific Treatment	
Organism	**Treatment**
Giardia	Metronidazole, tinidazole
Cryptosporidiosis	Treat underlying AIDS, nitazoxanide
Viral	Fluid support as needed
B. cereus, Staphylococcus	Fluid support as needed

HEPATITIS

Acute Hepatitis

DEFINITION/ETIOLOGY

Hepatitis is an infection or inflammation of the liver. Most cases of acute hepatitis are from viral hepatitis A or B. **Hepatitis C**, for unknown reasons, **rarely presents with an acute infection**, and is found as a "silent" infection on blood tests, or unfortunately, when patients present with cirrhosis. Hepatitis D exists exclusively in those who have active viral replication of hepatitis B.

Hepatitis E is typically the worst in pregnancy, especially among patients from East Asia.

Sex, blood, perinatal (parenteral): hepatitis B, C, and D.

Food and water (enteric): hepatitis A and E.

- You Ate hepatitis **A**; you Eat hepatitis **E**.

PRESENTATION

There is no way to detect the etiology or specific type of hepatitis from the acute symptoms. All forms of acute hepatitis present with:

- Jaundice
- Fever, weight loss, and fatigue
- Dark urine
- Hepatosplenomegaly
- Nausea, vomiting, abdominal pain

DIAGNOSTIC TESTS

Aplastic anemia is a rare complication of acute hepatitis.

- Increased direct bilirubin
- Increased ratio of alanine aminotransferase (ALT) to aspartate aminotransferase (AST)
- Increased alkaline phosphatase

Which of the following correlates the best with an increased likelihood of mortality?

a. Bilirubin
b. Prothrombin time
c. ALT
d. AST
e. Alkaline phosphatase

Answer: The correct answer is (B). All of these lab tests can be markedly elevated during acute hepatitis with little adverse significance except for prothrombin time (PT). If the PT is elevated, there is a markedly increased risk of fulminant hepatic failure and death.

Disease-Specific Diagnostic Tests

Hepatitis A, C, D, and E: The "best initial diagnostic test" for each of these is simply an IgM antibody for the acute infection and IgG antibody to detect resolution of infection. Disease activity of hepatitis C is assessed with PCR for RNA level, which tells the amount of active viral replication. Hepatitis C PCR levels are the first thing to change as an indication of improvement with treatment and are the best correlate of treatment failure if they rise.

Hepatitis B Diagnostic Tests

Serologic Patterns

Handwritten annotations above table:
HBSAg → INFECTION
HBE Ag → CORRELATES TO VIRAL LOAD → INFECTIOUS TO OTHERS
HBC Ab
HbS Ab

	Surface antigen	e-antigen	Core antibody	Surface antibody
Acute or chronic infection	Positive	Positive	Positive IgM or IgG	Negative
Resolved, old, past infection	Negative	Negative	Positive IgG	Positive
Vaccination	Negative	Negative	Negative	Positive
"Window period"	Negative	Negative	Positive IgM, then IgG	Negative

Most Likely Acute Hepatitis B Questions

Which of the following will become abnormal first after acquiring hepatitis B infection?

a. Bilirubin
b. e-antigen
c. Surface antigen
d. Core IgM antibody
e. ALT
f. Anti-hepatitis B e-antibody

Answer: The correct answer is (C). Surface antigen is a measure of actual viral particles. Bilirubin, ALT, and antibody production are a measure of the body's response to the infection.

Which of the following is the most direct correlate with the amount, or quantity, of active viral replication?

a. Bilirubin
b. e-antigen
c. Surface antigen
d. Core IgM antibody
e. ALT
f. Anti-hepatitis B e-antibody

Answer: The correct answer is (B). Although surface antigen is a measure of whether there is any viral replication or infection at all, surface antigen does not tell quantity. Hepatitis B e-antigen is directly correlated with the degree of DNA polymerase. E-antigen is present only when there is a high level of DNA polymerase activity.

Which of the following indicates that a patient is no longer a risk for transmitting infection to another person (active infection has resolved)?

a. Bilirubin normalizes
b. No e-antigen found
c. No surface antigen found
d. No core IgM antibody found
e. ALT normalizes
f. Anti-hepatitis B e-antibody

Answer: The correct answer is (C). As long as surface antigen is present, there is still some viral replication potentially occurring. Even if surface antibody was one of the choices, the correct answer would still be surface antigen. Transmissibility ceases when DNA polymerase ceases, not when surface antibody appears. Jaundice (increased bilirubin) and elevated ALT will all normalize long before viral replication stops. You can definitely have viral replication, elevated DNA polymerase, and positive surface antigen with a normal ALT.

*Hepatitis B e-antibody will appear **prior** to resolution of all DNA polymerase activity. It is an indication that the acute infection is moving toward resolution, but it does not conclusively prove resolution has occurred.*

Which of the following is the best indication of the need for treatment with antiviral medications in chronic disease?

a. Bilirubin
b. e-antigen
c. Surface antigen
d. Core IgM antibody
e. ALT
f. Anti-hepatitis B e-antibody

Answer: The correct answer is (B). The person most likely to benefit from antiviral medications is the one with the greatest degree of active viral replication. Hepatitis B e-antigen is the strongest indicator of active viral replication. Although surface antigen means there is at least some active disease, it might be on the way to spontaneous resolution and would not benefit. Everyone with e-antigen also has surface antigen. The person with the worst disease (highest DNA polymerase) will benefit the most from treatment.

Which of the following is the best indicator that a pregnant woman will transmit infection to her child?

a. Bilirubin
b. e-antigen
c. Surface antigen
d. Core IgM antibody
e. ALT
f. Anti-hepatitis B, e-antibody

*Answer: The correct answer is e-antigen. Your questions may offer DNA polymerase as a choice instead of e-antigen. Any time you would say e-antigen, you would also say DNA polymerase. The only difference is that e-antigen is a **qualitative** test, meaning it is simply positive or negative. DNA polymerase is a **quantitative** test, meaning you get a level that can have a lot of variability. It is like the gas tank in your car. Hepatitis B e-antigen tells you, "Gas present: yes or no." DNA polymerase is like the gauge on your tank: It tells an amount.*

*If a woman is positive for surface antigen, but the e-antigen is negative, only 10% of children will become infected with hepatitis B at birth. When both surface antigen and e-antigen are positive, 90% of children will be infected at birth. This is why **perinatal transmission is the most common method of transmission worldwide.***

TREATMENT

Hepatitis A and E resolve spontaneously over a few weeks and are almost always benign conditions. Hepatitis **B becomes chronic in 10%** of patients and no form of treatment has been found to alter this. Acute hepatitis C, in the few cases in which it is detected, should be treated with interferon and ribavirin. They decrease the likelihood of developing a chronic infection with hepatitis C.

> Only acute hepatitis C gets medical therapy.

Chronic Hepatitis

TREATMENT

By definition, **chronicity** for hepatitis B is defined as persistence of **surface antigen for more than 6 months**. If these patients are positive for e-antigen with an elevated level of DNA polymerase, treatment is any **one** of the following: entecavir, adefovir, lamivudine, telbivudine, interferon, or tenofovir.

Because interferon is an injection and has the most adverse effects, it is not the best first choice.

Adverse effects of interferon:

- Arthralgia/myalgia
- Leukopenia and thrombocytopenia
- Depression and flu-like symptoms

The goal of chronic hepatitis therapy is:

- Reduce DNA polymerase to undetectable levels
- Convert those patients with e-antigen to having anti-hepatitis e-antibody

---

Role of Liver Biopsy

The presence of fibrosis on biopsy is a strong indication to begin therapy for either hepatitis B or C right away. **If there is active viral replication, fibrosis will progress to cirrhosis.** Cirrhosis is not reversible. Older terms like "chronic active" or "chronic persistent" hepatitis have been irrelevant since the development of tests for DNA polymerase.

> ALT levels are not a good indication of the activity of chronic hepatitis. You can have significant infection with normal transaminase levels.

Treatment of Chronic Hepatitis C

There is no way to determine the duration of infection with hepatitis C, since there is no equivalent of the surface antigen test. **Most patients do not have acute symptoms.** If the PCR-RNA viral load is elevated, patients should be treated with interferon and ribavirin. If there is fibrosis on liver biopsy,

Ribavirin causes anemia.

initiating treatment becomes more urgent to prevent permanent hepatic insufficiency. **The goal of therapy is to achieve an undetectable viral load.**

SEXUALLY TRANSMITTED DISEASES

Urethritis

Look for urethral discharge to answer "What is the most likely diagnosis?" Both urethritis and cystitis give dysuria with urinary frequency and burning, but **cystitis does not give urethral discharge**.

DIAGNOSTIC TESTS

The best initial test is a urethral swab for Gram stain. Urine testing for nucleic acid amplification can also detect gonorrhea and *Chlamydia*. Urethritis gives an increased number of white blood cells. If intracellular gram-negative diplococci are seen, this is sufficient evidence of *Neisseria gonorrhoeae* to initiate treatment. The most accurate test is a urethral culture, DNA probe, or nucleic acid amplification test for *N. gonorrhoeae* and *Chlamydia trachomatis*. Other causes of urethritis are *Mycoplasma genitalium* and *Ureaplasma*.

TREATMENT

Use a combination of one drug for gonorrhea and one for *Chlamydia*. Quinolones are not the best initial therapy because of resistance.

Treatment of Urethritis	
Gonorrhea	***Chlamydia***
Cefixime	Azithromycin
Ceftriaxone	Doxycycline

Cervicitis

Cervicitis presents with cervical discharge and an inflamed "strawberry" cervix on physical examination. The testing and treatment are identical to that previously described for urethritis.

Pelvic Inflammatory Disease (PID)

PID presents with:

- Lower abdominal **tenderness**
- Lower abdominal **pain**
- Fever
- **Cervical motion tenderness**
- Leukocytosis

If all of these symptoms are present, the most appropriate next step in management is always to **exclude pregnancy first in a woman with lower abdominal pain or tenderness or cervical motion tenderness**.

DIAGNOSTIC TESTS

Cervical swab for culture, DNA probe, or nucleic acid amplification is done to confirm the etiology of PID. These tests clarify the need for treating the partner for an STD and make treatment more precise especially when organism may be resistant.

> Cervical testing is not the "most accurate test" for PID.

Laparoscopy in PID

The **most accurate** test for PID is **laparoscopy**, although it is only rarely needed. Laparoscopy is needed only if the diagnosis is unclear, symptoms persist despite therapy, or there are recurrent episodes for unclear reasons.

TREATMENT

PID is treated with a combination of medications for gonorrhea and *Chlamydia*.

Inpatient: Cefoxitin or cefotetan combined with doxycycline

Outpatient: Ceftriaxone and doxycycline (possibly with metronidazole)

Patients with anaphylaxis to penicillin: levofloxacin and metronidazole as an outpatient, or clindamycin and gentamicin as an inpatient.

Ulcerative Genital Disease

"WHAT IS THE MOST LIKELY DIAGNOSIS?"

▶ **TIP**

It is often impossible to determine the specific diagnosis of genital ulcers by physical examination characteristics alone, but if this issue appears on Step 2 CK, it means that the question must provide sufficient clues or evidence to give you the answer.

All ulcerative genital disease can have inguinal adenopathy.

Presentation of STDs	
History and physical findings	**Most likely diagnosis**
Pain**less** ulcer	Syphilis
Pain**ful** ulcer	Chancroid (*Haemophilus ducreyi*)
Lymph nodes tender and suppurating	Lymphogranuloma venereum
Vesicles prior to ulcer and painful	*Herpes simplex*

Diagnostic Tests	
Diagnosis	**Diagnostic Test**
Syphilis	Dark-field microscopy VDRL or RPR (75% sensitive in primary syphilis) FTA or MHA-TP (confirmatory)
Chancroid (*Haemophilus ducreyi*)	Stain and culture on specialized media
Lymphogranuloma venereum	Complement fixation titers in blood Nucleic acid amplification testing on swab
Herpes simplex	Tzanck prep is the best initial test Viral culture is the most accurate test

> If dark-field is positive for spirochetes, no further testing for syphilis is necessary.

Treatment	
Diagnosis	**Treatment**
Syphilis	Single dose of intramuscular benzathine penicillin Doxycycline if penicillin allergic
Chancroid (*Haemophilus ducreyi*)	Azithromycin (single dose)
Lymphogranuloma venereum	Doxycycline
Herpes simplex	Acyclovir, valacyclovir, famciclovir Foscarnet for acyclovir-resistant herpes

A woman comes to clinic with multiple painful genital vesicles.

What is the next step in management?

a. Acyclovir orally
b. Acyclovir topically
c. Tzanck prep
d. Viral culture
e. Serology
f. PCR

*Answer: The correct answer is (A). If the presentation is clear for herpes with multiple vesicles of the mouth or genitals, diagnostic testing is not necessary. Acyclovir, famciclovir, and valacyclovir are all equal in efficacy, so any one of them could be the right choice. **Topical acyclovir is worthless**. Viral culture is the most accurate test, but not necessary if the vesicles are clear. Serology is always worthless, since it cannot distinguish an acute genital infection from an oral herpes infection in the past.*

Syphilis

PRESENTATION

Primary Syphilis

- Painless genital ulcer with heaped-up **indurated edges** (it becomes painful if it becomes secondarily infected with bacteria)
- Painless adenopathy

Secondary Syphilis

- Rash (palms and soles)
- Alopecia areata
- Mucous patches
- Condylomata lata

Tertiary Syphilis

- Neurosyphilis

  - **Meningovascular** (stroke from vasculitis)
  - **Tabes dorsalis** (loss of position and vibratory sense, incontinence, cranial nerve)
  - **General paresis** (memory and personality changes)
  - **Argyll Robertson pupil**

- Aortitis (aortic regurgitation, aortic aneurysm)
- Gummas (skin and bone lesions)

> Chancres heal **spontaneously** even without treatment. Penicillin prevents later stages.

Sensitivity of Diagnostic Tests by Stage			
Test	**Primary**	**Secondary**	**Tertiary**
VDRL or RPR	75%–85%	99%	95%
FTA-ABS	95%	100%	98%

False positive VDRL:/RPR

- Infection, older age, injection drug use and AIDS, malaria, antiphospholipid syndrome, and endocarditis

> Titers of VDRL or RPR are reliable at greater than 1:8. Lower titer is more often falsely positive. High titers (greater than 1:32) are rarely false positive.

TREATMENT

Primary and secondary syphilis: single intramuscular injection of penicillin. Oral doxycycline if penicillin allergic.

Tertiary syphilis: intravenous penicillin. Desensitize to penicillin if penicillin allergic.

> **Jarisch-Herxheimer reaction**
> * Fever and worse symptoms after treatment
> * Give aspirin and antipyretics; it will pass.

▶ **TIP**

Desensitization is the answer for **neurosyphilis** and **pregnant women.**

Genital Warts (Condylomata Acuminata)

Condylomata acuminata from papillomavirus is diagnosed simply based on the visual appearance. Wrong answers include biopsy, serology, stain, smear, and culture. Remove them by physical means such as **cryotherapy with liquid nitrogen**, **surgery** for large ones, laser, or "melting" them with **podophyllin** or trichloroacetic acid. **Imiquimod is** a locally applied immunostimulant that leads to the sloughing off of the lesion.

Figure 1.2: Condylomata acuminata (genital warts).
Source: Farshad Bagheri, MD.

Pediculosis (Crabs)

* Found on hair-bearing areas (axilla, pubis)
* Causes itching
* Visible on the surface
* Treat with **permethrin**; lindane is equal in efficacy, but more toxic.

Scabies

- Found in **web spaces** between fingers and toes or at elbows
- Found around the nipples or near the genitals
- **Burrows** visible (they dig) but smaller than pediculosis
- **Scrape** and magnify
- Treat with **permethrin**
- Widespread disease responds to ivermectin; severe disease needs repeat dosing

Figure 1.3: Scabies burrow under the skin and must be scraped out to establish a diagnosis. *Source: Conrad Fischer, MD.*

URINARY TRACT INFECTIONS

All UTIs can present with **dysuria** (frequency, urgency, burning) and a **fever**. The urinalysis shows **increased WBCs** in all of them. *E. coli* is the most common cause. Quinolones are the best initial therapy.

Anatomic defects lead to UTIs, such as:

- Stones
- Strictures
- Tumor or prostate hypertrophy
- Diabetes

Any form of obstruction of or foreign body in the urinary system. Foley catheter is a foreign body. Neurogenic bladder is an obstruction.

> Frequency means multiple episodes of micturation. Polyuria is an increase in the volume of urine.

Cystitis

Presents with dysuria and:

- **Suprapubic pain**/discomfort
- Mild or absent fever

> Men with UTIs have anatomic abnormalities much more often than women.
>
> Best initial test: urinalysis with more than 10 WBCs
>
> Most accurate test: urine culture

Treat with:

> All beta-lactam antibiotics are considered safe in pregnancy.

- Trimethoprim/sulfamethoxazole **(TMP/SMZ)** if local resistance is low
- Ciprofloxacin
- Cephalexin
- **Nitrofurantoin** especially in pregnant women

A 36-year-old generally healthy woman comes to the office with urinary frequency and burning. The urinalysis shows more than 50 WBC per high power field.

What is the most appropriate next step in management?

a. TMP/SMZ for 3 days
b. TMP/SMZ for 7 days
c. Urine culture
d. Ultrasound of urinary system
e. CT scan of urinary system

Answer: The correct answer is (A). When symptoms of cystitis are clear and there are white cells in the urine, there is no need for urine culture or imaging studies. Urine culture and imaging are done if there are frequent episodes of cystitis or failure to respond to therapy. Three days is sufficient for uncomplicated cystitis. Seven days is used if there is an anatomic abnormality.

Pyelonephritis

Dysuria with:

- **Flank** or costovertebral angle tenderness
- High **fever**
- Occasionally with abdominal pain from an inflamed kidney

Urinalysis shows increased WBCs. Imaging studies (CT or sonogram) are not done to determine if there is an anatomic abnormality causing the infection.

Treat with:

> Any of the drugs for gram-negative bacilli would be effective for pyelonephritis.

- **Ampicillin and gentamicin** until culture results are known
- Ciprofloxacin

Acute Prostatitis

Acute prostatitis presents with dysuria with:

- **Perineal pain**
- **Tender prostate** on examination

The diagnostic yield of urine culture is greatly increased with **prostate massage**. Treat in the same way as you would for pyelonephritis. Long-term therapy with TMP/SMZ for **6 to 8 weeks** is used for chronic prostatitis.

[handwritten margin note: Amp! Gent or Cipro]

Perinephric Abscess

Look for pyelonephritis that does not resolve with appropriate therapy. When the choice of drug is correct and the dose is correct, failure of an infection to resolve is often from an anatomic problem. When pyelonephritis is associated with persistent fever after 5 to 7 days of therapy, perform an imaging study such as a sonogram or CT scan. **Drainage** of the fluid collection is **mandatory**. Culture of the infected fluid is essential to guide therapy.

ENDOCARDITIS

DEFINITION

Endocarditis is an infection of the valve of the heart leading to a **fever and a murmur**. It is diagnosed with vegetations seen on echocardiogram and positive blood cultures.

ETIOLOGY

It is very rare to have endocarditis develop on normal heart valves with the exception of injection drug users. The risk of endocarditis is directly proportional to the degree of damage of the valves. Regurgitant and stenotic lesions confer increased risk. Prosthetic valves are associated with the highest risk. Infection can develop on normal valves if there is severe bacteremia with highly pathogenic organisms such as occurs with injection drug use and *Staphylococcus aureus*.

Dental procedures confer an increased, but very small risk of endocarditis. Even surgery of the mouth or respiratory tract confers no risk unless there is a severe valvular disorder such as from an artificial valve or cyanotic heart disease. Less invasive procedures such as endoscopy confer no increased risk even with a biopsy.

PRESENTATION/"WHAT IS THE MOST LIKELY DIAGNOSIS?"

Look for:

- **Fever**
- New **murmur** or change in a murmur

- Complications of endocarditis
  - Splinter hemorrhages
  - Janeway lesions (flat and painless)
  - Osler nodes (raised and painful)
  - Roth spots in the eyes
  - Brain (mycotic aneurysm)
  - Kidney (hematuria, glomerulonephritis)
  - Conjunctival petechiae
  - Splenomegaly
  - Septic emboli to the lungs

DIAGNOSTIC TESTS

The best initial test:

- **Blood culture** (95%–99% sensitive)
- Transthoracic **echocardiogram** (60% sensitive but 95% specific)
- Transesophageal echocardiogram (95% sensitive and specific)

EKG rarely shows atrioventricular (AV) block if there is dissection of the conduction system (less than 5%–10% sensitive).

> Fever + murmur =
> endocarditis.

A man comes into the emergency department with fever and a murmur. Blood cultures grow Streptococcus bovis. Transthoracic echocardiography shows a vegetation.

What is the most appropriate next step in the management of this patient?

a. Colonoscopy
b. Transesophageal echocardiogram
c. CT of the abdomen
d. Repeat the blood cultures
e. Surgical valve replacement

Answer: The correct answer is (A). Streptococcus bovis is associated with colonic pathology ranging from diverticuli to polyps to colon cancer. If strep bovis grows, perform colonoscopy. CT scan will not show diverticuli. There is no point in repeating the blood culture if it is already positive. Valve replacement is premature.

Establishing a Diagnosis of Culture Negative Endocarditis

The diagnosis is based on:

1. Oscillating vegetation on echocardiography
2. Three minor criteria:
   - Fever
   - Risk such as injection drug use or prosthetic valve
   - Signs of embolic phenomena

TREATMENT

The best initial empiric therapy is vancomycin and gentamicin.

When culture results are available, treat as indicated in the table "Treatment of Endocarditis."

Treatment of Endocarditis	
Organism	**Treatment**
Viridans streptococci	Ceftriaxone for 4 weeks
Staphylococcus aureus (sensitive)	Oxacillin, nafcillin, or cefazolin
Fungal	Amphotericin and valve replacement
Staphylococcus epidermidis or resistant *Staphylococcus*	Vancomycin and gentamicin
Enterococci	Ampicillin and gentamicin

Treatment of Resistant Organisms

Add an aminoglycoside and extend the duration of treatment.

When Is Surgery the Answer?

- **CHF** or **ruptured valve** or chordae tendineae
- Prosthetic valves
- Fungal endocarditis
- Abscess
- AV block
- Recurrent emboli while on antibiotics

> Add rifampin for prosthetic valve endocarditis with *Staphylococcus*.

> The single strongest indication for surgery is acute valve rupture and CHF.

Treatment of Culture Negative Endocarditis

HACEK is an acronym for organisms that are difficult to culture that cause endocarditis.

- *Haemophilus aphrophilus*
- *Haemophilus parainfluenza*
- *Actinobacillus*
- *Cardiobacterium*
- *Eikenella*
- *Kingella*

Use ceftriaxone for the HACEK group of organisms.

Prophylaxis for Endocarditis

Two features are needed to establish the need for prophylaxis:

1. Significant cardiac defect
    - Prosthetic valve
    - Previous endocarditis
    - Cardiac transplant recipient with valvulopathy
    - Unrepaired cyanotic heart disease

and

2. Risk of bacteremia
    - Dental work **with blood**
    - Respiratory tract surgery that produces bacteremia

The best initial management is amoxicillin prior to the procedure. If the patient is penicillin allergic, then clindamycin, azithromycin, or clarithromycin is the answer.

Procedures and anatomic abnormalities that do **not** need prophylaxis are:

- Flexible endoscopies, even with biopsy
- Obstetrical and gynecologic procedures
- Urology procedures (including prostate biopsy)
- GI procedures including endoscopic retrograde cholangiopancreatography (ERCP)
- Valvular heart disease including mitral valve prolapse, even with a murmur
- Mitral regurgitation, mitral stenosis, aortic regurgitation, aortic stenosis, hypertrophic obstructive cardiomyopathy (HOCM), atrial septal defect (ASD)

LYME DISEASE

DEFINITION

Lyme disease is an arthropod-borne disease from the spirochete *Borrelia burgdorferi*. It results most often in a fever and a rash. Untreated infection can recur as joint pain, cardiac disease, or neurological disease.

ETIOLOGY

Lyme is transmitted by the deer tick (*Ixodes scapularis*). The tick is very small, and the bite is most often unnoticed. Only 20% of patients recall the bite of the tick. More often patients recall being outdoors; many cases will describe the patient as having recently been hiking or camping. In experimental models it has been determined that the tick must be attached for at least 24 hours in order to transmit the organism. The *Ixodes* tick is not present everywhere in the United States. Lyme typically occurs only in northeast states such as Connecticut (where the town of Lyme gave the disease its name), Massachusetts, New York, and New Jersey.

PRESENTATION

- **Rash** is the most common manifestation, occurring in 85% to 90% of patients. It usually occurs 5 to 14 days after, and may occur as much as a month after, the bite of the tick. Fever often accompanies the infection. The proper term for the rash is erythema migrans. It is a **round red lesion** with **a pale area in the center**; the lesion resembles a target or bull's-eye.
- **Joint pain** is the most common long-term manifestation. 60% of those without treatment will develop the joint pain. It is an oligoarthritis, which literally means that a "few joints" are affected. Joint fluid will have about 25,000 WBCs/μl. This would not distinguish it from other causes of joint inflammation or infection.
- **Neurological manifestations** occur in 10% to 15% of patients. They may present with symptoms of the CNS or peripheral nervous system such as meningitis, encephalitis, or cranial nerve palsy.
- **Cardiac** manifestations occur in 4% to 10% of patients. They present with damage to any part of the myocardium or pericardium such as myocarditis or ventricular arrhythmia.

> The knee is the most commonly affected joint in Lyme disease.

> Seventh cranial nerve or Bell palsy is the most common neurological manifestation of Lyme disease.

> Transient AV block is the most common cardiac manifestation in Lyme disease.

DIAGNOSTIC TESTS

If the lesion is typical, a rash consistent with Lyme does not need confirmatory testing with serology in order to initiate treatment.

Figure 1.6: Target-shaped rash of Lyme disease or erythema migrans. *Source: Nishith Patel.*

Serologic testing for Lyme is essential for all the other manifestations such as the joint, neurologic, and cardiac manifestations, since most causes of seventh cranial nerve palsy, arthralgia, and AV block are not caused by Lyme. Testing is with IgM, IgG, ELISA, Western blot, and PCR testing.

Treatment	
Manifestation	**Treatment**
Asymptomatic tick bite	No treatment routinely
Rash	• Doxycycline • Amoxicillin
Joint, seventh cranial nerve palsy	• Doxycycline • Amoxicillin
Cardiac and neurologic manifestations other than the seventh cranial nerve palsy	Intravenous ceftriaxone

Asymptomatic Tick Bite

Most patients with tick bite, but no symptoms of Lyme, do not need prophylactic treatment. A single dose of doxycycline is indicated within 72 hours of tick bite when:

• *Ixodes scapularis* clearly identified as the tick causing the bite
• Tick attached for longer than 24 to 48 hours
• Engorged nymph-stage tick
• Endemic area

HIV/AIDS

DEFINITION

HIV is a retrovirus infecting the CD4 (T-Helper) cell. CD4 cells drop from a normal level of 600 to 1000 per µl at a rate of 50 to 100 per year in a person who is untreated. Depletion of the CD4 cell count takes between 5 and 10 years before clinical manifestations generally occur. It is not HIV itself that leads to symptoms and death. Rather, the depletion of the CD4 count leads to opportunistic infections that lead to illness.

ETIOLOGY

HIV is transmitted through:

- Injection drug use with contaminated needles
- Sex, particularly men who have sex with men
- Transfusion (extremely rare since 1985)
- Perinatal
- Needle stick or blood-contaminated sharp instrument injury

Risk of Transmission of HIV Without Prophylactic Treatment	
Mode of transmission	**Percentage of risk with each event**
Vaginal transmission	1:3000–1:10,000 for insertive intercourse 1:1000 for receptive intercourse
Oral sex	1:1000 for receptive fellatio with ejaculation Unclear for insertive fellatio or cunnilingus
Needle stick injury	1:300
Anal sex	1:100 for receptive anal intercourse
Mother to child	25%–30% perinatal transmission without medication

Kissing is not proven to transmit HIV.

PRESENTATION

PRIMARY LOOKS LIKE FLU OR MONO

Infections occur with profound immunosuppresion when the CD4 count drops below 50/µl. PCP occurs at a CD4 below 200/µl or under 14%. When the CD4 count is above 200/µl, few infections occur. Infections at increased frequency with HIV but a CD4 above 200/µl are:

PCP < 200

- Varicella zoster (shingles)
- Herpes simplex
- Tuberculosis
- Oral and vaginal candidiasis
- Bacterial pneumonia

JC VIRUS

CRYPTOSPORIDIUM
CANDIDIASIS / THRUSH
PCP
KAPOSI'S

DIAGNOSTIC TESTS

The best initial test for HIV is the ELISA test. This is confirmed with Western blot testing. Infected infants are diagnosed with PCR or viral culture. ELISA testing is unreliable in infants because maternal HIV antibodies may be present for up to 6 months after delivery.

Viral Load Testing (PCR-RNA level)

Viral load testing is useful to:

- Measure response to therapy (decreasing levels are good)
- Detect treatment failure (rising levels are bad)
- Diagnose HIV in babies

The goal of therapy is to drive down the viral load. Undetectable levels (below 50/μl) indicate that the CD4 will most likely rise. When the viral load is driven to undetectable levels and the CD4 rises, opportunistic infections rarely occur. Life expectancy for a person with HIV whose viral load is undetectable by PCR-RNA is equal in duration to an HIV-negative person.

Viral Resistance Testing (Genotyping)

Viral resistance testing should be performed prior to initiating antiretroviral medications. This decreases the likelihood of starting medication to which the patient's virus is resistant. Resistance testing is also done if there is evidence of treatment failure. In the event of treatment failure, resistance testing guides the choice of medications to select 3 drugs from 2 different classes to which the patient's virus is susceptible.

> Treatment failure first manifests with a rising PCR-RNA viral load.

TREATMENT

Opportunistic infection treatment is discussed with each disease. For HIV itself, treatment is initiated when:

- CD4 drops below 500/μl in an asymptomatic patient

or

- Viral load is very high (greater than 100,000/μl)

or

- Opportunistic infection occurs

> The strongest indication for antiretroviral medication is a CD4 below 350/μl.

Choice of Initial Antiretroviral Medication

The best initial drug regimen is a combination of emtricitabine, tenofovir, and efavirenz. These 3 medications are combined in a single, once-a-day pill called Atripla (Bristol-Myers Squibb, New York, New York).

▶ **TIP**

USMLE Step 2 CK does not test dosing.

Treatment failure is detected by a rising viral load or failure of viral load to suppress to undetectable levels. CD4 count will decrease or fail to rise with a failing regimen, but changes in CD4 lag behind and are slower to occur than changes in viral load testing.

Alternate Drug Regimens

If emtricitabine/tenofovir/efavirenz cannot be used because of resistance, alternate regimens are based on a combination of 3 drugs from at least 2 different classes.

Antiretroviral First-line Medications by Class		
Nucleoside and nucleotide reverse transcriptase inhibitors (RTIs)	**Non-nucleoside RTIs**	**Protease inhibitors**
• Zidovudine • Didanosine • Stavudine • Lamivudine • Emtricitabine • Abacavir • Tenofovir	• Efavirenz • Etravirine • Nevirapine	• Ritonavir • Saquinavir • Nelfinavir • Amprenavir • Fosamprenavir • Lopinavir • Atazanavir • Indinavir • Tipranavir • Darunavir

[handwritten: LACTIC ACIDOSIS] *[handwritten: RASH]* *[handwritten: GI UPSET, METABOLIC SYNDROME]*

Additional Classes of Second-line Agents

These medications are used for those with drug resistance to multiple classes of first-line agents.

Entry inhibitors:

- Enfuvirtide
- Maraviroc

Integrase inhibitor:

- Raltegravir

▶ **TIP**

USMLE Step 2 CK will not require you to know details of efficacy differences between classes.

Postexposure Prophylaxis

All significant needle stick injuries and sexual exposures are given 4 weeks of therapy with combination therapy. The choice of therapy follows that described in "Choice of Initial Antiretroviral Medication." Exposures to urine and stool

> Postexposure prophylaxis is not routinely indicated for needle stick injury if the HIV status of the needle is unknown.

are not an indication for postexposure prophylaxis (PEP) unless blood is present in them. Bites from an HIV-positive person should initiate PEP.

Adverse Effects of HIV Medications	
Drug	**Adverse effect**
Zidovudine	Anemia
Stavudine and didanosine	Peripheral neuropathy and pancreatitis
Abacavir	Hypersensitivity, Stevens-Johnson reaction
Protease inhibitors	Hyperlipidemia, hyperglycemia
Indinavir	Nephrolithiasis
Tenofovir	Renal insufficiency

Prevention of Perinatal Transmission

HIV-positive pregnant women have special, unique treatment indications. If the patient is HIV positive and already on antiretroviral medications that are effective at the time of pregnancy, the answer is just to continue the same regimen of treatment. If the person is pregnant and not already on medications, she should be treated for the same indications as a nonpregnant person. The only exception is the use of efavirenz, which should be avoided in pregnancy because it is associated with teratogenicity in animals. Protease inhibitors are considered a safe alternative to efavirenz during pregnancy.

If the pregnant woman has a high CD4 (350 or higher) and does not need antiretroviral medications for her own health, treatment with combination antiretrovirals should still be given to prevent perinatal transmission. With a high CD4 and low viral load, antiretroviral medications are given in the second and third trimesters just to prevent perinatal transmission. The medications for the mother can be stopped after delivery if she does not need them for herself.

The baby should receive zidovudine during delivery (intrapartum) and for 6 weeks afterward to help prevent transmission.

Indications for Antiretrovirals During Pregnancy	
Condition	**Action**
Patient on antiretrovirals at the time of pregnancy	Continue same medications, except switch efavirenz to a protease inhibitor
Not on antiretrovirals, CD4 **low** or viral load **high**	Initiate antiretrovirals immediately
Not on antiretrovirals, CD4 **high** and viral load **low**	Antiretrovirals during second and third trimesters, stopping them in the mother after birth

Cesarean Delivery for HIV-Positive Mothers

Cesarean delivery is performed to prevent transmission of virus if the CD4 is low (below 350) or the viral load is high. There is a special cutoff for what is considered an elevated viral load in pregnancy: If the viral load is above 1000/µl at the time of delivery, a cesarean delivery is performed.

Most transmission from mother to child occurs during delivery. Make sure the viral load is controlled by the time of parturition. If the viral load is above 1000 µl, perform cesarean delivery.

Intrapartum antiretrovirals with zidovudine are routinely administered in every pregnant HIV-positive patient.

> Fully controlled HIV (viral load undetectable) gives less than 1% transmission.

TB PROPHYLAXIS	– ISONIAZID	
PCP	– TMP-SMX	< 200 CD4
TOXO	– TMP-SMX	< 100 CD4
MAC	– AZITHRO	< 50

Allergy and Immunology 2

Anaphylaxis

Definition

Anaphylaxis is defined as the worst form of allergic condition or acute event. It is synonymous with the term **immediate hypersensitivity**. The patient must already have been sensitized to the antigen. IgE binds to mast cells, leading to the release of their granules (eg, histamine, prostaglandins, and leukotrienes), which results in the abnormalities that essentially define anaphylaxis. Anaphylactoid reactions are non-IgE related, are clinically identical and treated the same way, and do not need preceding sensitization to the antigen.

- Respiratory

and

- Hemodynamic

> Anaphylaxis is defined by the **severity, not the cause,** of the reaction.

Etiology

The causes of anaphylaxis are the same as the causes of any allergic event, such as:

- Insect **bites** and stings
- **Medications**: penicillin, phenytoin, lamotrigine, quinidine, rifampin, sulfa
- **Foods**

> Latex is a very important cause of anaphylaxis in healthcare workers.

Presentation

In addition to the **rash** that would be present in any form of allergic reaction, anaphylaxis is characterized by:

- **Hypotension**, tachycardia
- **Respiratory**: shortness of breath; wheezing; swelling of the lips, tongue, or face; stridor

> Urticaria is considered part of anaphylaxis, not just an allergy.

Figure 2.1: Urticaria is localized anaphylaxis with a "wheal and flare." *Source: Farshad Bagheri, MD.*

TREATMENT

The best initial therapy is with:

- Epinephrine
- Antihistamines such as diphenhydramine (H1-blocker) and ranitidine (H2-blocker)
- Glucocorticoids such as methylprednisolone or hydrocortisone
- Emergent airway protection if needed: intubation or cricothyroidotomy

> There is no specific test to define anaphylaxis.

ANGIOEDEMA

DEFINITION

Angioedema is sudden swelling of the:

- Face
- Tongue
- Eyes
- Airway

> Look for recent start of ACE inhibitors preceding symptoms.

This can be from deficiency of C1 esterase inhibitor. There is a characteristic association with the onset with minor physical trauma. Angioedema often has an idiopathic origin.

PRESENTATION

Hereditary angioedema is characterized by sudden facial swelling and stridor with the **absence of pruritus** and urticaria. Hereditary angioedema **does not respond to glucocorticoids**.

Figure 2.2: Angioedema can often swell the eyes shut. *Source: Nishith Patel.*

DIAGNOSTIC TESTS

The best initial test is for decreased levels of C2 and C4 in the complement pathway as well as deficiency of C1 esterase inhibitor.

TREATMENT

1. Acute therapy with fresh frozen **plasma**
2. Long-term management with **androgens**: danazol and stanazol
3. Ensure airway protection first; can be a rapidly evolving process

URTICARIA

This is a form of allergic reaction that causes sudden swelling of the superficial layers of the skin. In addition to being caused by insects and medications, urticaria can also be caused by physical agents such as:

- **Pressure** (dermatographism)
- **Cold**
- **Vibration**

TREATMENT

1. Antihistamines: hydroxyzine, diphenhydramine, fexofenadine, loratidine, or cetirizine: ranitidine
2. Leukotriene receptor antagonists: monteleukast or zafirlukast

ALLERGIC RHINITIS

ETIOLOGY

Seasonal allergies such as "hay fever" are common. This is an IgE-dependent triggering of mast cells.

PRESENTATION

Allergic rhinitis presents with recurrent episodes of:

- Watery eyes, sneezing, itchy nose, and itchy eyes
- Inflamed, boggy nasal mucosa
- Pale or violaceous turbinates
- Nasal polyps

DIAGNOSTIC TESTS

Nasal smear may show large numbers of eosinophils.

Allergic rhinitis is most often a clinical diagnosis with recurrent episodes of the presentation previously described. Skin testing and blood testing for reactions to antigens may be useful to identify a specific etiology. Allergen-specific IgE levels may be elevated.

TREATMENT

1. Prevention with avoidance of the precipitating allergen:
   - Close the windows and use air conditioning to avoid pollen.
   - Get rid of animals to which the patient is allergic.
   - **Cover mattresses and pillows.**
   - Use air purifiers and dust filters.
2. Intranasal corticosteroid sprays
3. Antihistamines: loratidine, clemastine, fexofenadine, brompheniramine
4. Intranasal anticholinergic medications: ipratropium
5. Desensitization to allergens that cannot be avoided

PRIMARY IMMUNODEFICIENCY DISORDERS

USUALLY SHOW UP AFTER 3-months OF LIFE

Common Variable Immunodeficiency

ETIOLOGY

B cells are present in normal numbers but they do not make effective amounts of immunoglobulins. There is a decrease in all the subtypes: IgG, IgM, and IgA.

PRESENTATION

Common variable immunodeficiency (CVID) presents with **recurrent sino-pulmonary** infections in **adults** with an equal gender distribution. There are frequent episodes of bronchitis, pneumonia, sinusitis, and otitis media.

Other manifestations are:

- Giardiasis
- Spruelike intestinal malabsorption
- Increase in autoimmune diseases such as pernicious anemia and seronega-tive rheumatic diseases

> CVID gives a marked increase in the **risk of lymphoma.**

DIAGNOSTIC TESTS

Immunoglobulin levels are decreased and there is a **decreased response to antigen stimulation** of B cells.

▶ **TIP**

The clue to CVID is a **decrease in the output of B lymphocytes** with a normal number of B cells as well as normal amounts of lymphoid tissue such as nodes, adenoids, and tonsils.

TREATMENT

Antibiotics are used for each infection as it develops. Chronic maintenance is with regular **infusions of intravenous immunoglobulins.**

X-linked (Bruton) Agammaglobulinemia

X-linked agammaglobulinemia presents in **male children** with increased sino-pulmonary infections. B cells and lymphoid tissues are diminished. There is a decrease or **absence of the tonsils, adenoids, lymph nodes**, and spleen. T cells are normal. Treat the infections as they arise. Long-term regular administra-tion of intravenous immunoglobulin (IVIG) keeps these children healthier.

*BRUTON'S
BOYS
B-CELL DEFICIENCY*

*CD3 = T LYMPH
CD19 = B LYMPH*

45

Severe Combined Immunodeficiency

The word "combined" in severe combined immunodeficiency (SCID) means that there is **deficiency in both B and T cells**. This results in infections related to both deficiencies.

No THYMIC SHADOW

B cells: Decreased immunoglobulin production leads to **recurrent sinopulmonary infection** beginning as early as 6 months of age.

SEVERE RECURRENT INFXN
CHRONIC DIARRHEA
FAILURE TO THRIVE

T cells: Markedly decreased numbers of T cells gives many of the infections that you would see in someone with AIDS, such as PCP, varicella, and *Candida*.

Besides treating the infections as they arise, these patients should undergo bone marrow transplant, which can be curative.

IgA Deficiency

These patients also present with recurrent sinopulmonary infections. The difference between this syndrome and the others is:

- **Atopic** diseases
- **Anaphylaxis** to blood transfusion when blood is given from a patient who has normal levels of IgA
- Spruelike condition with fat malabsorption
- Increase in the risk of vitiligo, thyroiditis, and rheumatoid arthritis

Treat infections as they arise and only use blood that is from IgA-deficient donors or that has been washed. IVIG injections will **not** work because the amount of IgA in the product is too insignificant to be therapeutic. The trace amounts of IgA in IVIG may provoke anaphylaxis in the same way that a blood transfusion does.

Hyper IgE Syndrome   *JOB SYNDROME*

ECZEMA
BOILS
COARSE FEATURES
TWO ROWS OF TEETH

This presents with recurrent **skin infections** with *Staphylococcus*. Treat these infections as they arise and consider prophylactic antibiotics such as dicloxacillin or cephalexin.

Wiskott-Aldrich Syndrome

W ISKOTT
A LDRICH
I mmunodeficiency
T HROMBOCYTOPENIA
E czema
R ecurrent pyogenic INFXN

This is an **immunodeficiency** combined with **thrombocytopenia** and **eczema**. T lymphocytes are markedly deficient in the blood and the lymph nodes. Bone marrow transplantation is the only definitive treatment.

Chronic Granulomatous Disease

Chronic granulomatous disease (CGD) is a genetic disease resulting in extensive inflammatory reactions. This leads to **lymph nodes with purulent material** leaking out. Aphthous ulcers and inflammation of the nares is common. Granulomas may become obstructive in the GI or urinary tract.

"WHAT IS THE MOST LIKELY DIAGNOSIS?"

Look for infections with the odd combination of:

- *Staphylococcus*
- *Burkholderia*
- *Nocardia*
- *Aspergillus*

DIAGNOSTIC TESTS

Abnormal **nitroblue tetrazolium testing** detects the decrease in the respiratory burst that produces hydrogen peroxide. This is a decrease in NADPH oxidase, which generates superoxide.

TMP/SMX & INTERFERON GAMMA

ATAXIA - TELANGIECTASIA

↓ IMMUNITY

ATAXIA | TELAGECTASIAS

↑ AFP

SUPPORTIVE

CHEDIAK - HIGASHI

ALBINISM

PYOGENIC INFECTIONS

DELAYED UMBILICAL CORD

GIANT INCLUSION BODIES ON SMEAR

BM TRANSPLANT

CARDIOLOGY

3

CORONARY ARTERY DISEASE

DEFINITION

Coronary artery disease (CAD) can also be used interchangeably with the terms **atherosclerotic heart disease** or **ischemic heart disease**. All of these terms imply insufficient perfusion of the coronary arteries from an abnormal narrowing of the vessels, leading to insufficient oxygen delivery to the myocardial tissue.

A 48-year-old woman comes to the office with chest pain that has been occurring over the last several weeks. The pain is not reliably related to exertion. She is comfortable now. The location of the pain is retrosternal. The pain is sometimes associated with nausea. There is no shortness of breath and the pain does not radiate beyond the chest. She has no past medical history.

What is the most likely diagnosis?

a. Gastroesophageal reflux disease (GERD)
b. Unstable angina
c. Pericarditis
d. Pneumothorax
e. Prinzmetal angina

Answer: The correct answer is (A). When a patient has chest pain, and the etiology is not likely to be cardiac ischemia, the most likely cause is some type of gastrointestinal (GI) disorder such as GERD. Other common GI disorders that are associated with chest pain are:

- *Ulcer disease*
- *Cholelithiasis*
- *Duodenitis*
- *Gastritis*

*If a 48-year-old woman had chest pain with **no** risk factors it would be very unlikely that her chest pain was related to ischemic heart disease. By the time a woman is 55 to 60, the protective effect of menstruation and naturally-occurring estrogen have worn off, and the rates of CAD will at least equal the rates in men.*

49

Understanding risk factors for CAD is most important in establishing a diagnosis in cases of chest pain with equivocal or uncertain histories.

▶ **TIP**

Menstruating women virtually never have myocardial infarctions.

Which of the following is most likely to benefit a patient's risk of coronary disease?

a. Administration of estrogen replacement at the time of menopause
b. Stopping tamoxifen
c. Stopping aromatase inhibitors
d. Regular exercise
e. Relaxation methods such as meditation

Answer: The correct answer is (D). Increasing heart rates through regular exercise or even taking the stairs instead of using an elevator show clear benefit in cardiac outcome.

*Although myocardial infarction is extremely rare in women before the age of 50, which is the average age of menopause, this does **not** translate into a beneficial effect of administering estrogen replacement. While it may make intuitive sense that relaxation methods such as yoga, meditation, and tai chi should work, measurable evidence of their benefit has, as of yet, not been obtained. This may be from a difficulty in measuring "relaxation." Weight, LDL, and heart rates are measurable and reproducible.*

▶ **TIP**

Overall, more women will eventually die of heart disease than men.

Risk Factors for Coronary Artery Disease

The most clearly agreed-upon risk factors for CAD are:

- **Diabetes** mellitus
- **Tobacco** smoking
- Hypertension
- **Hyperlipidemia**
- Family history of **premature** coronary artery disease
- Age above 45 in men and above 55 in women

The **worst** risk factor for CAD is diabetes mellitus, but the most **common** risk is hypertension.

Patients with diabetes have the highest rates of CAD when followed over a long period of time such as 10 years. Hypertension, defined as a blood pressure above 140/90, is more **common** than diabetes with about 20% of the total population, or 60 million people, suffering from hypertension. Nearly half of these people do not currently know that they are hypertensive.

Family History

Family history does **not** convey a risk for the patient if CAD developed in **elderly** relatives or if the relatives were grandparents, cousins, or aunts and uncles. **First-degree** relatives are siblings and parents.

Premature coronary disease is defined as being in a family member who is:

- Male relative under 55
- Female relative under 65

Family History

- Only CAD in **first-degree** relatives conveys a risk of CAD for the patient.
- Only **premature** CAD in a family member is a risk for the patient.

Hyperlipidemia

Which of the following is the most dangerous to a patient in terms of risk for CAD?

a. Elevated triglycerides
b. Elevated total cholesterol
c. Decreased high density lipoprotein (HDL)
d. Elevated low density lipoprotein (LDL)
e. Obesity

*Answer: The correct answer is **(D)**. Marked elevation in LDL is by far the most dangerous portion of a lipid profile for a patient. A low HDL is also associated with a poor long-term prognosis, but is not as dangerous as an elevated LDL. Although elevations in triglyceride levels are potentially dangerous, this is not as reproducible in terms of poor outcome as the elevated LDL. The proper treatment of an isolated elevation of triglyceride level is not as clearly beneficial as treatment of an elevated LDL level. Obesity, particularly that resulting in increasing abdominal girth, is associated with increased cardiac mortality. However, much of the danger of obesity is from its association with other abnormalities such as hyperlipidemia, diabetes, and hypertension.*

Less Reliable but Probable Risk Factors for CAD

- Physical inactivity
- Excess alcohol ingestion
- Insufficient fruits and vegetables in the diet
- Emotional stress
- Elevated electron-beam CT scan calcium scores
- Positron emission tomography (PET) scanning

Increased physical activity and exercise reliably lower all-cause mortality, but physical inactivity is not as severe a risk for coronary disease as diabetes and hypertension.

Calcium scores on a CT scan of the heart are still considered experimental. It is not clear what to do differently with this information in addition to standard risk factors.

▶ **TIP**

New disease entity: **Tako-Tsubo cardiomyopathy**

A postmenopausal woman develops chest pain immediately on hearing the news of her son's death in a war. She develops acute chest pain, dyspnea, and ST segment elevation in leads V2 to V4 on electrocardiogram. Elevated levels of troponin confirm an acute myocardial infarction. Coronary angiography is normal including an absence of vasospasm on provocative testing. Echocardiography reveals apical left ventricular "ballooning."

What is the presumed mechanism of this disorder?

a. Absence of estrogen
b. Massive catecholamine discharge
c. Plaque rupture
d. Platelet activation
e. Emboli to the coronary arteries

Answer: The correct answer is **(B)**. Tako-Tsubo cardiomyopathy is acute myocardial damage most often occurring in postmenopausal women immediately following an overwhelming, emotionally stressful event. Examples are earthquake, lightning strike, and hypoglycemia. This leads to "ballooning" and left ventricular dyskinesis. As with ischemic disease, manage with beta blockers and ACE inhibitors. Revascularization will not help, since the coronary arteries are normal.

> Sudden, overwhelming emotional stress and anger can cause chest pain and sudden death.

Unreliable (Unproven) Risk Factors for CAD

Several disease markers such as elevated homocysteine levels, *Chlamydia* infection, and elevated C-reactive protein levels have **not** proven to be reliable. There is **no** benefit to measuring, following, or attempting to therapeutically intervene on these factors. They are the **wrong** answers.

> Frequently used **wrong** answers are **just as important** to learn as the right answer. Know which answer to select, and which choices to avoid.

▶ **TIP**

Most Common Wrong Answer on Risk Factor Questions

The most frequent mistake in risk factor questions involves family history: mistaking CAD in **elderly** relatives, even if they are the patient's parents, as a risk for the patient. When the question asks "Which of the following is the most important element in evaluating/assessing this patient?" students most commonly answer "CAD in the parents," despite the fact that the age of the parents presented is outside the risk factor guidelines, such as a mother in her late 60s.

> The presence of CAD risk factors can help answer the question "Which of the following is the most likely diagnosis?" when the patient is **young** or the presentation is equivocal.

Correcting which of the following risk factors for CAD will result is the most immediate benefit for the patient?

a. Diabetes mellitus
b. Tobacco smoking
c. Hypertension
d. Hyperlipidemia
e. Weight loss

Answer: The correct answer is (B). Smoking cessation results in the greatest immediate improvement in patient outcomes for CAD. Within a year after stopping smoking, the risk of CAD decreases by 50%. Within 2 years after stopping smoking, the risk is reduced by 90%.

STOPPING SMOKING IS MOST IMPORTANT IMMEDIATE INTERVENTION

Chest Pain Presentation

"WHAT IS THE MOST LIKELY DIAGNOSIS?"

Ischemic pain is described as:

- **Dull** or "sore"

- **Squeezing** or pressure-like

The heart is a muscle, and like any muscle, when it is starved for oxygen, it will produce a sore-muscle type of pain when ischemic.

Qualities of the pain that go **against** ischemia are:

- Sharp ("knifelike") or pointlike

- Lasts for a few seconds

Three features of chest pain tell whether or not the pain is ischemic in nature:

1. Changes with **respiration (pleuritic)**
2. Changes with **position** of the body
3. Changes with **touch** of the chest wall **(tenderness)**

Each of these features (pleuritic, positional, tender) will exclude ischemia as a cause of the chest pain with about a 95% negative predictive value. In real life, a 95% negative predictive value would not be enough to exclude ischemia as a cause of chest pain—it would mean that 1 out of 20 patients presenting with chest pain would be misdiagnosed. However, on board exams like the USMLE, a 95% negative predictive value is generally enough to allow you to answer the question correctly. When the pain is described as *changing with respiration, changing with bodily position,* or *touching the chest wall*, do **not** answer ischemia or CAD as the cause of the chest pain.

For every 100 people presenting to the emergency department with chest pain, less than 10% end up having a myocardial infarction as a cause of the chest pain. Fifty percent or more have no cardiac disease at all.

> The most common cause of chest pain that is **not** ischemic in nature is from **gastrointestinal** disorders.

Causes of Chest Pain		
If the case describes....	Answer as "most likely diagnosis"	Answer as "most accurate test"
Chest wall tenderness	Costochondritis	Physical examination
Radiation to back, unequal blood pressure between arms	Aortic dissection	Chest x-ray with widened mediastinum, chest CT, MRI, or TEE confirms the disease
Pain worse with lying flat, better when sitting up	Pericarditis	Electrocardiogram with ST elevation everywhere, PR depression
Epigastric discomfort, pain better when eating	Duodenal ulcer disease	Endoscopy
Bad taste, cough, hoarseness	Gastroesophageal reflux	Response to PPIs; aluminum hydroxide and magnesium hydroxide; viscous lidocaine
Cough, sputum, hemoptysis _FEVER_	Pneumonia	Chest x-ray
Sudden-onset _FEVER sometimes_ shortness of breath, tachycardia, hypoxia	Pulmonary embolus	Spiral CT, V/Q scan _X-RAY USUALLY NORMAL_
Sharp, pleuritic pain, tracheal deviation	Pneumothorax	Chest x-ray

Features of the Chest Pain That Will Not Help Determine a Diagnosis

These additional symptoms can be associated with **multiple** diagnoses, and are therefore **nonspecific**. Their presence will **not** help establish a diagnosis.

- Nausea
- Fever
- Shortness of breath (dyspnea)
- Sweating (diaphoresis)
- Anxiety

Shortness of breath in the setting of chest pain has the worst prognostic significance. Fever suggests PE or pneumonia as the cause.

DIAGNOSTIC TESTS

Electrocardiogram

The "best initial test" for all forms of chest pain is certainly an electrocardiogram (EKG). The results of the EKG are entirely dependent on the setting of the case.

In the **office-based**, **ambulatory setting**, you can expect the EKG to be normal the majority of the time, yet you cannot go on to other forms of testing until the EKG is performed.

Enzymes: (CK-MB/Troponin)

Cardiac enzymes are **not** the answer in the office/ambulatory case in which you are being asked to evaluate chronic or stable chest pain. Cardiac enzymes are not an appropriate answer for the office/clinic. If the patient has acute chest pain in that setting, the answer is "Transfer to the emergency department." Enzymes are the answer when you are evaluating acute cases of chest pain in the emergency department. The key to the right answer is:

- **Office (ambulatory clinic) chest pain for days to weeks:** NO enzymes
- **Emergency department chest pain for minutes to hours:** YES enzymes, after an EKG is performed

Stress (Exercise Tolerance) Testing

Exercise tolerance testing (ETT) is the **indispensible** tool to evaluate chest pain **when the etiology is not clear** and the EKG is not diagnostic.

ETT is based on **2** factors:

1. You can read the EKG.
2. The patient can exercise.

"Exercise" means that the patient can get his or her heart rate up above 80% of maximum.

▶ **TIP**

Maximum heart rate = 220 minus the age of patient

Ischemia is detected by ST segment depression on the EKG.

1. Cannot read the EKG: If you **cannot** read the EKG because of a baseline EKG abnormality, you must find a **different** way of detecting ischemia in the heart. The 2 best methods of detecting ischemia without the use of EKG are:
   - Nuclear isotope uptake: thallium or sestamibi
   - Echocardiographic detection of wall motion abnormalities

> Stress testing is the answer when the etiology of chest pain is **uncertain** and the EKG is **not** diagnostic.

▶ **TIP**

Reasons for baseline EKG abnormalities include left bundle branch block, left ventricular hypertrophy, pacemaker use, or the effect of digoxin.

Normal myocardium **will pick up thallium** in the same way that potassium is picked up by the sodium/potassium ATPase. If the myocardium is **alive** and **perfused**, thallium or other nuclear isotopes will be picked up. **Abnormalities** will be detected by seeing **decreased thallium uptake**.

Normal myocardium will move on contraction. Abnormalities will be detected by seeing **decreased** wall motion. This is also referred to as **dyskinesis**, **akinesis**, or **hypokinesis**.

▶ **TIP**

Ischemia versus infarction: Ischemia, or simply decreased perfusion, will be detected by seeing a **reversal** of the decrease in thallium uptake or wall motion that will **return to normal** after a period of rest.

> Ischemia gives **reversible** wall motion or thallium uptake between rest and exercise. Infarction is irreversible or "fixed."

2. Cannot exercise: If the patient **cannot** exercise, then an alternate method of increasing myocardial oxygen consumption must be performed.

   - Persantine (dipyridamole) or adenosine in combination with the use of nuclear isotopes such as thallium or sestamibi

   - Dobutamine in combination with the use of echocardiography: Dobutamine will increase myocardial oxygen consumption and provoke ischemia detected as decreased wall motion on an echocardiogram.

> Dipyridamole may provoke bronchospasm. Avoid in asthmatics.

Use of Exercise Tolerance Testing					
Test	**Exercise tolerance**	**Exercise thallium**	**Exercise echo**	**Dipyridamole thallium**	**Dobutamine echo**
Indication	Determine presence of ischemia	Inability to read the EKG, baseline ST segment abnormalities	Same as exercise thallium	Inability to exercise to target heart rate	Same as dipyridamole thallium
Ischemia detected	ST segment depression	Decreased uptake of nuclear isotope	Decreased wall motion	Decreased uptake of nuclear isotope	Decreased wall motion

▶ **TIP**

The 2 different methods of detecting ischemia in terms of using nuclear isotopes or echocardiography are essentially equal in terms of sensitivity and specificity.

Exercise Thallium = Exercise Echo
Dipyridamole Thallium = Dobutamine Echo

Coronary Angiography

Angiography is used to detect the anatomic location of coronary artery disease. Angiography is predominantly a test to detect the presence of narrowing that is best managed with **surgery**, **angioplasty**, or other methods

> Angiography determines bypass **surgery** versus **angioplasty**.

of revascularization. Sometimes angiography is used if noninvasive tests such as EKG or stress testing are equivocal. **Angiography** is the **most accurate** method of detecting coronary artery disease.

Stenosis (narrowing) less than 50% of the diameter is **insignificant**. Surgically correctable disease generally begins with at least 70% stenosis.

Holter Monitoring

The **Holter** monitor is a continuous **ambulatory EKG monitor** that records the rhythm; it is usually used for a 24-hour period, but may be continued for 48 to 72 hours. **Holter** monitoring **detects rhythm disorders** including atrial fibrillation, flutter, ectopy such as premature beats, or ventricular tachycardia. Holter monitor does **not detect ischemia** and is **not** accurate for evaluating the ST segment.

> Holter monitoring is used **only** for rhythm evaluation.

A 48-year-old woman comes to the office with chest pain that has been occurring over the last several weeks. The pain is not reliably related to exertion. She is comfortable now. The location of the pain is retrosternal. She has no past medical history and the EKG is normal.

What is the most appropriate next step in management?

a. CK-MB
b. Troponin
c. Echocardiogram
d. Exercise tolerance testing
e. Angiography
f. CT angiography
g. Cardiac MRI
h. Holter monitor

*Answer: The correct answer is (**D**). Enzymes are to evaluate acute coronary syndromes. Serial troponin measurements are done prior to stress test. Echocardiography is to evaluate valve function, wall motion, and ejection fraction. Exercise tolerance testing is to evaluate stable patients with chest pain whose diagnoses are not clear. ETT is **not** used in acute coronary syndrome cases in which the patient is **currently** having pain and the diagnosis is already clear. Also, **don't put patients on a treadmill to exercise if they are currently having chest pain**.*

TREATMENT

USMLE Step 2 CK is most concerned that you know the medications that will **lower mortality**. For a patient with chronic angina (**not** an acute coronary syndrome), the therapeutic options are easier. There are only a few right choices:

- Aspirin
- Beta blockers
- Nitroglycerin

USMLE Step 2 CK, like most board examinations, will **not** test dosing, although the **route** of administration is **important** to know. Knowing that nitroglycerin can be used either **orally** or by transdermal patch in chronic angina is important, but knowing the specific dose is **not**. Knowing that sublingual, paste, and intravenous forms of nitroglycerin are used in **acute** coronary syndromes, but not in chronic angina, is important. Knowing **how much** paste is **not** important.

▶ **TIP**

Nonspecific beta blockers such as propranolol are **not** used routinely in cardiology.

Clopidogrel is used in:

- **Aspirin intolerance** such as allergy
- Recent angioplasty with stenting

Clopidogrel is rarely associated with thrombotic thrombocytopenic purpura.

Prasugrel

A new thienopyridine medication in the same class as clopidogrel and ticlopidine, **prasugrel** is indicated as an **antiplatelet medication** that has its best evidence for use in those undergoing **angioplasty and stenting**. Prasugrel is dangerous in patients 75 and older because of an increased risk of hemorrhagic stroke.

Ticlopidine

- Used to inhibit platelets in the rare patient who is intolerant of **both** aspirin **and** clopidogrel. You cannot use ticlopidine if the reason for aspirin and clopidogrel intolerance is bleeding, since **ticlopidine will inhibit platelets** as well.
- Ticlopidine causes **neutropenia**.

Ranolazine

- Additional therapy for angina refractory or persistent through other treatment.

ACE Inhibitors/Angiotensin Receptor Blockers

- **Low ejection fraction**/systolic dysfunction (best mortality benefit)
- **Regurgitant** valvular disease
- Cough is the most common adverse effect of ACE inhibitors, occurring in up to 7% of patients.

A 64-year-old man is placed on lisinopril as part of managing CAD in association with an ejection fraction of 24% and symptoms of breathlessness. Although he sometimes has rales on lung examination, the patient is asymptomatic today. Physical examination reveals minimal edema of the lower extremities. Blood tests reveal an elevated level of potassium that is present on a repeat measurement. EKG is unchanged.

How would you best manage the patient?

> **Best** mortality benefit in **chronic** angina: aspirin and beta blockers.

a. *Add kayexalate (potassium-binding resin)*

b. *Insulin and glucose*

c. *Stop lisinopril*

d. *Switch lisinopril to candesartan*

e. *Switch lisinopril to hydralazine and nitrates*

*Answer: The correct answer is **(E)**. Although **cough** may be the most common **adverse effect of ACE inhibitors (ACEi)**, they may also cause **hyperkalemia**. You cannot just switch the ACEi to an angiotension receptor blocker, since **both** classes of medications lead to hyperkalemia because of their effect on inhibiting aldosterone. **Aldosterone** normally functions **to excrete potassium** from the distal tubule.*

*Hydralazine is a direct-acting arterial vasodilator. Hydralazine will decrease afterload and has been shown to have a **clear** mortality benefit in patients with systolic dysfunction. Hydralazine should be used in association with nitrates to dilate the coronary arteries so that blood is not "stolen" away from coronary perfusion when afterload is decreased with the use of hydralazine.*

Lipid Management

▶ **TIP**

Statins (HMG CoA Reductase inhibitors)

- CAD with an LDL above 100 mg/dL

The guideline of using statins when the LDL is above 100 mg/dL is very carefully selected, since recommendations vary. The National Cholesterol Education Program recommends statins for those with CAD and an LDL above 100 to 130. There are groups that recommend statins in **any** patient with CAD, regardless of LDL level. The American College of Cardiology recommends a goal of LDL below 70 for those with coronary disease **and** diabetes.

How are you, a student at the level of a USMLE Step 2 CK exam, supposed to get a bottom-line answer when you may hear may different recommendations? Remember that you are being tested on **national** guidelines from nonbiased federal organizations, not private organizations like the ACC.

Everyone will agree that with CAD, the **goal of LDL** should be at least **less than 100 mg/dL**.

▶ **TIP**

CAD equivalents (goal of LDL is below 100 and statins should be used to bring the LDL down if above 100):

- Peripheral artery disease (PAD)
- Carotid disease (**not** stroke)
- Aortic disease (the aortic **artery**, not the valve)
- Diabetes mellitus

Which of the following is the most common adverse effect of statin medications?

a. Rhabdomyolysis
b. Liver dysfunction
c. Renal failure
d. Encephalopathy
e. Hyperkalemia

Answer: The correct answer is (B). At least 1% of patients taking statin medications will develop elevation of transaminases to the level where you will need to discontinue the medication. Myositis, elevation of CPK levels, or rhabdomyolysis will occur in less than 0.1% of patients. It is very rare to have to stop statins because of myositis. There is no recommendation to routinely test all patients for CPK levels in the absence of symptoms. On the other hand, all patients started on statins should have their AST and ALT tested as a matter of routine monitoring, even if no symptoms are present.

Other Lipid-Lowering Therapies

Niacin, gemfibrozil, cholestyramine, and ezetimibe all have beneficial effects on lipid profiles. However, **none** of them is the best initial therapy because none of them has the clear mortality benefit in CAD that statins provide. Niacin and fibric acid derivatives such as gemfibrozil have some mortality benefit, but not as much as the statins. **Statins have an antioxidant effect on the endothelial lining** of the coronary arteries that gives a benefit that transcends simply lowering the LDL number.

PROSTAGLANDIN INDUCED- VASODILATION

Niacin: Associated with glucose intolerance, elevation of uric acid level, and an uncomfortable "itchiness" from a transient relief of histamine, niacin is an excellent drug to **add** to statins if full lipid control is not achieved with statins. Although statins, exercise, and cessation of tobacco use will all raise the HDL level, niacin will raise HDL somewhat more.

Gemfibrozil: Fibric acid derivatives lower triglyceride levels somewhat more than statins; however, the benefit of **lowering triglycerides** alone has **not** proven to be as useful as the straightforward mortality benefit of statins. Use caution in combining **fibrates with statins because of an increased risk of myositis.**

Cholestyramine: This bile acid sequestrant also has significant **interactions** with **other medications** in the gut, potentially blocking their absorption. In addition, cholestyramine can be associated with uncomfortable gastrointestinal complaints such as constipation and flatus.

Ezetimibe: This agent definitely lowers LDL level without any evidence of actual benefit to the patient. LDL levels are an imperfect marker of benefit with cholesterol-lowering therapies. Ezetimibe is no better than a placebo in terms of clinical endpoints such as myocardial infarction, stroke, or death.

▶ **TIP**

Lipid-lowering therapy: What is clear?

- Statins **lower mortality** the most.
- Adverse effects of other agents are well established.

Since USMLE Step 2 CK must ask questions that are clear, you are **most likely** to get questions about **adverse effects**. Besides the benefit of statins in CAD with LDL levels above 100 mg/dL, the only truly clear aspect of the other therapies is their adverse effects.

Lipid-lowering Medications and Their Adverse Effects	
Agent	**Adverse effect**
Statins	Elevations of transaminases (liver function tests), myositis
Niacin	Elevation in glucose and uric acid level, pruritus
Fibric acid derivatives	Increased risk of myositis when combined with statins
Cholestyramine	Flatus and abdominal cramping
Ezetimibe	Well tolerated and nearly useless

> Check AST and ALT when using statins.

Calcium Channel Blockers

Dihydropyridine calcium channel blockers (CCBs) such as nifedipine, nitrendipine, nicardipine, and nimodipine may actually **increase** mortality in patients with CAD because of their effect in raising heart rates. The best example of an increased heart rate is the "reflex tachycardia" developing from the use of nifedipine. This is probably the best explanation for the failure of the CCBs to decrease mortality. Although CCBs are negative inotropes which should decrease myocardial oxygen consumption via that mechanism, the **increased heart rate** in the aggregate will **increase** myocardial oxygen consumption.

Bottom line: Do **not** routinely use CCBs in CAD.

The CCBs verapamil and diltiazem, which do **not** increase heart rate, are used in those who cannot tolerate beta blockers because of severe asthma. However, 70% of patients with reactive airway diseases such as asthma can still tolerate the use of beta-1 specific beta blockers.

Use CCBs (verapamil/diltiazem) in CAD **only** with:

- **Severe asthma** precluding the use of beta blockers
- **Prinzmetal** variant angina
- **Cocaine**-induced chest pain (beta blockers thought to be contraindicated)

> **None** of the calcium channel blockers have been shown to lower mortality in CAD.

> When studying medications, you **must** know the clear adverse effects. These USMLE Step 2 CK questions do **not** change over time.

Adverse Effects of CCBs

- Edema
- Constipation
- Heart block (rare)

Revascularization

Angiography is indispensible in evaluating a patient for the possibility of revascularization, which is either coronary bypass surgery or angioplasty. Symptoms alone **cannot** tell the number of vessels involved, **what** vessels are involved, or the degree or percentage of stenosis.

Coronary artery bypass grafting (CABG) lowers mortality only in a few specific circumstances with **very** severe disease such as:

- **Three vessels** with at least 70% stenosis in each vessel
- **Left main** coronary artery occlusion
- Two-vessel disease in a patient with diabetes
- Persistent symptoms despite maximal medical therapy

Long-term mortality benefit is greater with the most severe disease such as those with left ventricular dysfunction. The immediate operative mortality may be greater in patients with an ejection fraction (EF) below 35%, but in the long term, those surviving the procedure will do better in those with 3-vessel disease and left ventricular dysfunction.

Internal mammary **artery grafts last on average for 10 years** before they occlude, whereas saphenous **vein grafts remain patent reliably for only 5 years**.

Percutaneous coronary intervention (PCI) is commonly referred to as **angioplasty**. The term *intervention* is more precise, because there are other interventions besides angioplasty. PCI is unquestionably the **best** therapy in **acute coronary syndromes**, particularly those **with ST segment elevation**. The mortality benefit of PCI has been much harder to demonstrate in chronic stable angina. Maximal medical therapy with aspirin, beta blockers, ACEi/ARBs, and statins has proven to have equal or even superior benefit compared to PCI in stable CAD. PCI is more definitive in terms of decreasing dependence on medication and decreasing frequency of painful angina episodes.

> PCI is the best in **acute coronary syndromes**, particularly with ST segment elevation. PCI does **not** provide clear mortality benefit for stable patients.

ACUTE CORONARY SYNDROMES

DEFINITION

It is **impossible** to determine the precise etiology of acute coronary syndromes (ACS) from history and physical examination alone. The risk factors (eg, hypertension, diabetes mellitus, tobacco) are the same as those described previously for CAD.

A 70-year-old woman comes to the emergency department with crushing substernal chest pain for the last hour. The pain radiates to her left arm and is associated with anxiety, diaphoresis, and nausea. She describes the pain as "sore" and "dull" and clenches her fist in front of her chest. She has a history of hypertension.

Which of the following is most likely to be found in this patient?

a. >10 mm Hg decrease in blood pressure on inhalation
b. Increase in jugular venous pressure on inhalation
c. Triphasic scratchy sound on auscultation
d. Continuous "machinery" murmur
e. S4 gallop
f. Point of maximal impulse displaced towards the axilla

Answer: The correct answer is (E). Acute coronary syndromes are associated with an S4 gallop because of ischemia leading to noncompliance of the left ventricle. The S4 gallop is the sound of atrial systole as blood is ejected from the atrium into a stiff ventricle. A decrease of blood pressure of greater than 10 mm Hg on inhalation is a pulsus paradoxus and is associated with cardiac tamponade.

An increase in jugulovenous pressure on inhalation is the **Kussmaul sign** and is most often **associated with constrictive pericarditis** or restrictive cardiomyopathy. A triphasic "scratchy" sound is a pericardial friction rub. Although pericarditis can occur as a complication of myocardial infarction (Dressler syndrome), this would not occur for several days after an MI and is **much** rarer than simple ventricular ischemia.

▶ TIP

A continuous "machinery" murmur is what would be found with a patent ductus arteriosus.

A displaced point of maximal impulse (PMI) is characteristic of left ventricular hypertrophy (LVH) as well as dilated cardiomyopathy. A displaced PMI is an anatomic abnormality that could **not** possibly occur with an acute coronary syndrome.

A 70-year-old woman comes to the emergency department with crushing substernal chest pain for the last hour.

Which of the following EKG findings would be associated with the worst prognosis?

a. ST elevation in leads II, III, aVF
b. PR interval >200 milliseconds
c. ST elevation in leads V2-V4
d. Frequent premature ventricular complexes (PVCs)
e. ST depression in leads V1 and V2
f. Right bundle branch block (RBBB)

> There are no specific physical findings to allow you to answer a "most likely diagnosis" question in terms of ST elevation or depression without an EKG.

> Do not walk into your USMLE Step 2 CK exam without knowing when you will expect each of the cardiac physical findings described here.

*Answer: The correct answer is **(C)**. Leads V2 to V4 correspond to the anterior wall of the left ventricle. ST segment elevation most often signifies an acute myocardial infarction.*

*ST elevation in leads **II, III, and aVF** is also consistent with an acute myocardial infarction, but of the **inferior** wall. Untreated, the **mortality associated with an IWMI is less than 5%** at 1 year after the event. With an **AWMI**, mortality untreated is closer to **30% to 40%**.*

*PR interval greater than 200 milliseconds is first-degree atrioventricular (AV) block. **First-degree AV block has little pathologic potential** and, when isolated, requires no additional therapy.*

Ectopy such as PVCs and atrial premature complexes (APCs) are associated with the later development of more severe arrhythmias, but no additional therapy is needed for them if magnesium and potassium levels are normal. We don't like to see PVCs, but their presence does not require any changes in management.

ST depressions in leads V1 and V2 are suggestive of a posterior wall myocardial infarction. These leads are read in the opposite direction of the rest of the leads. In other words, ST depression in leads V1 and V2 would be like ST elevation elsewhere—an acute infarction. Infarctions of the posterior wall are associated with a very low mortality, and again, there is no additional therapy to give because of it.

*Right bundle branch block **(RBBB) is relatively benign** compared to a new left bundle branch block.*

> PVCs should **not** be treated, even when associated with an acute infarction. Treatment of PVCs only **worsens** outcome.

A 70-year-old woman comes to the emergency department with crushing substernal chest pain for the last hour. An EKG shows ST segment elevation in V2 to V4.

What is the most appropriate next step in the management of this patient?

a. CK-MB level
b. Oxygen
c. Nitroglycerin sublingual
d. Aspirin
e. Thrombolytics
f. Metoprolol
g. Atorvostatin
h. Angioplasty
i. Consult cardiology
j. Transfer the patient to the intensive care unit
k. Troponin level
l. Morphine
m. Angiography
n. Clopidogrel

*Answer: The correct answer is **(D)**. Aspirin lowers mortality with acute coronary syndromes, and it is critical to administer it as rapidly as possible. With only 1 hour since the onset of pain, neither the CK-MB level nor the troponin level would be elevated yet. Morphine, oxygen, and nitroglycerin should all be administered, but they do not lower mortality and are therefore not as important as aspirin. Aspirin should be given simultaneously with activating the catheterization lab.*

Clopidogrel is indicated when the patient has an intolerance of aspirin or has undergone angioplasty with stenting.

The patient should be transferred to an intensive care unit (ICU), but you must always **initiate therapy** *and testing* **before you** *simply* **move the patient** *to another part of the hospital. It is much more important to start proper care than to move the patient, even if it is a movement to an area of increased observation and potential treatment. Thrombolytics or angioplasty should be done and it is critical to do them quickly; however, aspirin is simply recommended to be given* **first**. *Aspirin is then followed with another form of acute revascularization.*

▶ **TIP**

On USMLE Step 2 CK, consultation is almost **never** the correct choice. Do everything yourself.

A 70-year-old woman comes to the emergency department with crushing substernal chest pain for the last hour. An EKG shows ST segment elevation in V2 to V4. Aspirin has been given to the patient to chew.

What is the most appropriate next step in the management of this patient?

a. CK-MB level
b. Oxygen
c. Nitroglycerin sublingual
d. Morphine
e. Thrombolytics
f. Metoprolol
g. Atorvostatin
h. Angioplasty
i. Troponin level
j. Lisinopril

Answer: The correct answer is **(H)**. *Angioplasty is associated with the greatest mortality benefit of all the steps listed in this question. All of the answers are partially correct in that all of them should be done for the patient. Again, morphine, oxygen, and nitrates should be given to the patient immediately, but they do not clearly lower mortality.*

Enzyme tests should be done, but within the first 4 hours of the onset of chest pain, they will certainly be normal. Even if they are elevated, CK-MB and troponin levels would not alter the management.

Beta blockers *are associated with a decrease in mortality, but they are* ***not critically dependent upon time***. *As long as the patient receives metoprolol sometime during the hospital stay and at discharge, she will derive benefit. The same is true of the use of statins and ACE inhibitors.*

One of the **most** critical points of preparation is to learn the **order** in which to do things. It is not enough simply to know which tests and treatments must be done at some point. You **must** be able to prioritize what is **first**.

The key issues in the management of acute coronary syndromes are:

- Does the intervention/treatment lower mortality?
- Which management is most important to do **first**?

Diagnostic Tests		
Test	**Time to becoming abnormal**	**Duration of abnormality**
EKG	Immediately at onset of pain	ST elevation progresses to Q-waves over several days to a week
Myoglobin	1–4 hours	1–2 days
CK-MB	4–6 hours	1–2 days
Troponin	4–6 hours	10–14 days

The use of the troponin level is not without its difficulties:

- Troponin cannot distinguish a reinfarction occurring several days after the first event.
- Renal insufficiency can result in false positive tests since troponin is excreted through the kidney.

Reinfarction

When a patient has a new episode of pain within a few days of the first cardiac event, the management is:

1. Perform an EKG to detect **new** ST segment abnormalities.
2. Check CK-MB levels.

After 2 days, the CK-MB level from the initial infarction should have returned to normal. A CK-MB level that is elevated several days after an initial myocardial infarction is indicative of a new ischemic event.

Intensive Care Unit Monitoring

After the initial management is put in place, the patient should be monitored in an ICU. Continuous rhythm monitoring is essential to an improved survival and outcome. Multiple factors contribute to the lowering of mortality through ICU monitoring:

- The most common cause of death in the first several days after a myocardial infarction is ventricular arrhythmia (ventricular tachycardia, ventricular fibrillation).
- Rapid performance of electrical cardioversion or defibrillation is available.

TREATMENT

ST Segment Elevation Myocardial Infarction

ACS is best managed initially with aspirin, either orally or chewed. Clopidogrel is often used if there is an allergy to aspirin, but prasugrel is an alternative to clopidogrel that seems to have superior benefit.

Angioplasty versus Thrombolytics

Angioplasty (PCI) is **superior to thrombolytics** in terms of:

- Survival and mortality benefit
- Fewer hemorrhagic complications
- Likelihood of developing complications of MI (less arrhythmia, less CHF, fewer ruptures of septum, free wall [tamponade] and papillary muscles [valve rupture])

The standard of care is that **PCI** is expected to be performed within **90 minutes** of the patient arriving in the emergency department with chest pain.

> "Door to balloon time": under 90 minutes

Complications of PCI

Complications include:

- **Rupture** of the coronary artery on inflation of the balloon
- **Restenosis** of the vessel after the angioplasty
- **Hematoma** at the site of entry into the artery (eg, femoral area hematoma)

Only 20% of U.S. hospitals are equipped to perform primary angioplasty because many lack a catheterization laboratory. It is important to have the ability to perform emergency cardiac surgery to repair the vessel.

Which of the following is most important in decreasing the risk of restenosis of the coronary artery after PCI?

a. Multistage procedure: ie, doing 1 vessel at a time, with multiple procedures
b. Use of heparin for 3–6 months after the procedure
c. Warfarin use after the procedure
d. Placement of bare metal stent
e. Placement of drug-eluting stent (paclitaxel, sirolimus)

Answer: The correct answer is (E). The placement of drug-eluting stents that inhibit the local T cell response has markedly reduced the rate of restenosis. Heparin is used at the time of the procedure, but is not continued long term. Warfarin has no place in the management of coronary disease. Warfarin is useful for clots on the venous side of the circulation such as DVT or pulmonary embolus.

Rates of Restenosis within 6 Months of PCI

- No stenting: 30%–40%
- Bare metal stent: 15%–30%
- Drug-eluting stent: 10%

If there is a contraindication to the use of thrombolytics, the patient should be transferred to a facility performing PCI.

Absolute Contraindications to Thrombolytics

- Major bleeding into the bowel (melena) or brain (**any** type of CNS bleeding)
- Recent surgery (within the last 2 weeks)

> Heme-positive **brown** stool is **not** an absolute contraindication to the use of thrombolytics.

- Severe hypertension (above 180/110)
- Nonhemorrhagic stroke within the last 6 months

A patient comes to a small rural hospital without a catheterization laboratory. The patient has chest pain and ST segment elevation. What is the most appropriate next step in the management of the patient?

a. Transfer for angioplasty
b. Administer thrombolytics now
c. Consult cardiology

Answer: The correct answer is (B). Immediate thrombolytics is far more beneficial to the patient than angioplasty delayed by several hours. Remember that consultation is almost never the right answer on USMLE Step 2 CK.

The mortality benefit of thrombolytics extends out to 12 hours from the onset of chest pain. In other words, you can answer "thrombolytics" in any patient with chest pain and ST segment elevation within the first 12 hours of the onset of chest pain. The mortality benefit is as much as a 50% relative risk reduction within the first 2 hours of the onset of pain. This is why a patient with chest pain who arrives in the emergency department should receive thrombolytics within 30 minutes of coming through the door.

> Time is **muscle**. Delay = death.

> "Door to needle time": under 30 minutes

TREATMENT

All of the treatments listed in this table are used in patients with ACS. The **benefit** of each treatment depends on the specific circumstance.

WARFARIN USED IN A-FIB

Treatment Indications and Benefits	
Therapy	**In what cases is effect greatest?**
Aspirin	Everyone, as the best initial therapy
Clopidogrel	Aspirin not tolerated, those undergoing angioplasty and stenting
Beta blockers	Everyone, effect is **not** dependent on time; started any time during admission
ACEi/ARB	Everyone, benefit best with ejection fraction below 40%
Statins	Everyone, benefit best with LDL >100 mg/dL
Oxygen, nitrates	Everyone, no clear mortality benefit
Heparin	After thrombolytics/PCI to prevent restenosis, initial therapy with ST depression and other NON-ST elevation events (unstable angina)
Calcium channel blockers	Can't use beta blockers, cocaine-induced pain, Prinzmetal or vasospastic variant angina

ST Segment Depression ACS

A man comes to the emergency department with chest pain for the last hour that is crushing in quality and does not change with respiration or the position of his body. An EKG shows ST segment depression in leads V2 to V4. Aspirin has been given.

What is the most appropriate next step in the management of this patient?

a. Low molecular-weight heparin
b. Thrombolytics
c. Glycoprotein IIb/IIIa inhibitor (abciximab)
d. Nitroglycerin
e. Morphine
f. Angioplasty
g. Metoprolol

*Answer: The correct answer is (A). Heparin will prevent a clot from forming in the coronary arteries. Heparin does **not** dissolve clots that have already formed. When the patient has ACS and there is **no** ST segment elevation, there is **no** benefit of thrombolytic therapy.*

Nitroglycerin, morphine, and oxygen are not associated with a clear reduction in mortality.

ACE inhibitors and statins are used, but the mortality benefit is, again, based on either a low ejection fraction or increased LDL respectively.

*Metoprolol should be used, but it has not been proven that it matters whether we give the beta blockers immediately, or at any time before hospital discharge. In other words, there is **no** urgency in terms of time for metoprolol. There is tremendous urgency to give heparin immediately because we want to prevent the clot from growing further and closing off the coronary artery.*

Glycoprotein IIb/IIIa Inhibitors (Abciximab, Tirofiban, Eptifibitide)

These agents (**GPIIb/IIIa inhibitors**) are used in acute coronary syndromes in those who are to **undergo angioplasty and stenting**. They are **not** beneficial in acute ST elevation infarctions separate from the use of angioplasty and stenting. GPIIb/IIIa inhibitors inhibit the aggregation of platelets. They lead to a reduction in mortality in those with ST depression, particularly in patients whose troponin or CK-MB levels rise and who then develop a myocardial infarction requiring PCI with stenting.

ANGIOPLASTY IF INFARCTION
WITHIN LAST 90 MIN

Summary of Treatment Differences between Cardiac Events			
	Stable angina	Unstable angina/ non-ST elevation MI	ST elevation MI
Aspirin	Yes	Yes	Yes
Beta blockers	Yes	Yes	Yes
Nitrates	Yes	Yes	Yes
Heparin	No	Yes	Yes, but only after thrombolytics
GPIIb/IIIa meds	No	Yes	No
Thrombolytics	No	No	Yes, but not as good as PCI
CCBs	No	No	No
Warfarin	No	No	No

Bottom Line:

1. tPA (thrombolytics) are beneficial **only** with ST elevation MI.

2. Heparin is **best** for **non**-ST elevation MI.

3. GP IIb/IIIa inhibitors are **best** for **non**-ST elevation MI and those undergoing PCI and stenting.

▶ **TIP**

Calcium channel blockers and warfarin have **no** clear mortality benefit in ACS.

▶ **TIP**

Low molecular-weight heparin is **superior** to unfractionated heparin in terms of mortality benefit.

In non-ST elevation ACS, when all medications have been given, and the patient is **not** better, urgent angiography and possibly angioplasty (PCI) should be done.

"Not better" means:

- Persistent pain
- S3 gallop or CHF developing
- Worse EKG changes
- Rising troponin levels

Complications of Acute Myocardial Infarction

▶ TIP

Complications of acute myocardial infarction are an **excellent** source of "What is the most likely diagnosis?" questions, the most common type of question on USMLE Step 2 CK.

All the complications of myocardial infarction can result in hypotension, so the presence of hypotension will **not** help you determine the diagnosis.

Bradycardia

Heart rate is key to establishing the diagnosis.

Sinus bradycardia is **very common** in association with MI because of vascular insufficiency of the sinoatrial (SA) node.

Third-degree (complete) AV block will have **cannon A waves**. They are the best way to distinguish third-degree AV block from sinus bradycardia before you obtain an EKG. Cannon A waves are produced by atrial systole against a closed tricuspid valve. The tricuspid valve is closed because the very essence of third-degree block is that the atria and ventricles are contracting separately and **out of coordination with each other**.

The cannon is the bounding jugulovenous wave bouncing up into the neck. Look for an association with right ventricular infarction and third-degree AV block. All symptomatic bradycardias are treated first with atropine and then by placing a pacemaker if the atropine is not effective.

Tachycardia

Right Ventricular Infarction

Look for the association with a **new inferior** wall MI and **clear lungs** on auscultation. You cannot get blood into the lungs if the blood cannot get into the heart. You can diagnose by flipping the EKG leads from the usual left side of the chest to the **right** side of the chest. ST elevation in RV4 is the most specific finding.

The right coronary artery supplies:

- Right ventricle (RV)
- AV node
- Inferior wall of the heart

This is why up to 40% of those with an inferior wall myocardial infarction (IWMI) will have a right ventricular infarction. Treat RV infarctions with high-volume fluid replacement. Avoid nitroglycerin to RV infarctions. They markedly worsen cardiac filling.

Tamponade/Free Wall Rupture

It usually takes several days after an infarction for the wall to scar and weaken enough for it to rupture. Look for "sudden loss of pulse" in the case. Lungs are clear. It is a cause of pulseless electrical activity.

You can diagnose with emergency echocardiography. Emergency pericardiocentesis is done on the way into the operating room to repair it.

Ventricular Tachycardia/Ventricular Fibrillation

Both ventricular tachycardia and ventricular fibrillation can cause **sudden death** and there is **no way to distinguish them without an EKG** if they cause loss of pulse. Both are treated with emergency electrical shock (cardioversion/defibrillation).

Valve or Septal Rupture

Both valve rupture and septal rupture present with **new onset of a murmur** and pulmonary **congestion**. Mitral regurgitation murmur is best heard at the apex with radiation to the axilla. Ventricular septal rupture is best heard at the lower left sternal border.

> ▶ **TIP**
>
> Most accurate test: Echocardiogram for both valve rupture and septal rupture.

> ▶ **TIP**
>
> You can't always depend on buzzwords like "step-up" for oxygenation. Often, the numbers are simply presented to you: "42% oxygen saturation is found on a sample of blood from the right atrium. 85% saturation is found on the right ventricular sample."

Intraaortic Balloon Pump

Intraaortic balloon pump (IABP) is the answer when there is acute pump failure from an anatomic problem that can be fixed in the operating room. IABP contracts and relaxes in sync with natural heartbeat. It helps give a "push" forward to the blood.

> ▶ **TIP**
>
> IABP is **never** a permanent device. Like valve replacement or transplant, it serves as a bridge to surgery.

Extension of the Infarction/Reinfarction

When a patient presents with either an inferior or anterior infarction, it is common for a second event to infarct a **second** geographic area of the heart.

Look for recurrence of pain, new rales on exam, a new bump up in CK-MBs, and even sudden onset of pulmonary edema.

These complications are the reason patients with acute MI are monitored in an ICU for the first several days after the infarction.

Look for a **step-up in oxygen saturation** as you go from the right atrium to the right ventricle to hand you the diagnosis of **septal rupture**.

Repeat the EKG and re-treat with angioplasty and sometimes thrombolytics in addition to the usual medications (aspirin, metoprolol, nitrates, ACE, statins).

Aneurysm/Mural Thrombus

Aneurysm or mural thrombus is detected with echocardiography. Most aneurysms do not need specific therapy. Mural thrombi, like all thrombi, are treated with heparin followed by warfarin.

"What Is the Most Likely Diagnosis?"	
Diagnosis	**Key feature**
Third-degree AV block	Bradycardia, cannon A waves
Sinus bradycardia	No cannon A waves
Tamponade/wall rupture	Sudden loss of pulse, jugulovenous distention
RV infarction	IWMI in history, clear lungs, tachycardia, hypotension with nitroglycerin
Valve rupture	New murmur, rales/congestion
Septal rupture	New murmur, increase in oxygen saturation on entering the right ventricle
Ventricular fibrillation	Loss of pulse, need EKG to answer question

Preparation for Discharge from Hospital

Detection of Persistent Ischemia

Everyone gets a stress test prior to discharge. The **stress test determines if angiography is needed**. Angiography determines the need for revascularization such as angioplasty or bypass surgery.

▶ **TIP**

Do **not** do a stress test if the patient remains symptomatic. These people clearly need angiography.

Do **not** do angiography if reversible signs of myocardial ischemia are **absent**. There is no point in revascularizing to myocardium that is dead (infarcted).

Post-MI Stress Test

Identify those with residual ischemia **prior** to leaving the hospital. Do **not** just cath (angiography) everyone.

Postinfarction Routine Medications

Everyone should go home on:

- Aspirin
- Beta blockers (metoprolol)
- Statins
- ACE inhibitors

ACE inhibitors are **best for anterior wall infarctions** because of the high likelihood of developing systolic dysfunction.

- **Clopidogrel**: those **intolerant of aspirin** or post-stenting
- **ARBs**: those with a **cough on ACE inhibitor**
- Ticlopidine: the rare person intolerant of both aspirin and clopidogrel

> Dipyridamole is **never** the right choice for coronary artery disease.

Prophylactic antiarrhythmic medications:

Do **not** use amiodarone, flecainide, or **any** rhythm-controlling medication to **prevent** the development of ventricular tachycardia or fibrillation. Do **not** be fooled by the question describing "frequent PVCs and ectopy." Prophylactic antiarrhythmics **increase** mortality.

Sexual Issues Postinfarction

This is a **very** frequently tested subject. The 4 most commonly tested facts are:

1. **Do not combine nitrates with sildenafil**; hypotension can result because they are both vasodilators.
2. Erectile dysfunction postinfarction is **most commonly from anxiety**; however, of all the medications that cause erectile dysfunction, the most common is beta blockers.
3. The **patient does not have to wait after an MI to reengage in sexual activity**. If the patient is symptom-free, sexual activity may begin immediately. This is because sexual activity usually does not last long enough to constitute an excessive increase in myocardial oxygen consumption.
4. If the post-MI stress test is described as normal, the patient can reengage in any form of exercise program as tolerated, including sex.

ED Post M.I MCC = ANXIETY

CONGESTIVE HEART FAILURE

DEFINITION

Shortness of breath **(dyspnea)** is the essential feature of congestive heart failure (CHF). CHF is a dysfunction of the heart as a pump of blood. This results in insufficient oxygen delivery to tissues accompanied by the accumulation of fluid in the lungs. This can be either from systolic dysfunction, which is a low ejection fraction and dilation of the heart, or from diastolic dysfunction. Diastolic dysfunction is the inability of the heart to "relax" and receive blood. **In diastolic dysfunction, the ejection fraction is preserved** and sometimes even above normal.

Causes of Systolic Dysfunction

Hypertension resulting in a cardiomyopathy or abnormality of the myocardial muscle is the most common cause of CHF. Initially, when caused by hypertension, there is preservation of the ejection fraction. Over time, the heart dilates, resulting in systolic dysfunction and low ejection fraction. Valvular heart disease of all types results in CHF.

Myocardial infarction (MI) is a very common cause of dilated cardiomyopathy and decreased ejection fraction. When the heart is "dead" or infarcted, it will not pump. In U.S. adults, **CHF is the most common cause of being admitted to the hospital**. Those with CHF are admitted repeatedly for exacerbations. The use of thrombolytics, beta blockers, angioplasty, and aspirin has lead to an enormous decrease in the risk of death from MI. Many are normal and many are living with CHF.

▶ **TIP**

Infarction → Dilation → Regurgitation → CHF

Infarction, cardiomyopathy, and valve disease account for the vast majority of cases (over 95%). Less common causes are:

- Alcohol
- Postviral (idiopathic) myocarditis
- Radiation
- Adriamycin (doxorubicin) use
- Chagas disease and other infections
- Hemochromatosis (also causes restrictive cardiomyopathy)
- Thyroid disease
- Peripartum cardiomyopathy
- Thiamine deficiency

PRESENTATION

Dyspnea (shortness of breath) is the indispensible clue to the diagnosis of CHF. CHF, especially its worst form, pulmonary edema, is a **clinical** diagnosis. That means you should be able to answer the "What is the most likely diagnosis?" question essentially from the history and physical examination and without the use of lab tests.

In addition to dyspnea on exertion, look for:

- **Orthopnea** (worse when lying flat, relieved when sitting up or standing)
- Peripheral **edema**
- **Rales** on lung examination
- Jugulovenous distention (**JVD**)
- Paroxysmal nocturnal dyspnea (**PND**) (sudden worsening at night, during sleep)
- S_3 gallop rhythm (Be prepared to identify the **sound** on USMLE Step 2 CK. It may be played.)

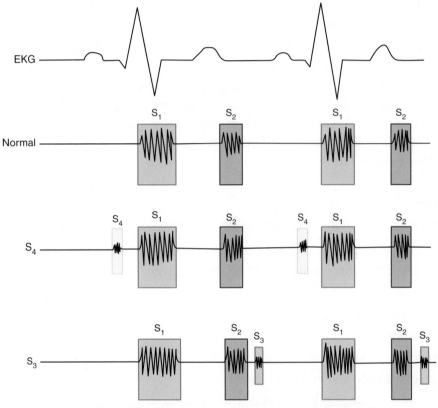

Figure 3.1: Timing of S_3 and S_4 gallops in the cardiac cycle. *Source: Andrew Peredo.*

▶ **TIP**

The most frequently asked USMLE Step 2 CK question is "What is the most likely diagnosis?"

| "What Is the Most Likely Diagnosis?" for Dyspnea ||
Key feature	Most likely diagnosis is...
Sudden onset, clear lungs (*even on x ray*)	Pulmonary embolus
Sudden onset, wheezing, increased expiratory phase	Asthma
Slower, fever, sputum, unilateral rales/rhonchi	Pneumonia
Decreased breath sounds unilaterally, tracheal deviation	Pneumothorax
Circumoral numbness, caffeine use, history of anxiety	Panic attack
Pallor, gradual over days to weeks	Anemia
Pulsus paradoxus, decreased heart sounds, JVD	Tamponade
Palpitations, syncope	Arrhythmia of almost any kind
Dullness to percussion at bases	Pleural effusion
Long smoking history, barrel chest	COPD
Recent anesthetic use, **brown blood** not improved with oxygen, clear lungs on auscultation, cyanosis	Methemoglobinemia
Burning building or car, **wood-burning stove** in winter, suicide attempt	Carbon monoxide poisoning

All of these will **lack**:

- Orthopnea/PND
- S$_3$ gallop

DIAGNOSTIC TESTS

There is an **enormous** difference in the management of chronic, office, or ambulatory-based cases of CHF and pulmonary edema questions. The key to the right answer is:

- Setting (emergency department versus office or clinic)
- Presence of acute symptoms of dyspnea **at the time of presentation**

Echocardiography

Echocardiography is unquestionably the **most important** of all the tests of CHF. There is **no** reliable way to distinguish systolic from diastolic dysfunction by history, physical examination, or other tests such as the EKG, chest x-ray, or brain (atrial) natriuretic peptide (BNP) levels.

> Every patient with CHF **must** undergo echocardiography to evaluate ejection fraction.

Ejection Fraction

What is the **best initial test**? Trans**thoracic** echo.

What is the most **accurate** test? Multiple-gated acquisition scan (MUGA) or **nuclear ventriculography**.

Transesophageal echocardiography (TEE) is more accurate than either of these tests in evaluating heart valve function and diameter. TEE is **not** necessary for evaluating CHF.

When should you answer "nuclear ventriculography"? **Nuclear** testing for the **best** precision is rarely needed. An example of when it is necessary would be a person receiving chemotherapy with doxorubicin; you are trying to give the maximum amount of chemotherapy to cure the lymphoma, but need to make sure you are not causing cardiomyopathy.

Nuclear ventriculogram gives precise evaluation of **wall motion** abnormalities.

When should you answer BNP? Answer "**BNP** level" in a patient with **acute shortness of breath** in whom the **etiology** of the dyspnea **is not clear** and you cannot wait for an echo to be done. A normal BNP excludes CHF as a cause of the shortness of breath.

Other Diagnostic Tests

Other tests that are used are **not** to diagnose CHF. They are used to diagnose the **cause** of CHF. The diagnosis of CHF is a clinical diagnosis (history and physical as described) with the **type** of CHF determined by transthoracic echo (TTE).

Tests Used to Determine Etiology of CHF	
Test	**Etiology of CHF**
EKG	MI, heart block
Chest x-ray	Dilated cardiomyopathy
Holter monitor	Paroxysmal arrhythmias
Cardiac catheterization	Precise valve diameters, septal defects
CBC	Anemia
Thryoid function (T4/TSH)	Both high and low thyroid levels cause CHF
Endomyocardial biopsy	Rarely done; excludes infiltrative disease such as sarcoid or amyloid when other sites for biopsy inconclusive; biopsy is "most accurate test" for some infections
Swan-Ganz right heart catheterization	Distinguishes CHF from ARDS; not routine

TREATMENT

Systolic Dysfunction (Low Ejection Fraction)

- ACE inhibitors or angiotensin receptor blockers (ARBs)
- Beta blockers
- Spironolactone
- Diuretics
- Digoxin

ACE Inhibitors and ARBs

These agents should be given to **all** patients with systolic dysfunction at any stage of disease. The beneficial effects of ACEi and ARBs occur with **any** drug in the class.

Beta Blockers

Unlike ACEi and ARBs, it is **not** clear that the benefit from beta blockers will occur with any drug in the class. There is evidence **only** for:

- Metoprolol $\beta 1$
- Bisoprolol $\beta 1$
- Carvedilol $\beta 1 / \beta 2$

Metoprolol and bisoprolol are beta-1 specific antagonists. **Carvedilol** is a **nonspecific beta blocker** that also has alpha-1 receptor blocking activity.

BETA BLOCKERS ARE:
- ANTIISCHEMIC
- $\downarrow O_2$ NECESSITY OF $\heartsuit$
- ANTIARRHYTHMIC

The benefit of beta blockers likely stems from:

- Antiischemic effect
- Decrease in heart rate leading to decreased oxygen consumption
- Antiarrhythmic effect

Which of the following is the most common cause of death from CHF?

a. Pulmonary edema
b. Myocardial infarction
c. Arrhythmia/sudden death
d. Emboli
e. Myocardial rupture

Answer: The correct answer is (C). Ischemia provokes ventricular arrhythmias leading to sudden death. Over 99.9% of patients with CHF are at home, not acutely short of breath. If they die of sudden death, the physician never sees them. Beta blockers are antiarrhythmic and antiischemic, so they prevent sudden death. Do not give beta blockers in the acute treatment of CHF.

Spironolactone

Spironolactone's beneficial effect is directly related to its ability to inhibit the effects of aldosterone. Spironolactone is only proven effective for more advanced and serious stages of CHF (class III and IV) in which the patient is

What is the management of a patient with severe CHF who develops gynecomastia? Switch spironolactone to eplerenone.

Diuretics control symptoms of CHF. They do **not** lower mortality.

short of breath either with minimal exertion or at rest. **Adverse effects include hyperkalemia and gynecomastia.**

Eplerenone is an alternative to spironolactone that inhibits aldosterone and has a proven mortality benefit, but does **not have the antiandrogenic effects** that lead to gynecomastia.

Diuretics

Initial therapy of CHF with low ejection fraction often includes a loop diuretic in combination with an ACEi or ARB. It does not matter whether the diuretic is furosemide, torsemide, or bumetanide. Spironolactone, although a diuretic, is **not** used at the doses where it has a diuretic effect.

Digoxin

Digoxin has **never** been proven to lower mortality in CHF. This is often the **single most important question** concerning CHF on USMLE Step 2 CK.

Digoxin is used to control symptoms of dyspnea and will decrease the frequency of hospitalizations. In fact, **no positive inotropic agent (digoxin, milrinone, amrinone, dobutamine) has been proven to lower mortality.**

A 74-year-old African American man with a history of dilated cardiomyopathy secondary to MI in the past is seen in the office for routine evaluation. He is asymptomatic and is maintained on lisinopril, furosemide, metoprolol, aspirin, and digoxin. Lab tests reveal a persistently elevated potassium level. The EKG is unchanged.

What is the best management?

a. Switch lisinopril to candesartan
b. Stop lisinopril
c. Start kayexalate
d. Refer for dialysis
e. Switch lisinopril to hydralazine and nitroglycerin

Answer: The correct answer is (E). Hydralazine is a direct-acting arteriolar vasodilator. There is a definite survival advantage with the use of hydralazine in combination with nitrates in systolic dysfunction. Candesartan is associated with hyperkalemia as well. Dialysis is sometimes used in hyperkalemia, but only if associated with renal failure as the cause.

▶ TIP

Don't walk into the USMLE Step 2 CK exam without being 100% clear on which drugs lower mortality in CHF.

Devices for CHF Treatment

Two other treatments are associated with a mortality benefit in CHF.

1. **Implantable defibrillator:** For those with **ischemic cardiomyopathy and an ejection fraction below 35%**, these devices have as much as a 25% relative reduction in the risk of death. Remember that arrhythmia and sudden death is the most common cause of death in CHF.

2. **Biventricular pacemaker:** The biventricular pacemaker is indicated in those with dilated cardiomyopathy and an **ejection fraction under 35% and** a wide **QRS above 120 milliseconds** who have persistent symptoms.

Do **not** confuse the biventricular pacemaker with a dual-chamber pacemaker with a wire in both an atrium and a ventricle.

The biventricular pacemaker resynchronizes the heart when there is a conduction defect. Many patients who would otherwise be heading to a cardiac transplantation have had their symptoms markedly improved with the biventricular pacemaker.

Transplantation

When maximal medical therapy (ACE, BB, spironolactone, diuretics, digoxin) and possibly the biventricular pacemaker fail to control symptoms of CHF, then the only alternative is to seek cardiac transplantation.

Routine anticoagulation with warfarin **is always wrong** in the absence of a clot in the heart.

> Calcium channel blockers (CCBs) provide **no** clear benefit in systolic dysfunction. Some CCBs can actually **raise** mortality.

Mortality Benefit in Systolic Dysfunction

- ACEi/ARBs
- Beta blockers
- Spironolactone
- Hydralazine/nitrates
- Implantable defibrillator

TREATMENT

Diastolic Dysfunction (CHF with Preserved Ejection Fraction)

The management of CHF with a preserved ejection fraction is **much** less clear. **Beta blockers have clear benefits** and are indicated. Digoxin clearly has **no benefit** and should **not be used** in diastolic dysfunction.

Diuretics are used to control symptoms of fluid overload as they are in any CHF patient. Do not confuse diastolic dysfunction from hypertrophic cardiomyopathy with hypertrophic **obstructive** cardiomyopathy (HOCM). HOCM is a congenital disease with an asymmetrically enlarged (hypertrophic) septum leading to an obstruction of the left ventricular outflow tract. Diuretics are contraindicated in HOCM because they will increase the obstruction.

ACEi and ARBs have unclear benefit in diastolic dysfunction.

> Clearly beneficial: beta blockers and diuretics
> Clearly **not** beneficial: digoxin and spironolactone
> Uncertain: ACEi , ARBs, and hydralazine

ACUTE PULMONARY EDEMA

DEFINITION

Pulmonary edema is the worst, or most severe, form of CHF. Pulmonary edema is the rapid onset of fluid accumulating in the lungs.

PRESENTATION

Pulmonary edema presents with the acute onset of shortness of breath associated with:

- Rales
- JVD
- S_3 gallop
- Edema
- Orthopnea

There may also be ascites and enlargement of the liver and spleen if there has been sufficient time for the chronic passive congestion of the right side of the heart to prevent filling of the heart.

DIAGNOSTIC TESTS

Brain Natriuretic Peptide

This is used **if the diagnosis of the etiology of the shortness of breath is not clear**. A normal BNP level excludes pulmonary edema.

Chest X-ray

You will see vascular congestion with filling of the blood vessels towards the head (cephalization of flow). Ordinarily, most flow in the lungs is at the bases because of simple gravity. In more chronic cases, there will be enlargement of the heart and pleural effusions.

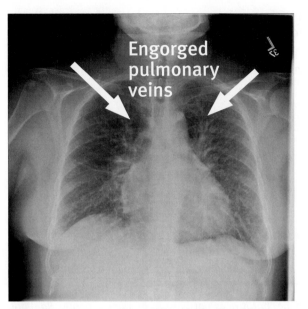

Figure 3.2: Pulmonary edema with cephalization of flow and engorged pulmonary veins. *Source: Saba Ansari, MD.*

Oximetry/Arterial Blood Gases

Hypoxia is expected. Until the acute disease is extremely severe, there is also respiratory alkalosis because of hyperventilation. Because of the increased respiratory rate, **carbon dioxide leaves more easily than oxygen enters** the bloodstream.

EKG

This is the most important test to do acutely, because the EKG can lead to a change in immediate therapy.

If atrial fibrillation, atrial flutter, or ventricular tachycardia is the cause of pulmonary edema, the first thing to do is to perform rapid, synchronized cardioversion in order to restore atrial systole and to return the atrial contribution to cardiac output. Normally, atrial systole contributes only 10% to 20% of cardiac output. If the heart is diseased from dilated cardiomyopathy, decreased ejection fraction, or valvular heart disease, then the atrial contribution to cardiac output can be as much as 40% to 50% of cardiac output. **If acute pulmonary edema is from an arrhythmia, the fastest way to fix it is with cardioversion**.

Echocardiography

This should be **done in all patients** to determine if there is systolic or diastolic dysfunction. This makes no difference acutely if there is pulmonary edema because the initial therapy does not differ.

A 74-year-old woman comes to the emergency department with the acute onset of shortness of breath, respiratory rate of 38 per minutes, rales to her apices, S_3 gallop, and jugulovenous distension.

What is the best initial step in the management of this patient?

a. Oximeter
b. Echocardiography
c. Intravenous furosemide
d. Ramipril
e. Metoprolol
f. Nesiritide

*Answer: The correct answer is **(C)**. All of the answers are partially correct because they can all be used in the management of CHF at some point. However, the best **initial** therapy for acute pulmonary edema is to remove a large volume of fluid from the vascular space with a loop diuretic. Oximetry should be done, but should not alter acute management because we now must give oxygen because the patient complains of shortness of breath, and she is hyperventilating.*

Echocardiography should be done, but it does not have to be done urgently. Ramipril, or any other form of ACEi or ARB, should be used if there is systolic dysfunction with a low ejection fraction, but it does not make a difference in an acutely unstable patient. The same is true of metoprolol.

*Nesiritide is a therapeutic, intravenous form of atrial natriuretic peptide. Nesiritide functions in much the same way as nitrates. Because it is only a weak diuretic, **there is no proven mortality** benefit.*

TREATMENT

Preload Reduction

Initial therapy of acute pulmonary edema is with:

- Oxygen
- Loop diuretics such as furosemide or bumetinide
- Morphine
- Nitrates

The majority of patients in acute pulmonary edema can be managed with preload reduction. Removing 1 to 2 liters of fluid from the vascular space and the lungs is the best thing that can be done acutely to decrease symptoms. **Nesiritide** can be used as part of this therapy, but it is **not clear that it works** better than standard agents.

Positive Inotropic Agents

Dobutamine can be used in the acute setting of patients placed in the ICU when their shortness of breath did not respond to therapy acutely with preload reduction. Amrinone and milrinone are phosphodiesterase inhibitors that perform the same role. They increase contractility and decrease afterload.

Digoxin is a positive inotrope that increases contractility, but it will not have this effect for several weeks after starting its use. There is no benefit of using digoxin in the acute setting.

Afterload Reduction

ACEi and ARBs are used on discharge for long-term use in all patients with systolic dysfunction and low ejection fraction. In an acute setting, nitroprusside and intravenous hydralazine can be used.

VALVULAR HEART DISEASE

DEFINITION/PRESENTATION

All valvular heart disease can be **congenital** in nature. **Rheumatic fever** can lead to **any form of valve disease**, but mitral stenosis is most common. Aging can automatically be associated with aortic stenosis. Regurgitant disease is most commonly caused by hypertension and ischemic heart disease. Infarction automatically leads to regurgitation, which automatically leads to dilation.

All forms of valvular heart disease are associated with shortness of breath and many of the signs and symptoms of CHF. Only the murmurs are specific in terms of presentation. Lesions on the right side of the heart (tricuspid and pulmonic valve) increase in intensity or loudness with inhalation. Inhalation will increase venous return to the right side of the heart. Left-sided lesions (mitral and aortic valve) increase with exhalation. Exhalation will "squeeze" blood out of the lungs and into the left side of the heart.

Heparin is always wrong for acute pulmonary edema management in the absence of a clot.

DIAGNOSTIC TESTS

All of the following statements can be made in general for all valvular heart disease.

The best initial test for all valvular heart disease is the **echocardiogram**. **Transesophageal** echo is generally both **more sensitive and more specific** than transthoracic echo. Catheterization is the most accurate test. Catheterization allows the most precise measurement of valvular diameter, as well as the exact pressure gradient across the valve.

There is nothing specific about the EKG in those with valvular heart disease. The EKG is expected to show hypertrophy of chambers, but you cannot confirm a diagnosis of valvular heart disease from an EKG alone.

Chest x-ray will also show hypertrophy and enlargement of various cardiac chambers, but the precise anatomic correlation with the chest x-ray is poor. Since the advent of echocardiography, **x-ray evaluation of cardiac chamber size is neither "the most accurate test" nor "the best initial test."**

TREATMENT

Since all forms of valvular heart disease are associated with fluid overload in the lungs, all of them will benefit from diuretics.

Medicine alone can do very little to improve stenotic lesions of the mitral and aortic valves. Nearly all patients with symptoms will need correction of the anatomy of the heart. **Mitral stenosis is dilated with a balloon.** Aortic stenosis needs surgical removal.

Regurgitant lesions seem to **respond best to vasodilator therapy** with ACEi/ARBs, nifedipine, or hydralazine. Surgical replacement of regurgitant lesions must be done before the heart dilates too much. If the heart dilates excessively, then valve replacement will **not** be able to correct the decrease in systolic function. If the myocardium "stretches" too much, it will not return to normal size and shape. Assessment of ventricular size is based on the end-**systolic** diameter and the ejection fraction. When the end-systolic diameter expands, you must replace the valve.

Mitral Stenosis

DEFINITION/ETIOLOGY

Mitral stenosis (MS) is most often caused by **rheumatic fever**. MS is extremely uncommon in the United States because of the very low incidence of acute rheumatic fever. Critical narrowing is defined as a valve surface area less than 1 cm^2; however, the main indication for treatment is the presence of symptoms. There is not much point in treating MS that is asymptomatic.

> ▶ **TIP**
>
> Look for **pregnancy** and **immigrant** in the history as a clue to answering "What is the most likely diagnosis?"

Pregnancy is associated with a 50% increase in plasma volume which must traverse a narrow valve. In addition, during delivery, contraction of the uterus can "squeeze" as much as 500 mL extra of blood into the central circulation, thereby inducing pregnancy-related cardiomyopathy. Most patients with mitral stenosis are immigrants to the United States coming from geographic regions in which acute rheumatic fever is still common.

PRESENTATION

Besides the usual shortness of breath and CHF associated with all forms of valvular heart disease, MS has a number of relatively unique features of presentation:

- **Dysphagia** from left atrium (LA) pressing on the esophagus
- **Hoarseness** (LA pressing on laryngeal nerve)

Endocarditis prophylaxis is **not** indicated for **any** of these valve disorders unless the valve has actually been replaced or there has been previous endocarditis.

Mitral stenosis often presents in **young adult** patients.

- **Atrial fibrillation** and stroke from enormous LA
- **Hemoptysis**

Figure 3.3: Enlarged left atrium in mitral stenosis compresses the esophagus, causing dysphagia. *Source: Andrew Peredo.*

Physical Findings

Murmur is in diastole, just after an opening snap. Squatting and leg raising increase the intensity from increased venous return to the heart.

DIAGNOSTIC TESTS

Echo

TTE is the best initial test, with TEE **more** accurate than TTE. However, catheterization is the **most** accurate diagnostic test. This is the same for **all** valve diseases.

EKG

Atrial rhythm disturbance, particularly atrial fibrillation, is **very** common. Left atrial hypertrophy shows up as a biphasic P wave in leads V1 and V2.

Chest X-ray: Left Atrial Hypertrophy

- Straightening of the left heart border
- Elevation of the left main-stem bronchus
- Second "bubble" behind the heart

Figure 3.4: Enlarged left atrium compresses and displaces the left main-stem bronchus. *Source: Andrew Peredo.*

TREATMENT

1. **Diuretics and sodium restriction** when fluid overload is present in the lungs
2. **Balloon valvuloplasty** done with a catheter
3. Valve replacement only when a catheter procedure cannot be done, or fails
4. **Warfarin for atrial fibrillation** to an INR of 2 to 3
5. **Rate control** of atrial fibrillation with digoxin, beta blockers, or diltiazem/verapamil

Aortic Stenosis

DEFINITION/ETIOLOGY

Aortic stenosis (AS) can be caused by a congenital bicuspid valve or with increasing calcification as people age.

PRESENTATION

- **Angina:** most common presentation
- **Syncope**
- **CHF:** poorest prognosis with 2-year average survival

Murmur

A systolic, crescendo-decrescendo murmur peaking in a diamond-shape in mid-systole. The murmur of AS is heard best at the second right intercostal space, and radiates to the carotid artery. Valsalva and standing improve or decrease the intensity of the murmur from decreased venous return to the heart. Handgrip softens the murmur because of decreased ejection of blood.

DIAGNOSTIC TESTS

TTE, then TEE, then catheterization.

Chest X-ray: Left Ventricular Hypertrophy

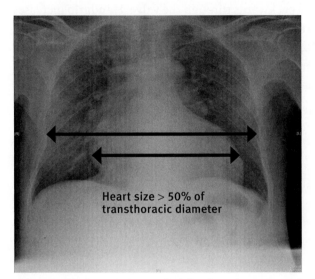

Heart size > 50% of transthoracic diameter

Figure 3.5: Cardiac enlargement is defined as a heart greater in diameter than 50% of the total transthoracic diameter. *Source: Nihar Shah, MD.*

EKG

Left ventricular hypertrophy (LVH). S wave in V1 plus an R wave in V5 greater than 35 millimeters.

TREATMENT

Valve replacement is the only truly effective therapy for AS. Diuretics can be used to decrease CHF, but patients do not tolerate volume depletion very well.

Balloon valvuloplasty is not routinely done for AS. This is because the main mechanism for developing AS is calcification, which does not improve very well with balloon valvuloplasty. Balloon/catheter procedures are done only if surgery is not an option secondary to the instability or fragility of the patient.

Mitral Regurgitation

DEFINITION/ETIOLOGY

Mitral regurgitation (MR) is an abnormal backward flow of blood through a mitral valve that does not fit together. Hypertension, endocarditis, myocardial infarction with papillary muscle rupture, or **any other reason that the heart dilates will lead to MR.**

PRESENTATION

MR presents with the same signs and symptoms as CHF. The only unique finding is the murmur, which is pansystolic (holosystolic), obscuring both S1 and S2. **The murmur of MR radiates to the axilla.** Handgrip will worsen the murmur of MR by pushing more blood backwards through the valve. Handgrip increases afterload and will worsen the murmurs of both aortic regurgitation (AR) and MR. Squatting and leg raising will also worsen MR by increasing venous return to the heart. All left-sided murmurs except mitral valve prolapse (MVP) and hypertrophic obstructive cardiomyopathy will increase with expiration.

As with all murmurs, MR is diagnosed with echocardiography.

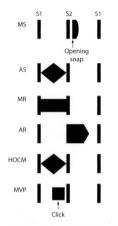

Figure 3.6: Timing of each of the murmurs in the cardiac cycle. *Source: Shawn Christian.*

TREATMENT

1. Vasodilators: **ACE or ARBs are best**. They decrease the rate of progression of regurgitant lesion.
2. Digoxin and diuretics may be used sometimes as they would be in any form of CHF.
3. Valve replacement is indicated when the heart starts to dilate. Do **not** wait for left ventricular end **systolic** diameter (LVESD) to become too large because the damage will be irreversible. When LVESD is above 40 mm or the ejection fraction drops below 60%, surgical valve repair or replacement is indicated. Valve repair means either operatively, or with a catheter placing a clip or sutures across the valve to tighten it up.

Aortic Regurgitation

DEFINITION/ETIOLOGY

AR is caused by anything that makes the heart or aorta dilate in size:

- Myocardial infarction
- Hypertension
- Endocarditis
- Marfan syndrome or cystic medial necrosis

- Inflammatory disorders such as ankylosing spondylitis or Reiter syndrome
- Syphilis

PRESENTATION

Besides CHF, AR has a large array of relatively unique physical findings such as:

- Wide pulse pressure
- Water-hammer (wide, bounding) pulse
- Quincke pulse (pulsations in the nail bed)
- Hill sign (BP in legs as much as 40 mm Hg above arm BP)
- Head bobbing (de Musset sign)

Murmur

AR gives a diastolic, decrescendo murmur heard best at the lower left sternal border. Valsalva and standing make it better. Handgrip, which increases afterload by compressing the arteries of the arms, makes it worse.

DIAGNOSTIC TESTS

Same as previous diagnostic tests mentioned. EKG and chest x-ray may show left ventricular hypertrophy.

TREATMENT

1. ACEi/ARBs or nifedipine as vasodilators will increase forward flow of blood and delay progression.
2. Digoxin and diuretics have a little benefit.
3. Surgical valve replacement is used when there is acute valve rupture such as with a myocardial infarction. Replace the valve before the left ventricle dilates excessively. EF less than 55% or left ventricular end systolic diameter greater than 55 mm.

Mitral Valve Prolapse

DEFINITION/ETIOLOGY

MVP is so common as to be considered a normal anatomic variant occurring in as much as 2% to 5% of the population, particularly in women. Other causes are Marfan and Ehlers-Danlos syndrome.

PRESENTATION

MVP is most often asymptomatic. When symptoms do occur, it is **different** from the other forms of valvular heart disease. The **symptoms of CHF** are usually **absent**. The most common presentation is:

- Atypical chest **pain**
- **Palpitations**
- **Panic** attack

MURMUR

MVP presents with a midsystolic click that, when severe, is associated with a murmur just after the click from mitral regurgitation. Auscultory maneuvers have the **opposite** effect from the murmurs of the valvular disease described so far. Valsalva and standing, which decrease venous return to the heart, will **worsen** MVP. Anything that **increases** left ventricular chamber size, such as squatting or handgrip, will **improve** or diminish the murmur of MVP.

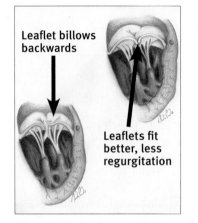

Figure 3.7: Redundant mitral valve leaflet does not seal, allowing regurgitation. *Source: Andrew Peredo.*

DIAGNOSTIC TESTS

Echocardiography is the best choice. Catheterization should rarely, if ever, be done. This is largely because an exact pressure gradient does **not** need to be determined, since valve replacement is rarely needed.

TREATMENT

1. Beta blockers are used when the patient is symptomatic.
2. Valve repair can be performed with a catheter by placing a clip to tighten up the valve.
3. A few stitches into the valve can markedly tighten up the leaflets, but surgical repair of the valve is rarely necessary.
4. Endocarditis prophylaxis is **not** recommended even in the presence of a murmur of mitral regurgitation.

CARDIOMYOPATHY

DEFINITION

Cardiomyopathy is an abnormal function of the heart muscle. Although there are frequently valvular or auscultory abnormalities, the origins of all the defects are in an abnormally contracting or relaxing myocardium.

ETIOLOGY

Cardiomyopathy can be dilated, hypertrophic, or restrictive. The terms *dilated cardiomyopathy*, *systolic dysfunction*, and *low ejection fraction* are often used interchangeably. Hypertrophic cardiomyopathy is often interchanged with the phrase *diastolic dysfunction*. An even more accurate phrase is "cardiac failure with preserved ejection fraction."

PRESENTATION/DIAGNOSTIC TESTS/TREATMENT

All forms or cardiomyopathy present with shortness of breath, particularly worsened by exertion. Edema, rales, and JVD, as previously described, are found in all types of cardiomyopathy. Echocardiography is the best initial test and often the most accurate test for all of them. Although an EKG and chest x-ray should be performed, there is nothing specific on these tests to confirm the diagnosis. **All of them are treated with diuretics**. Other treatment is based on the type of cardiomyopathy. In fact, besides the etiology and the physiology of the heart, the only real functional difference in the management of the patients and the answers to the questions is the treatment.

Murmurs that do not increase with expiration:

- HOCM
- MVP

DILATED CARDIOMYOPATHY

ETIOLOGY/PRESENTATION/DIAGNOSTIC TESTS

In addition to previous MI and ischemia, dilated cardiomyopathy can be from:

- Alcohol
- Postviral myocarditis
- Radiation
- Toxins such as doxorubicin
- Chagas disease

All the other aspects of the dyspnea, gallop, edema, and other symptoms are described in the section on CHF. The same is true for the evaluation of EF, first with echocardiography and the nonspecificity of the EKG and chest x-ray.

TREATMENT

Dilated cardiomyopathy has the greatest number of medications to lower mortality. ACEi, ARBs, and beta blockers such as metoprolol or carvedilol and spironolactone all lower mortality. Diuretics and digoxin are used to control symptoms. If the QRS is wide (more than 120 milliseconds), a biventricular pacemaker can be placed that will improve both symptoms and survival. Automated implantable cardioverter/defibrillator has mortality benefit in some patients.

HYPERTROPHIC CARDIOMYOPATHY

DEFINITION/ETIOLOGY

Hypertension is, by far, the most common cause. It is **very** important to distinguish between hypertrophic cardiomyopathy (HCM) and HOCM. HCM is a reaction to stressors on the heart such as increased blood pressure. The heart hypertrophies to carry the load, but then develops difficulty "relaxing" in diastole. If the heart can't relax to receive blood, the patient becomes short of breath.

HOCM is a genetic disorder with an abnormal shape to the septum of the heart. The asymmetrically hypertrophied septum will literally form an anatomic obstruction between the septum and the valve leaflet to block blood leaving the heart.

Differences Between HCM and Other Forms of Cardiomyopathy

- S_4 gallop
- Fewer signs of right heart failure such as ascites and enlargement of the liver and spleen

Hypertrophic Obstructive Cardiomyopathy

- Dyspnea, like any other form of cardiomyopathy
- Chest pain
- Syncope and lightheadedness
- Sudden death, particularly in healthy athletes
- Symptoms worsened by anything that **increases heart rate**, eg, exercise, dehydration, and diuretics
- Worsened by anything that **decreases left ventricular chamber size**, eg, ACEi, ARBs, digoxin, hydralazine, Valsalva, and standing suddenly

Narrow outflow tract

Figure 3.8: Thickened asymmetric septum obstructs left ventricular outflow tract as the chamber becomes smaller. *Source: Andrew Peredo.*

DIAGNOSTIC TESTS

Echo is the best initial test. The septum is 1.5 times the thickness of the posterior wall.

TREATMENT

1. **Beta blockers** are the "best initial therapy" for both HOCM and ordinary HCM.
2. Agents with strong negative inotropic qualities such as verapamil and disopyramide can also be useful.
3. Diuretics may help in HCM, but they are **contraindicated** in HOCM.

HOCM: Specific Therapy

1. **Implantable defibrillators** should be used in any HOCM patient with syncope.
2. **Ablation of the septum** should first be tried with a catheter placing absolute alcohol in the muscle causing small infarctions. If symptoms persist, surgical myomectomy removing part of the septum is the ultimate therapy.

Differences in Therapy between Hypertrophic Cardiomyopathy and Dilated Cardiomyopathy		
	Hypertrophic	**Dilated**
Beta Blockers	Yes	Yes
Diuretics	Yes	Yes
ACEi/ARB	Unclear benefit	Yes
Spironolactone	No	Yes
Digoxin	No	Yes

Systolic anterior motion (SAM) of the mitral valve is classic for HOCM. It contributes to obstruction.

Catheterization is the **most** accurate test to determine precise gradients of pressure across the chamber.

EKG: Nonspecific ST and T wave changes are common. LVH is common. EKG can be normal in a quarter.

Septal Q waves in the inferior and lateral leads are common in HOCM. They are **not** in MI.

Digoxin and spironolactone are definitely **always** wrong in hypertrophic cardiomyopathy.

Surgical myomectomy is the therapy **only** if all medical and catheter procedures fail.

In HOCM, ACEi and diuretics definitely do **not** help. This is the major difference between HOCM and HCM.

RESTRICTIVE CARDIOMYOPATHY

DEFINITION/ETIOLOGY

Restrictive cardiomyopathy combines the worst aspects of both dilated and hypertrophic cardiomyopathy. The heart neither contracts nor relaxes normally because it is infiltrated with substances creating immobility. Causes are:

- Sarcoidosis
- Amyloid
- Hemochromatosis
- Endomyocardial fibrosis
- Scleroderma

PRESENTATION

Dyspnea is the most common complaint with signs of right heart failure such as ascites, edema, JVD, and enlargement of the liver and spleen.

Pulmonary hypertension is common because of an increase in wedge pressure.

▶ **TIP**

Kussmaul sign: An increase in jugulovenous pressure on inhalation is common.

DIAGNOSTIC TESTS

Echocardiography is the best initial test. Ejection fraction may be normal or elevated. EKG shows low voltage. Amyloid presents with speckling of the septum on echo or cardiac MRI. The most accurate test is an endomyocardial biopsy, but this is rarely done because the diagnosis is made from biopsies elsewhere in the body.

TREATMENT

Treat the underlying cause. Diuretics may relieve some of the pulmonary hypertension and signs of right heart failure. There is no other clear therapy.

> More blood increases all murmurs except MVP and HOCM.

Murmurs and the Effects of Maneuvers		
Lesion	Squatting/ leg raising	Standing/ Valsalva
Mitral and aortic stenosis	Increases both	Decreases both
Mitral and aortic regurgitation	Increases both	Decreases both
Mitral valve prolapse	Decrease	Increase
HOCM	Decrease	Increase

Effects of Maneuvers

These effects simulate medical treatments.

Standing and Valsalva

Standing suddenly from a squatting position will open the venous capacitance vessels of the legs.

Valsalva is exhalation against a closed glottis, increasing intrathoracic pressure. When intrathoracic pressure is increased, it will make it harder for blood to return to the right side of the heart.

▶ **TIP**

Standing or Valsalva = diuretic use.

Standing and Valsalva are similar to using a diuretic. Stenotic and regurgitant murmurs are all treated with diuretics and/or salt restriction, so the maneuvers of standing and Valsalva will improve them.

MVP and HOCM have worsening of their cardiac physiology with diuretics. Diuretics decrease left ventricular chamber size, and worsen the regurgitation of MVP and the obstruction of HOCM. Hence, standing and Valsalva will worsen them.

Handgrip and Amyl Nitrate

Handgrip is performed by having the patient squeeze the examiner's hand. The contraction of the muscles of the arms will compress the arteries of the upper extremity such as the brachial, radial, and ulnar arteries. The main effect of handgrip is to increase afterload by obstructing the ability of blood to empty the heart.

Amyl nitrate is a direct arteriolar vasodilator. Amyl nitrate simulates the effect of ACE inhibitors or ARBs on the heart. Any valvular disease that is treated with an ACEi/ARB will improve with amyl nitrate. "Improve" means a softer murmur.

▶ **TIP**

Handgrip = fuller left ventricle.

Amyl nitrate = ACEi = emptier left ventricle.

Effect of Maneuvers on Intensity (Loudness) of Murmurs		
Lesion	**Handgrip**	**Amyl nitrate**
Aortic stenosis	Decreases	Increases
Mitral stenosis	No effect	No effect
Aortic regurgitation	Increases	Decreases
Mitral regurgitation	Increases	Decreases
Mitral valve prolapse	Decreases	Increases
HOCM	Decreases	Increases

Standing and Valsalva **decrease** venous return to the heart.

Less blood decreases **all** murmurs except MVP and HOCM.

Handgrip **decreases** left ventricular emptying; amyl nitrate **increases** emptying.

Handgrip and amyl nitrate have no meaningful effect on mitral stenosis, in the same way ACEi has no meaningful effect on MS.

Maneuvers Are Like Treatment

Since regurgitant lesions are treated with ACEi, ARBs, and nifedipine as vaso-dilators, it is understandable that amyl nitrate decreases the intensity of these lesions, since it increases the forward flow of blood and decreases the regurgitant, backward flow of blood.

Handgrip decreases ventricular emptying by increasing afterload. This will improve the lesions of MVP and HOCM. A bigger, fuller heart improves the obstruction of HOCM. With amyl nitrate, the emptier heart is smaller such as would occur with diuretics, dehydration, and tachycardia. That is why amyl nitrate will worsen MVP and HOCM.

> Handgrip improves HOCM because the heart is larger (more full), which decreases the obstruction.

PERICARDIAL DISEASE

The causes of pericarditis, pericardial tamponade, and constrictive pericarditis have considerable overlap. If the etiology of pericarditis is associated with the extravasation of a great deal of fluid, then tamponade can occur. If the cause of pericarditis is chronic, then patients can develop the fibrosis and calcification of the pericardium that leads to constrictive pericarditis.

Pericarditis

Coxsackie B

Any infection, inflammatory disorder, connective tissue disorder, trauma to the chest, or cancer of an organ anatomically near the heart can cause pericarditis. The most common infection is viral; however, *Staphylococcus*, *Streptococcus*, fungi, and other agents can cause pericarditis in the same way that virtually any infection can cause pneumonia. Systemic lupus erythematosus is the most common connective tissue disorder, but Wegener granulomatosis, Goodpasture syndrome, rheumatoid arthritis, polyarteritis nodosa, and other disorders can cause pericarditis.

"WHAT IS THE MOST LIKELY DIAGNOSIS?"

Pericarditis is associated with sharp chest pain that changes in intensity with respiration as well as the position of the body. The pain is worsened by lying flat and improved by sitting up. This is probably from a change in the level of tension or "stretch" of the pericardium.

EKG shows ST segment elevation in all leads, but the most specific finding is PR segment depression.

Figure 3.9: Pericarditis with ST segment elevation and PR segment depression everywhere.
Source: Alejandro E. de la Cruz, MD.

Treat the underlying cause. For the majority, no clear cause is identified, and these "idiopathic" cases are generally presumed to be viral in etiology with Coxsackie B virus. These cases are treated with NSAIDs such as ibuprofen, naproxen, indomethacin, or any other drug in the class.

MUST RULE OUT M.I. STILL

Pericardial Tamponade

DEFINITION/ETIOLOGY

Any of the causes of pericarditis can extravasate enough fluid to cause tamponade. Compression of the chambers of the heart starts on the right side because the walls are thinner. As little as 50 mL of fluid accumulating acutely can cause tamponade. If accumulating over weeks to months, the pericardium will stretch to accommodate as much as 2 liters of fluid. Tamponade can also be from trauma with a bleed into the pericardium; it requires emergent thoracotomy.

> Which of the following physical findings is most likely to be associated with this patient? Pulsus paradoxus. This is a decrease of more than 10 mm Hg in blood pressure on inhalation.

"WHAT IS THE MOST LIKELY DIAGNOSIS?"

- Hypotension
- Tachycardia
- Distended neck veins
- Clear lungs

BECK'S TRIAD
DISTENDED NECK VEINS
HYPOTENSION
DISTANT HEART SOUNDS

Figure 3.10: Pericardial effusion. *Source: Birju Shah, MD.*

A 78-year-old man with a history of lung cancer comes to the emergency department with several days of increasing shortness of breath. He became somewhat lightheaded today, and that is what has brought him to the hospital. On physical examination, he has a blood pressure of 106/70; pulse of 112; jugulovenous distention; and the lungs are clear to auscultation. The blood pressure drops to 92/58 on inhalation.

Which of the following is the most appropriate to confirm the diagnosis?

a. EKG
b. Chest x-ray
c. Echocardiogram
d. Right heart catheterization
e. Cardiac MRI

*Answer: The correct answer is (C). The phrase "most appropriate" can be very difficult to interpret. It is not always clear whether "appropriate" means "first," "best," or "most accurate." In this case, the reason the echo is "most appropriate" is because the EKG often shows nothing except sinus tachycardia. The chest x-ray is normal in an acute tamponade (x-ray can show a "globular heart"), and although right heart catheterization is the most accurate to determine precise pressures, it would **never** be appropriate to do a catheterization to evaluate for tamponade without having done an echocardiogram first.*

DIAGNOSTIC TESTS

EKG: electrical alternans (different heights of QRS complexes between beats) found on the EKG

Chest x-ray: enlarged cardiac shadow expanding in both directions ("globular heart")

Echocardiogram: **right atrial and ventricular diastolic collapse**

Right heart catheterization: equalization of pressures in diastole

TREATMENT

1. Pericardiocentesis: Needle drainage will rapidly reexpand the heart
2. Intravenous fluids
3. A hole or "window" placed into the pericardium for recurrent cases

> Diuretics will decrease intracardiac filling pressure and may markedly worsen the collapse of the right side of the heart.

Constrictive Pericarditis

Any cause of pericarditis can result in sufficient calcification and fibrosis to prevent filling of the right side of the heart if it is chronic, such as tuberculosis.

M.C.C. → RADIATION & CARDIAC SURGERY

"WHAT IS THE MOST LIKELY DIAGNOSIS?"

Signs of right heart failure such as:

- Edema
- Ascites
- Enlargement of the liver and spleen
- JVD

Constrictive pericarditis is a combination of the physical findings described above with calcification on chest x-ray.

"Which of the Following Physical Findings Is Most Likely to Be Associated with This Patient?"

★ EQUAL PRESSURES IN ALL CHAMBERS ★

- **Kussmaul sign**: increase in JVD on inhalation (normally the neck veins should go **down** on inhalation)
- **"Knock"**: This is an extra heart sound in diastole from ventricular filling. As the heart fills to its maximum, it hits the stiff, rigid pericardium with a "knock."

DIAGNOSTIC TESTS

The **best initial test is a chest x-ray** that shows calcification and fibrosis.

CT scan and MRI are both more accurate, but would not be done if a chest x-ray were not done first.

An echocardiogram is often indispensible in order to exclude right ventricular hypertrophy or cardiomyopathy as a cause of the presentation. The myocardium moves normally in those with constrictive pericarditis.

TREATMENT

1. **Diuretics: used first** to decompress the filling of the heart and relieve edema and organomegaly
2. **Surgical removal** of the pericardium

Peripheral Artery Disease

Peripheral artery disease (PAD) is the stenosis of peripheral arteries with the same causative factors as coronary and carotid disease such as:

- Diabetes mellitus
- Hyperlipidemia
- Hypertension
- Tobacco smoking

"What Is the Most Likely Diagnosis?"

The key to this question is **leg pain in the calves on exertion**, relieved by rest. PAD pain occurs when walking up or down hills. Severe disease is associated with loss of:

- Hair follicles
- Sweat glands
- Sebaceous glands

The skin becomes smooth and shiny.

Spinal stenosis pain is worse when walking **down** hills, because of leaning back.

Diagnostic Tests

The **best initial test is the ankle-brachial index (ABI)**. This is the ratio of the blood pressure in the ankles to the brachial arteries. Normally BP is equal between them, or slightly greater in the ankles because of gravity. If the difference between them is greater than 10% (ABI less than 0.9), then disease is present.

The most accurate test is an angiogram, but this is not necessary unless specific revascularization will be done.

Treatment

The best initial therapy is:

- Aspirin
- Stopping smoking
- Cilostazol

There is **no** routine screening for PAD since there is no mortality benefit to be obtained.

The **single most effective medication is cilostazol**. Surgery is done to bypass stenosis if these medical therapies are not effective.

> **In all major vascular disease, control each of the following:**
>
> - BP
> - LDL below 100
> - Diabetes

AORTIC DISEASE

▶ **TIP**

The most frequently tested points regarding aortic disease are:

- Diagnosis and treatment of acute dissection
- Screening recommendations

A 67-year-old man comes to the emergency department with the sudden onset of chest pain. He also has pain between his scapulae. He has a history of hypertension and tobacco smoking. His blood pressure is 169/108.

What is the best initial test?

a. Chest x-ray
b. Chest CT
c. MRA
d. Transesophageal echocardiogram
e. Transthoracic echocardiogram
f. CT angiogram
g. Angiography

Answer: The correct answer is (A). Although not as sensitive as the other tests, the chest x-ray might show widening of the mediastinum, which is an excellent clue as to the presence of aortic dissection.

> **Key points for presence of aortic dissection**
>
> - Pain in between the scapulae
> - Difference in blood pressure between the arms

A 67-year-old man comes to the emergency department with the sudden onset of chest pain. He also has pain between his scapulae. He has a history of hypertension and tobacco smoking. His blood pressure is 169/108.

What is the most accurate test?

a. MRA
b. Transesophageal echocardiogram
c. Transthoracic echocardiogram
d. CT angiogram
e. Angiogram

> There is no difference in the accuracy of the MRA, CT angiogram, or TEE. MRA = CTA = TEE

Answer: The correct answer is (E). Angiography is more accurate than any of the other choices. It is the most invasive and has the potential allergic complications of contrast as well as renal failure, but it is the most sensitive and specific.

TREATMENT

In aortic dissection, the most important step is to control the blood pressure. This can be done with:

1. Beta blockers
2. Nitroprusside
3. Surgical correction

Beta blockade will decrease the "shearing forces" that are worsening the dissection. Beta blockers must be started before nitroprusside to protect against reflex tachycardia of nitro prusside, which will worsen shearing forces.

Which of the following is the most appropriate screening for aortic aneurysm?

a. Everyone above 50 with CT angiography
b. Men who ever smoked above 65 with ultrasound
c. Everyone above 50 with ultrasound
d. Everyone above 65 with ultrasound
e. Men above 65 with ultrasound

*Answer: The correct answer is (B). When the width of the abdominal aortic aneurysm (AAA) exceeds 5 cm in diameter, surgical or catheter-directed repair of the lesion is indicated. The incidence of AAA is less in both nonsmokers and in women, so there is **no** recommendation for screening in those groups. New-onset back pain in elderly patients (above 65) should have ultrasound of aorta to rule out AAA.*

HEART DISEASE IN PREGNANCY

Which of the following is the most dangerous to a pregnant woman?

a. Mitral stenosis
b. Peripartum cardiomyopathy
c. Eisenmenger phenomenon
d. Mitral valve prolapse
e. Atrial septal defect

*Answer: The correct answer is (B). The **worst** form of heart disease in pregnancy is peripartum cardiomyopathy with persistent ventricular dysfunction. If a woman with peripartum cardiomyopathy and persistent LV dysfunction becomes pregnant again, she has a **very** high chance of markedly worsening her cardiac function.*

Peripartum Cardiomyopathy

It is unknown why there are antibodies made against the myocardium in some pregnant women. The LV dysfunction is often reversible and short term. If the LV dysfunction does **not** improve, then the person must undergo cardiac transplantation.

The medical therapy consists of the same drugs as used for dilated cardiomyopathy of any cause, namely:

- ACEi/ARB
- Beta blockers
- Spironolactone
- Diuretics
- Digoxin

Repeat pregnancy in a woman with peripartum cardiomyopathy will provoke enormous antibody production against the myocardium.

> Peripartum cardiomyopathy develops **after** delivery in most cases; that is why ACEi/ARBs are acceptable to use.

Eisenmenger Syndrome

This is the development of a **right-to-left shunt from pulmonary hypertension**. Eisenmenger develops in a person with a ventricular septal defect who has significant left-to-right shunting that eventually leads to the development of pulmonary hypertension. When the pulmonary hypertension becomes very severe, then the shunt reverses and right-to-left shunting develops.

> Pregnancy increases plasma volume by 50%. Mitral stenosis will worsen in pregnancy, but **not** as much as peripartum cardiomyopathy or Eisenmenger syndrome.

▶ **TIP**

If peripartum cardiomyopathy is not one of the choices in asking, "What is the worst cardiac disease in pregnant women?" then look for Eisenmenger as one of the choices.

ENDOCRINOLOGY

4

PITUITARY DISORDERS

Panhypopituitarism

ETIOLOGY

Panhypopituitarism is caused by any condition that **compresses** or **damages** the pituitary gland. **Tumors** of many types can compress the gland, such as metastatic cancer, adenomas, Rathke cleft cysts, meningiomas, craniopharyngiomas, or lymphoma. Trauma and radiation are damaging to the pituitary. Conditions such as hemochromatosis, sarcoidosis, and histiocytosis X or infection with fungi, TB, and parasites infiltrate the pituitary, destroying its function. Finally, autoimmune and lymphocytic infiltration can damage the gland.

PRESENTATION

The symptoms of panhypopituitarism are based on the deficiencies of the specific hormone.

Symptoms of hypothyroidism and hypoadrenalism will be covered in the sections devoted to those glands.

> Ultimately, anything that damages the brain, from tumor to stroke to infection to trauma, can cause panhypopituitarism.

Specific Deficiencies

Prolactin deficiency: There are never any symptoms of prolactin **deficiency** in men. In women, prolactin deficiency inhibits lactation after childbirth. **Pro**lactin literally means "in favor of" or "pro" lactation. If deficient, the patient cannot lactate normally.

Luteinizing hormone (LH) and follicle-stimulating hormone (FSH): Women will not be able to ovulate or menstruate normally and will become **amenorrheic. Men** will not make testosterone or sperm. Both will have **decreased libido** and decreased axillary, pubic, and body hair. Men will have **erectile dysfunction** and decreased muscle mass.

Kallman Syndrome

- Decreased FSH and LH from decreased GnRH
- Anosmia
- Renal agenesis in 50%

Growth hormone (GH) deficiency: Children present with **short stature** and dwarfism. **Adults have few symptoms** of GH deficiency because several other hormones, such as catecholamines, glucagon, and cortisol, act as stress hormones.

Adults deficient in GH have subtle findings such as:

- Central obesity
- Increased LDL and cholesterol levels
- Reduced lean muscle mass

DIAGNOSTIC TESTS

Hyponatremia is common secondary to hypothyroidism and isolated glucocorticoid underproduction. Potassium levels remain normal because aldosterone is not affected and aldosterone excretes potassium.

MRI detects compressing mass lesions on the pituitary.

Specific Diagnostic Tests for Each Hormone	
Standard blood tests	**Abnormality confirmed with**
Low thyroid-stimulating hormone (TSH) and low thyroxine levels	Decreased TSH response to thyrotropin-releasing hormone (TRH)
Decreased adrenocorticotropic hormone (ACTH) and decreased cortisol level	Normal response to cosyntropin stimulation of the adrenal. Cortisol will rise (adrenal is normal) in recent disease, but abnormal in chronic disease because of adrenal atrophy. No response (rise) in ACTH level with corticotropin-releasing hormone (CRH). An elevated baseline cortisol level excludes pituitary insufficiency.
Decreased LH and FSH levels Decreased testosterone level	No confirmatory test
GH levels low, but this finding is not helpful since GH is pulsatile and maximum at night.	No response to arginine infusion No response to GH releasing hormone (GHRH)
Prolactin level low, but not helpful	No response to TRH

Older, Less Useful Tests

- **Metyrapone:** Metyrapone inhibits 11-beta hydroxylase. This decreases the output of the adrenal gland. **Metyrapone should normally cause ACTH levels to rise** because cortisol goes down. Cortisol is the feedback inhibition on the pituitary.

- **Insulin stimulation:** When insulin decreases glucose levels, GH should usually rise. **Failure of GH to rise** in response to insulin indicates pituitary insufficiency.

TREATMENT

Replace deficient hormones with:

- Thyroxine
- Cortisone
- Testosterone and estrogen
- Recombinant human growth hormone

Posterior Pituitary

The 2 products of the posterior pituitary are antidiuretic hormone (ADH) and oxytocin. There is **no deficiency disease described for oxytocin.** Oxytocin helps uterine contraction during delivery, but delivery still occurs even if it is absent. ADH deficiency is also known as central diabetes insipidus.

Diabetes Insipidus

DEFINITION

Diabetes insipidus (DI) is a decrease in either the amount of ADH from the pituitary (central DI) or its effect on the kidney (nephrogenic DI).

ETIOLOGY

Central DI (CDI): Any destruction of the brain from stroke, tumor, trauma, hypoxia, or infiltration of the gland from sarcoidosis or infection can cause CDI.

Nephrogenic DI (NDI): A few kidney diseases such as chronic pyelonephritis, amyloidosis, myeloma, or sickle cell disease will damage the kidney enough to inhibit the effect of ADH. **Hypercalcemia** and **hypokalemia** also inhibit ADH's effect on the kidney.

> Lithium is a classic cause of NDI.

PRESENTATION

DI presents with extremely high-volume urine and excessive thirst resulting in volume depletion and hypernatremia. When **hypernatremia** is severe, there will be neurological symptoms such as confusion, disorientation, lethargy, and eventually seizures and coma. Neurological symptoms occur only when volume losses are not matched with drinking enough fluid.

DIAGNOSTIC TESTS

Serum sodium is elevated when oral replacement is insufficient. Urine osmolality and urine sodium are decreased. Serum osmolality, which is largely a function of serum sodium, is elevated. Urine volume is enormous.

The **difference between central and nephrogenic DI is determined by the response to vasopressin**. In central DI, urine volume will decrease and urine osmolality will increase. With nephrogenic DI, there is no effect of vasopressin use on urine volume or osmolality.

TREATMENT

Central DI is treated with long-term **vasopressin** (desmopressin) use. Nephrogenic DI is managed by trying to **correct the underlying cause** (eg, hypokalemia or hypercalcemia). Nephrogenic DI also responds to hydrochlorothiazide, amiloride, and prostaglandin inhibitors such as NSAIDs (eg, indomethacin).

Acromegaly

DEFINITION

Acromegaly is the overproduction of growth hormone leading to soft tissue overgrowth throughout the body.

ETIOLOGY

Acromegaly is almost always caused by a pituitary **adenoma**. This can be in association with one of the multiple endocrine neoplasias when it is combined with parathyroid and pancreatic disorders like gastrinoma or insulinoma. Rarely, acromegaly is caused by ectopic GH or GHRH production from a lymphoma or bronchial carcinoid.

PRESENTATION/"WHAT IS THE MOST LIKELY DIAGNOSIS?"

Acromegaly enlarges soft tissue like cartilage and bone, resulting in:

- Increased **hat, ring, and shoe size**
- **Carpal tunnel** syndrome and obstructive sleep apnea from soft tissues enlarging
- Body **odor** from sweat gland hypertrophy
- **Coarsening facial features** and teeth widening from jaw growth
- **Deep voice** and macroglossia (big tongue)
- **Colonic polyps** and skin tags
- **Arthralgias** from joints growing out of alignment
- **Hypertension** for unclear reasons in 50%
- Cardiomegaly and CHF

> Abuse of GH can give the same presentation as acromegaly. ARNOLD

- Erectile dysfunction from increased prolactin cosecreted with the pituitary adenoma

DIAGNOSTIC TESTS

Laboratory tests will show glucose intolerance and hyperlipidemia, which contribute to the cardiac dysfunction. The **best initial test is a level of insulinlike growth factor (IGF)**. The most accurate test is the glucose suppression test. Normally, glucose should suppress growth hormone levels.

MRI should be done **only after** the laboratory identification of acromegaly.

CHECK IGF

GIVE GLUCOSE ↓ SHOULD SUPPRESS GH

> Prolactin levels are tested because of cosecretion with growth hormone.

TREATMENT

1. Surgery: Acromegaly responds to **transphenoidal resection** of the pituitary in 70% of cases. Larger adenomas are harder to cure.
2. Medications:
   - Cabergoline: Dopamine will inhibit GH release.
   - Octreotide or lanreotide: Somatostatin inhibits GH release.
   - **Pegvisomant:** A GH receptor antagonist, it inhibits IGF release from the liver.
3. Radiotherapy: Radiation is used only in those who do not respond to surgery or medications.

> If GH is an **anti**insulin, why does it make **insulin**like growth factor? Only the effect on proteins and amino acids is insulinlike.

Hyperprolactinemia

ETIOLOGY

High prolactin levels can seem confusing because so many causes have nothing to do with a pituitary adenoma. **Prolactin can be cosecreted with GH**, and increase simply because of acromegaly. Hypothyroidism leads to hyperprolactinemia because extremely high TRH levels will stimulate prolactin secretion.

Physiologic causes: Pregnancy, intense exercise, and increased chest wall stimulation all raise prolactin levels. Cutting the pituitary stalk eliminates dopamine delivery to the anterior pituitary. Dopamine inhibits prolactin release.

Drugs: Antipsychotic medications, methyldopa, metoclopromide, opioids, tricyclic antidepressants, and SSRIs all raise the prolactin level.

↑GH = ↑ PROLAC
↑TRH = ↑ PROLAC
↑ DOPA = ↓ PROLAC

PRESENTATION

Women present with galactorrhea, amenorrhea, and infertility. **Men** experience erectile dysfunction and decreased libido. Although there is gynecomastia, galactorrhea is very rare.

> Do **not** do an MRI of the head first in any endocrine disorder.

DIAGNOSTIC TESTS

After the prolactin level is found to be high, perform:

- **Thyroid function tests**
- **Pregnancy test**
- BUN/creatinine (**kidney disease elevates prolactin**)
- Liver function tests (cirrhosis elevates prolactin)

MRI is done after:

1. High prolactin level is confirmed;
2. Secondary causes like medications are excluded; **and**
3. Patient is not pregnant.

> Always **exclude pregnancy first** in any woman with a high prolactin level.

TREATMENT

↑ DOPA = ↓ PROLACTIN

1. **Dopamine agonists:** Cabergoline is better tolerated than bromocriptine.
2. Transphenoidal surgery is appropriate for those not responding to medications.
3. Radiation is rarely needed.

THYROID DISORDERS

Hypothyroidism

ETIOLOGY

Hypothyroidism is almost always from a single cause: failure of the thyroid gland from burnt-out Hashimoto thyroiditis. The acute phase is rarely perceived. Occasionally patients have hypothyroidism from:

- Dietary deficiency of iodine
- Amiodarone

"WHAT IS THE MOST LIKELY DIAGNOSIS?"

Hypothyroidism is characterized by almost all bodily processes being slowed down—except menstrual flow, which is increased.

HASHIMOTO'S IS M.C. CAUSE

CONGENITAL HYPOTHYROIDISM
→ LETHARGY | LARGE FONTANELLE'S | LARGE TONGUE | UMBILICAL HERNIA

What to Look for in Hypothyroidism and Hyperthyroidism	
Hypothyroidism	**Hyperthyroidism**
Bradycardia	Tachycardia, palpitations, arrhythmia (atrial fibrillation)
Constipation	Diarrhea (hyperdefecation)
Weight gain	Weight loss
Fatigue, lethargy, coma	Anxiety, nervousness, restlessness
Decreased reflexes	Hyperreflexia
Cold intolerance	Heat intolerance
Hypothermia (hair loss, edema)	Fever

DIAGNOSTIC TESTS

All thyroid disorders are **best tested first with a TSH**. If the TSH level is suppressed, measure **T4 levels**. TSH levels are markedly elevated if the gland has failed.

TREATMENT

Replacing thyroid hormone with thyroxine (synthroid) is sufficient.

[handwritten note: HYPO CAN GET LYMPHOMA OF THYROID]

Hyperthyroidism

Etiology/"What Is the Most Likely Diagnosis?"	
Diagnosis	**Unique feature**
Graves disease	Eye (proptosis) (20%–40%) and skin (5%) findings
Subacute thyroiditis	Tender thyroid
Painless "silent" thyroiditis *(DE QUARVAIN'S)*	Nontender, normal exam results
Exogenous thyroid hormone use	Involuted gland is not palpable
Pituitary adenoma	High TSH level

[handwritten note: AFIB → MS. ARRYTHMIA]

[handwritten note: SELF LIMITED]

Only Graves disease has eye and skin abnormalities.

DIAGNOSTIC TESTS

All forms of hyperthyroidism have an elevated T4 (thyroxine) level.

Only pituitary adenomas will have a high TSH level. In all the others, the pituitary release of TSH is inhibited.

Only Graves disease has TSH receptor antibodies.

[handwritten notes:
PIT ADENOMA = ↑TSH
ALL OTHERS = ↓TSH
ONLY GRAVES HAVE EYE & SKIN CHANGES]

113

Lab Findings in Hyperthyroidism			
Diagnosis	**TSH**	**RAIU***	**Confirmatory**
Graves disease	Low	Elevated	Positive antibody testing
Subacute thyroiditis	Low	Decreased	Tenderness
Painless "silent" thyroiditis	Low	Decreased	None
Exogenous thyroid hormone use	Low	Decreased	History and involuted, nonpalpable gland
Pituitary adenoma	High	Not done	MRI of head

*RAIU = radioactive iodine uptake

[handwritten: PTU → BLOCKS PERIPH CONVERSION / METHIMAZOLE]

Treatment	
Diagnosis	**Treatment**
Graves disease	Radioactive iodine
Subacute thyroiditis	Aspirin
Painless "silent" thyroiditis	None
Exogenous thyroid hormone use	Stop use
Pituitary adenoma	Surgery

Treatment of Acute Hyperthyroidism and "Thyroid Storm"

[handwritten: HIGH FEVER / TACHY / ↑ BP / A.MS.]

1. Propranolol: blocks target organ effect, inhibits peripheral conversion of T4→T3
2. Thiourea drugs (methimazole and propylthiouracil): blocks hormone production
3. Iodinated contrast material (iopanoic acid and ipodate): blocks the peripheral conversion of T4 to the more active T3; also blocks the release of existing hormone
4. Steroids (hydrocortisone)
5. Radioactive iodine: ablates the gland for a permanent cure

Graves Ophthalmopathy

Steroids are the best initial therapy. Radiation is used in those not responding to steroids. Severe cases may need decompressive surgery.

Thyroid Nodules

These are incredibly common, and are palpable in as much as 5% of women and 1% of men. Ninety-five percent are benign (adenoma, colloid nodule, cyst). Thyroid nodules are rarely associated with clinically apparent hyperfunctioning or hypofunctioning.

A 46-year-old woman comes to the office because of a small mass she found on palpation of her own thyroid. A small nodule is found in the thyroid. There is no tenderness. She is otherwise asymptomatic and uses no medications.

What is the most appropriate next step in the management of this patient?

a. Fine-needle aspiration
b. Radionuclide iodine uptake scan
c. T4 and TSH levels
d. Thyroid ultrasound
e. Surgical removal (excisional biopsy)

Answer: The correct answer is (C). If the patient has a hyperfunctioning gland (ie, the T4 is elevated or the TSH is decreased), the patient does not need immediate biopsy. Malignancy is not hyperfunctioning. Ultrasound of thyroid is done to evaluate the size of the lesion, but does not change the need for either thyroid function testing or needle aspiration.

DIAGNOSTIC TESTS

Thyroid **nodules** must be **biopsied** with a **fine-needle aspirate** if there is normal thyroid function (T4/TSH). Nodules in those who are euthyroid should be biopsied. There is no need to ultrasound or do radionuclide scanning because these tests cannot exclude cancer.

When a patient has a nodule:

1. Perform thyroid function tests (TSH and T4).
2. If tests are normal, biopsy the gland.

> Needle biopsy is the mainstay of thyroid nodule management.

A 46-year-old woman with a thyroid nodule is found to have normal thyroid function testing. The fine-needle aspirate comes back as "indeterminant for follicular adenoma."

What is the most appropriate next step in the management of this patient?

a. Neck CT
b. Surgical removal (excisional biopsy)
c. Ultrasound
d. Calcitonin levels

Answer: The correct answer is (B). A follicular adenoma is a histologic reading that cannot exclude cancer. The only way to exclude thyroid malignancy is to remove the entire nodule. This is an indeterminant finding on fine-needle aspiration. A sonogram cannot exclude cancer. Calcitonin levels are useful if the biopsy shows medullary carcinoma.

CALCIUM DISORDERS

Hypercalcemia

ETIOLOGY

The **most common cause** of hypercalcemia is **primary hyperparathyroidism** (PTH). Most of the patients are asymptomatic. For those with severe, acute symptomatic hypercalcemia, there is a high prevalence of cancer and the hypercalcemia of malignancy which is from a PTH-like particle. Other causes are:

- Vitamin D intoxication
- Sarcoidosis and other granulomatous diseases
- Thiazide diuretics
- Hyperthyroidism
- Metastases to bone and multiple myeloma

PRESENTATION

Acute, symptomatic hypercalcemia presents with confusion, stupor, lethargy, and constipation.

Cardiovascular
- **Short QT syndrome** and hypertension

Bone lesions
- Osteoporosis

Renal
- Nephrolithiasis
- Diabetes insipidus
- Renal insufficiency

TREATMENT

Acute hypercalcemia is treated with:

1. **Saline hydration** at high volume with a loop diuretic such as **furosemide**
2. Bisphosphonates: pamidronate, zoledronic acid

> *A 75-year-old man with a history of malignancy is admitted with lethargy, confusion, and abdominal pain. He is found to have a markedly elevated calcium level. After 3 liters of normal saline and pamidronate, his calcium level is still markedly elevated the following day.*

Primary hyperparathyroidism and cancer account for 90% of hypercalcemia patients.

The mechanism of hypertension in hypercalcemia is not clear.

What is the most appropriate next step in management?

a. Calcitonin
b. Zolendronic acid
c. Plicamycin
d. Gallium
e. Dialysis
f. Cinacalcet

*Answer: The correct answer is (A). Calcitonin inhibits osteoclasts. The onset of action of calcitonin is very rapid, and it wears off rapidly. Bisphosphonates take several days to work. Plicamycin and gallium are older therapies for hypercalcemia that no longer have any place in management. When they are given as choices for therapy, **plicamycin and gallium are always wrong.** Zolendronic acid is a bisphosphonate and does not add anything to the use of Pamidronate. Cinacalcet is an inhibitor of PTH release. If the hypercalcemia is from malignancy, PTH should already be maximally suppressed. Dialysis would be used only for those in renal failure.*

> Prednisone controls hypercalcemia when it is from sarcoidosis or any granulomatous disease.

Hyperparathyroidism

Primary hyperparathyroidism is from:

- Solitary adenoma (80%–85%)
- Hyperplasia of all 4 glands (15%–20%)
- Parathyroid malignancy (1%)

$$PTH = \uparrow Ca^{2+} \mid \downarrow Phos \mid \uparrow Vit\ D \mid \downarrow Bone$$

PRESENTATION

Primary hyperparathyroidism often presents as an asymptomatic elevation in calcium levels found on routine blood testing. When there are symptoms, it can occasionally present with the signs of acute, severe hypercalcemia previously described. More often, there are slower manifestations such as:

- Osteoporosis   *BONES*
- Nephrolithiasis and renal insufficiency   *STONES*
- Muscle weakness, anorexia, nausea, vomiting, and abdominal pain
- Peptic ulcer disease (calcium stimulates gastrin)— *MOANS*
  PANCREATITIS

BONES
STONES
MOANS
PSYCHIC OVERTONES

DIAGNOSTIC TESTS

Besides high calcium and PTH levels, you will also find a low phosphate level, high chloride level, EKG with a short QT, and sometimes an elevated BUN and creatinine. Alkaline phosphatase may be elevated from the effect of PTH on bone.

> Bone x-ray is not a good test for bone effects of high PTH. DEXA densitometry is better.

▶ **TIP**

Preoperative **imaging** of the neck with sonography or nuclear scanning **may be helpful** in determining the surgical approach.

CHRONIC RENAL DISEASE
↳ NOT ENOUGH VIT D = ↑ PTH
↳ PHOSPHATE NOT WASTED

TREATMENT

Surgical removal of the involved parathyroid glands is the standard of care.

Hypocalcemia

ETIOLOGY

Primary hypoparathyroidism is most often a complication of **prior neck surgery**, such as for thyroidectomy, in which the parathyroids have been removed. Other causes are:

↓Mag = ↓PTH
↑Ca²⁺ IN URINE

- **Hypomagnesemia:** Magnesium is necessary for PTH to be released from the gland. Low magnesium levels also lead to increased urinary loss of calcium.
- **Renal failure:** This leads to hypocalcemia. The kidney converts **25** hydroxy-D to the more active **1,25** hydroxy-D. VIA VIT D

Other Causes

Other causes include vitamin D deficiency, genetic disorders, fat malabsorption, and low albumin states. For every point decrease in albumin, the calcium level decreases by 0.8.   1 POINT LOSS IN ALBUMIN = 0.8 LOSS IN Ca²⁺

> Low albumin causes a decrease in total calcium, but the free calcium level is normal; hence, no symptoms.

PRESENTATION

Signs of neural hyperexcitability in hypocalcemia:

- Chvostek sign (facial nerve hyperexcitability)
- Carpopedal spasm
- Perioral numbness
- Mental irritability
- Seizures
- Tetany (Trousseau sign)

DIAGNOSTIC TESTS

EKG shows a **prolonged QT** that may eventually cause arrhythmia.

Slit lamp exam shows early cataracts.

TREATMENT

Replace calcium and vitamin D. This is done orally if symptoms are mild or absent and intravenously if symptoms are severe.

> Low calcium = twitchy and hyperexcitable
> High calcium = lethargic and slow

ADRENAL DISORDERS

Hypercortisolism

DEFINITION

Cushing syndrome can be used interchangeably with the term *hypercortisolism*. **Cushing disease** is a term used for the pituitary overproduction of ACTH. Hypercortisolism can also be from the ectopic production of ACTH from carcinoid or cancer or from overproduction autonomously in the adrenal gland. Prednisone and other glucocorticoid use can cause the same manifestations.

Etiology of Hypercortisolism	
Cause of hypercortisolism	**Frequency**
Pituitary ACTH (Cushing disease)	70%
Adrenals	15%
Unknown source of ACTH	5%
Ectopic ACTH (cancer, carcinoid)	10%

PRESENTATION

- **Fat redistribution:** "Moon face," truncal obesity, "buffalo hump," thin extremities, increased abdominal fat
- **Skin:** striae, easy bruising, decreased wound healing, and thinning of skin
- **Osteoporosis**
- **Hypertension:** from increased sodium reabsorption in the kidney and increased vascular reactivity
- **Menstrual disorders** in women
- **Erectile dysfunction** in men
- **Cognitive disturbance:** from decreased concentration to psychosis
- **Polyuria:** from hyperglycemia and increased free water clearance

DIAGNOSTIC TESTS

1. *Establish the Presence of Hypercortisolism*

The **best initial test** for the presence of hypercortisolism is the **24-hour urine cortisol**. If this is not in the choices, then answer is the 1 mg overnight dexamethasone suppression test. The 1 mg overnight dexamethasone suppression test should normally suppress the morning cortisol level. If this suppression occurs, hypercortisolism can be excluded.

There are **false positive tests on the 1 mg overnight dexamethasone suppression test**.

The **24-hour urine** cortisol is a **more specific** test of hypercortisolism. If the 24-hour urine cortisol is elevated, the presence of hypercortisolism is confirmed.

Causes of false positive 1 mg overnight suppression testing:

- Depression
- Alcoholism
- Obesity

2. Establish the Cause of Hypercortisolism

ACTH testing is the best initial test to determine the **cause (source) or location** of hypercortisolism.

If the ACTH level is elevated, the source could be from:

- Pituitary
- Ectopic production: lung cancer, carcinoid

Once the **ACTH level is elevated**, scan the brain with an MRI. If the MRI shows a pituitary lesion, that is the source. If the MRI does not show a clear pituitary lesion, sample the inferior petrosal sinus for ACTH, possibly after stimulating the patient with corticotrophin releasing hormone (CRH). An elevated ACTH from the venous drainage of the pituitary confirms the pituitary as the source. The petrosal venous sinus must be sampled because **some pituitary lesions are too small to be detected on MRI.**

If the ACTH is elevated, and you cannot find a defect in the pituitary either by MRI or by sampling the petrosal sinus, scan the chest looking for an ectopic source of ACTH production. You must always **confirm the source of hypercortisolism with biochemical tests before you perform imaging studies.**

> **▶TIP**
>
> At least 10% of the population has an abnormality of the pituitary on MRI. If you start with a scan, you may remove the pituitary when the source is in the adrenals.

Other Laboratory Testing in Hypercortisolism

Cortisol is a stress hormone that is an **anti**insulin. In addition, there is some aldosteronelike effect of cortisol that has an effect on the kidney's distal tubule of excreting potassium and hydrogen ions.

Effects of hypercortisolism include:

- Hyperglycemia
- Hyperlipidemia
- Hypokalemia
- Metabolic alkalosis
- **Leukocytosis** from demargination of white blood cells. At least half of white cells in the blood are on the vessel wall waiting for an acute stress to come into circulation. They are like parked police cars waiting to be called.

Decreased ACTH level = adrenal source

TREATMENT

Surgically remove the source of the hypercortisolism. Transsphenoidal surgery is done for pituitary sources whereas laparoscopic removal is done for adrenal sources.

Evaluation of Adrenal "Incidentaloma"

How far should you go in the evaluation of an unexpected, asymptomatic adrenal lesion found on CT?

- Metanephrines of blood or urine to exclude pheochromocytoma
- Renin and aldosterone levels to exclude hyperaldosteronism
- 1 mg overnight dexamethasone suppression test

> 4% of the population has adrenal "incidentaloma." Do not start with a scan or you will remove the wrong organ.

Confirmatory Laboratory Findings in Adrenal Disorders			
	Adrenal	**Pituitary**	**Ectopic**
ACTH level	Low	High	High
Petrosal sinus	Not done	High ACTH	Low ACTH
High-dose dexamethasone	No suppression	Suppresses	No suppression

Hypoadrenalism

DEFINITION

Chronic hypoadrenalism is also called **Addison disease**. Acute adrenal insufficiency is an adrenal crisis. These conditions are different severities of the same disorder.

ETIOLOGY

Addison disease is caused by autoimmune destruction of the gland in more than 80% of cases. Less common causes are:

← 1° ↓ AT ADRENALS

- Infection (tuberculosis)
- Adrenoleukodystrophy
- Metastatic cancer to the adrenal gland

Acute adrenal crisis is caused by hemorrhage, surgery, hypotension, or trauma that rapidly destroys the gland. The sudden removal of chronic high-dose prednisone (steroid) use can precipitate acute adrenal crisis. It is less common to have an acute adrenal crisis from loss of the pituitary because aldosterone is not under the control of ACTH.

2° ↓ OF ACTH @ PITUITARY

3° ↓ OF CRH @ HYPOTHALAMUS
↳ USUALLY EXCESS GLUCOCORTICOIDS

PRESENTATION

Weakness, fatigue, altered mental status, nausea, vomiting, anorexia, hypotension, hyponatremia, and hyperkalemia are common in both acute and chronic

SKIN DARKENING ONLY IN 1°

→ 1° ONLY

presentations. Hyperpigmentation from chronic adrenal insufficiency develops over a longer period of time.

Acute adrenal crisis presents with profound hypotension, fever, confusion, and coma.

DIAGNOSTIC TESTS

Patients have the opposite of the tests previously described in hypercortisolism. Hypoadrenalism leads to: *↓BICARB | ↓ BG | ↓ Na⁺ | ↑ K⁺*
↓ pH

- Hypoglycemia
- Hyperkalemia *OPPOSITE OF ↑ ALDOSTERONE*
- Metabolic acidosis *OPPOSITE OF ↑ ALDO*
- Hyponatremia
- High BUN

> Eosinophilia is common in hypoadrenalism.

↳ DRUGS
NEOPLASM
ALLERGY
* ADDISON'S
AIN
COLLAGEN VASC. DISEASE
PARASITE

If hypoadrenalism is from pituitary failure, the ACTH level is low. A high ACTH level means the etiology of adrenal insufficiency is a primary adrenal failure.

Cosyntropin Stimulation Test

The most specific test of adrenal function is the cosyntropin test. Cosyntropin is synthetic ACTH. You measure the cortisol level before and after the administration of cosyntropin. In a patient whose health is otherwise normal, there should be a rise in cortisol level after giving cosyntropin.

▶ **TIP**

Treatment is more important than testing in acute adrenal crisis.

TREATMENT

HYDRO = CORTISOL
FLUDRO = ALDO

1. Replace steroids with hydrocortisone.
2. Fludrocortisone is a steroid hormone that is particularly high in mineralocorticoid or aldosterone-like effect. Fludrocortisone is most useful if the patient still has evidence of postural instability. Mineralocorticoid supplements should be used in primary adrenal insufficiency when the patient is on oral steroids such as cortisone.

IF SICK, LIKELY NEED HIGHER "STRESS" DOSES ESPECIALLY IF MISSED DOSES

A patient is brought to the emergency department after a motor vehicle accident in which he sustains severe abdominal trauma. On the second hospital day, the patient becomes markedly hypotensive without evidence of bleeding. There is fever, a high eosinophil count, hyperkalemia, hyponatremia, and hypoglycemia.

What is the most appropriate next step in management?

a. CT scan of the adrenals
b. Draw cortisol level and administer hydrocortisone
c. Cosyntropin stimulation testing
d. ACTH level
e. Dexamethasone suppression testing

Answer: The correct answer is (B). In a patient with suspected acute adrenal insufficiency, it is critical to administer hydrocortisone. This is more important than diagnosing the etiology. Hydrocortisone possesses sufficient mineralocorticoid activity to be life-saving. In addition, hydrocortisone will increase the blood pressure because there is a permissive effect of glucocorticoids on the vascular reactivity effect of catecholamines. BP will come up fast with steroids because norepinephrine will be more effective on constricting blood vessels.

Primary Hyperaldosteronism

ETIOLOGY

Primary hyperaldosteronism is the autonomous overproduction of aldosterone despite a high pressure with a low renin activity. Eighty percent are from **solitary adenoma**. Most of the rest is from **bilateral hyperplasia**. It is **rarely malignant**. ↓CONN'S SYNDROME

PRESENTATION/"WHAT IS THE MOST LIKELY DIAGNOSIS?"

All forms of secondary hypertension are more likely in those whose onset:

- Is under age 30 or above age 60   < 30 or > 60
- Is not controlled by 2 antihypertensive medications
- Has a characteristic finding on the history, physical, or labs

METABOLIC ALKALOSIS

In the case of primary hyperaldosteronism, there is high blood pressure in association with a low potassium level. The low potassium level is either found on routine lab testing or because of symptoms of muscular weakness or diabetes insipidus from the hypokalemia.

↑ BP + ↓ K⁺

High BP + hypokalemia = primary hyperaldosteronism

DIAGNOSTIC TESTS

The best initial test is to measure the ratio of plasma aldosterone to plasma renin. An elevated plasma renin excludes primary hyperaldosteronism.

IF RENIN ↑↑ = Ø Primary ↑ALDO
IF RENIN is ↓ = Primary

The most accurate test to confirm the presence of a unilateral adenoma is a sample of the venous blood draining the adrenal. It will show a high aldosterone level.

CT scan of the adrenals should only be done **after biochemical testing** confirms:

- Low potassium
- High aldosterone despite a high-salt diet
- Low plasma renin level

▶ **TIP**

Never start with a scan in endocrinology. There are too many incidental lesions of the adrenal.

TREATMENT

- Unilateral adenoma is resected by laparoscopy.
- Bilateral hyperplasia is treated with eplerenone or spironolactone.

CHF

Pheochromocytoma

DEFINITION/ETIOLOGY

Pheochromocytoma is a nonmalignant lesion of the adrenal medulla autonomously overproducing catecholamines despite a high blood pressure.

"WHAT IS THE MOST LIKELY DIAGNOSIS?"

Pheochromocytoma is the answer when there is:

- Hypertension that is episodic in nature
- Headache
- Sweating
- Palpitations and tremor

DIAGNOSTIC TESTS

The best initial test is the level of free metanephrines in plasma. This is confirmed with a 24-hour urine collection for metanephrines. This is more sensitive than the urine vanillylmandelic acid level. Direct measurements of epinephrine and norepinephrine are useful as well.

Imaging of the adrenal glands with CT or MRI is done only **after biochemical testing.**

MIBG scanning: This is a nuclear isotope scan that detects the location of pheochromocytoma that originates outside the adrenal gland.

TREATMENT

MUST GIVE
β BLOCKERS
AND
α BLOCKER

Phenoxybenzamine is an alpha blocker that is the best initial therapy of pheochromocytoma. Calcium channel blocker and beta blockers are used afterwards.

Pheochromocytoma is removed surgically or by laparoscopy.

DIABETES MELLITUS

DEFINITION/ETIOLOGY

Diabetes mellitus (DM) is defined as persistently high fasting glucose levels greater than 125 on at least 2 separate occasions.

Type 1 DM

AUTOIMMUNE DISEASE ATTACKING ISLET CELLS   HLA-DR3/4 DQ

- Onset in childhood   *POLYURIA/DIPSIA/PHAGIA   WEIGHT LOSS   DEHYDRATION*
- Insulin dependent from an early age
- Not related to obesity
- Defined as insulin deficiency

Type 2 DM

- Onset in adulthood   *GESTATIONAL DM   ACANTHOSIS NIGRICANS*
- Directly related to obesity
- Defined as insulin resistance

PRESENTATION

Polyuria, polyphagia, and polydipsia are the most common presentation. Type 1 diabetics are generally thinner than Type 2 diabetics. Type 2 DM is more resistant to diabetic ketoacidosis (DKA). Both types present with decreased wound healing. Type 2 diabetics are much less likely to present with polyphagia.

DIAGNOSTIC TESTS

Diabetes is defined/diagnosed as:

- Two fasting blood glucose measurements greater than 125 mg/dL   *2- FASTING >125mg/dL*
- Single glucose level about 200 mg/dL with above symptoms   *>200 1 TIME*
- Increased glucose level on oral glucose tolerance testing

>6.5%

Hemoglobin A_{1c} >6.5% is now one of the diagnostic criteria and is the best test to follow response to therapy over the last several months.

TREATMENT

Diet, Exercise, and Weight Loss

Weight loss can control as much as 25% of cases of Type 2 DM without the need for medications, since decreasing the amount of adipose tissue helps to decrease insulin resistance. Exercising muscle does not need insulin.

ALWAYS 1ST LINE FOR T2DM

Oral Hypoglycemic Medication

The best initial drug therapy is with oral metformin. Sulfonylureas are not used as first-line therapy because they increase insulin release from the pancreas, thereby driving the glucose and increasing obesity.

Metformin works by blocking gluconeogenesis. *→ G.I. SEs*

Thiazoladinediones (glitazones) provide no clear benefit over the other hypoglycemic medications. They are relatively contraindicated in CHF because they increase fluid overload. *ROSGLITAZONE → ↑MI*

> Metformin is contrainidicated in those with renal dysfunction because it can accumulate and cause metabolic acidosis. *LACTIC ACIDOSIS*

Nateglinide and repaglinide are stimulators of insulin release in a similar manner to sulfonylureas, but do not contain sulfa. They do not add any therapeutic benefit to sulfonylureas.

Alpha glucosidase inhibitors (acarbose, miglitol) are agents that block glucose absorption in the bowel. They add about half a point decrease in HgA_{1c}. They cause flatus, diarrhea, and abdominal pain.

Incretins (exenatide, sitagliptin) are part of the mechanism by which oral glucose normally produces a rise in insulin and decreases glucagon levels. These agents also decrease gastric motility and help in weight loss, decreasing Type 2 diabetes. Exenatide may cause pancreatitis.

↓ DPP4

Pramlintide is an analog of a protein called amylin that is secreted normally with insulin. Amylin decreases gastric emptying, decreases glucagon levels, and decreases appetite.

> Metformin does not cause hypoglycemia. It is the safest drug to start in newly diagnosed diabetics.

Insulin is added if the patient is not controlled with oral hypoglycemic agents. Insulin glargine gives a steady state of insulin for the entire day. Dosing is not tested. Glargine provides much more steady blood levels than NPH insulin, which is dosed twice a day. Long-acting insulin is combined with a short-acting insulin such as lispro, aspart, or glulisine. Regular insulin is sometimes used as the short-acting insulin.

DAWN (MORE COMMON)
↑ MORNING BG
HIGH ALL NIGHT

SOMOGYI
↑ MORNING BG
NIGHTTIME INSULIN IS TOO HIGH
DROPS LOW AT 3AM AND THEN SURGES
LOWER NIGHT DOSE

PREMEAL
PUMPS
DKA

Pharmacokinetics of Insulin Formulations			
Insulin formulation	**Onset**	**Peak action**	**Duration**
Lispro, aspart, and glulisine	5–15 minutes	1 hour	3–4 hours
Regular	30–60 minutes	2 hours	6–8 hours
NPH	2–4 hours	6–7 hours	10–20 hours
Glargine	1–2 hours	1–2 hours	24 hours

COMPLICATIONS
HYPOGLYCEMIA FROM INSULIN
CAD
NEPHROPATHY
NEUROPATHY

HONS (HNS) ↑OSM?
NON-KETOTIC
STATE

SAME AS DKA
DIFFERENCES → GLUCOSE IS HIGHER
→ NO ACIDOSIS
→ NOT IN T1DM

SAME TREATMENT

STOP

Diabetic Ketoacidosis

Although more common in those with Type 1 diabetes, diabetic ketoacidosis (DKA) can definitely present in those with Type 2 diabetes.

Patients present with:

- Hyperventilation KUSSMAUL'S
- Possibly altered mental status
- Metabolic acidosis with an increased anion gap
- Hyperkalemia in blood, but decreased total body potassium because of urinary spillage
- Increased anion gap on blood testing
- Serum is positive for ketones
- Nonspecific abdominal pain

CAUSES
INFECTION
MED CHANGES
MED ILLNESS (MI)
UNDIAGNOSED M
DEHYDRATION
ALCOHOL/DRUGS
STEROIDS

- "Acetone" odor on breath
- Polydipsia, polyuria

Treat with large-volume saline and insulin replacement. **Replace potassium when the potassium level comes down to a level approaching normal.** Correct the underlying cause: noncompliance with medications, infection, pregnancy, or any serious illness.

A 57-year-old man is admitted to the intensive care unit with altered mental status, hyperventilation, and a markedly elevated glucose level.

Which of the following is the most accurate measure of the severity of his condition?

a. Glucose level
b. Serum bicarbonate
c. Urine ketones
d. Blood ketones
e. pH level on blood gas

Answer: The correct answer is (B). Hyperglycemia is not the best measure of the severity of DKA. The glucose level can be markedly elevated without the presence of ketoacidosis. Urine ketones mean very little. Although blood ketones are important, they are not all detected. If the serum bicarbonate is very low, the patient is at risk of death. If the serum bicarbonate is high, it does not matter how high the glucose level is, in terms of severity. Serum bicarbonate level is a way of saying "anion gap." If the bicarbonate level is low, the anion gap is increased.

Health Maintenance

All patients with DM should receive:

- Pneumococcal vaccine
- Yearly eye exam to check for proliferative retinopathy, which needs laser therapy
- Statin medication if the LDL is above 100 mg/dL
- ACE inhibitors or ARBs if the blood pressure is **greater than 130/80** mm Hg
- ACEi or ARB if urine tests positive for microalbumuria
- Aspirin, used regularly in all diabetic patients above the age of 30
- Foot exam for neuropathy and ulcers

Complications of Diabetes

Cardiovascular Complications

Diabetic patients are at significantly increased risk of myocardial infarction, stroke, and CHF from premature atherosclerotic disease. This is why the goal of blood pressure in these patients (**below 130/80 mmHg**) is lower than in the general population. In addition, diabetes is considered an equivalent of

[handwritten margin notes:]
METABOLIC SYNDROME ♂ ♀
→ ABDOMINAL OBESITY >40 IN >35
→ TRIG >150
→ HDL <40
→ BLOOD PRESSURE >130/85
→ FASTING B.G. >100

HYPOGLYCEMIA
INSULINOMA
ADMINISTRATION of DRUGS
FASTING + MALNUTRITION
ALCOHOL + FASTING

β-BLOCKERS CAN BLOCK SYMPTOMS OF HYPOGLYCEMIA!!! AVOID IN DIABETICS coronary disease for treatment of LDL, and the goal is less than 100 mg/dL when initiating treatment with statins.

Diabetic Nephropathy

Diabetes leads to microalbuminuria early in the disease. The dipstick for urine becomes trace positive at 300 mg of protein per 24 hours. Microalbuminuria means levels of albumin between 30 and 300 mg per 24 hours. **Patients with DM should be screened annually for microalbuminuria** and started on an ACE inhibitor or ARB when it is present. These agents are proven to decrease the rate of progression of nephropathy by decreasing intraglomerular hypertension and decreasing damage to the kidney.

Gastroparesis

After several years, DM decreases the ability of the gut to sense the stretch of the walls of the bowel. Stretch is the main stimulant to gastric motility. Gastroparesis is an immobility of the bowels that leads to bloating, constipation, early satiety, vomiting, and abdominal discomfort. **Treatment is with metoclopromide and erythromycin**, which increase gastric motility.

(REGLAN)

Retinopathy _(NON PROLIFERATIVE & PROLIFERATIVE)_

DM's effect on microvasculature is especially apparent in the eye. In the United States, nearly 25,000 people go blind from DM each year. The only management for nonproliferative retinopathy is tighter control of glucose. Aspirin does not help retinopathy. When neovascularization and vitreous hemorrhages are present, it is called **proliferative retinopathy**. This is treated with laser photocoagulation, which markedly retards the progression to blindness.

Neuropathy

Damage to microvasculature damages the vasonervorum that surrounds large peripheral nerves. This leads to **decreased sensation in the feet**—the main **cause of skin ulcers** of the feet which lead to osteomyelitis. When the neuropathy leads to pain, treatment is with pregabalin, gabapentin, or tricyclic antidepressants. → ESPECIALLY w/ PSYCH/NEURO PROBLEMS AS WELL

PULMONARY

5

	OBSTRUCTIVE	RESTRICTIVE
TOTAL LUNG CAPACITY	↑	↓
FVC	↓	↓
FEV₁	↓	-/↓
FEV₁/FVC	↓↓	-/↑

ASTHMA

DEFINITION

Asthma, or reactive airway disease, is an abnormal bronchoconstriction of the airways. Asthma is a **reversible** obstructive lung disease, which is the main difference between this disorder and chronic obstructive pulmonary disease (COPD).

ETIOLOGY

Although asthma is extremely common, its **etiology is unknown**. There is an association with atopic disorders and obesity.

Causes of acute exacerbations of symptoms include:

- Allergens such as pollen, dust mites, cockroaches, and cat dander
- Infection and cold air
- Emotional stress or exercise
- Catamenial (related to menstrual cycle)
- Aspirin, NSAIDs, beta blockers, histamine, any nebulized medication, tobacco smoke
- Gastroesophageal reflux disease (GERD)

> Asthma prevalence, incidence, and hospitalization rates are all increasing.

PRESENTATION

The clear presence of **wheezing** with the acute onset of shortness of breath, cough, and chest tightness make a "What is the most likely diagnosis?" question unlikely. Increased sputum production is common although a fever is not always present.

> The oral temperature may **not be accurately measured** in patients breathing fast. Mouth breathing cools the thermometer.

"Which of the Following Is Most Likely to Be Associated with/Found in This Patient?"

- Symptoms worse at night
- **Nasal polyps**

129

> The answer to the "best initial test" question in asthma is based on the severity of presentation.

- Eczema or atopic dermatitis on physical examination
- **Increased length of expiratory phase** of respiration
- Increased use of accessory respiratory muscles (eg, intercostals)

▶ **TIP**

Make sure you can identify the sound of wheezing. This is a good multi-media question.

DIAGNOSTIC TESTS

The best initial test in an acute exacerbation: **arterial blood gas (ABG)** or **peak expiratory flow (PEF)**.

Chest x-ray is most often **normal in asthma**, but may show hyperinflation. Chest x-ray is used to:

- Exclude pneumonia as a cause of exacerbation
- Exclude other diseases such as pneumothorax or CHF in cases that are not clear

The **most accurate diagnostic test** is **pulmonary function testing (PFTs)**. Spirometry will show a decrease in the ratio of forced expiratory volume in 1 second (FEV1) to forced vital capacity (FVC). The FEV1 decreases **more** than the FVC.

$FEV_1 / FVC = \downarrow$

A 15-year-old boy comes to the office because of occasional shortness of breath every few weeks. Currently he feels well. He uses no medications and denies any other medical problems. Physical examination reveals a pulse of 70 and a respiratory rate of 12 per minute. Chest examination is normal.

Which of the following is the single most accurate diagnostic test at this time?

a. Peak expiratory flow
b. Increase in FEV1 with albuterol
c. Diffusion capacity of carbon monoxide
d. >20% decrease in FEV1 with use of methacholine
e. Increased alveolar-arterial oxygen difference (A-a gradient)
f. Increase in FVC with albuterol
g. Flow-volume loop on spirometry
h. Chest CT scan
i. Increased pCO_2 on ABG

Answer: The correct answer is (D). When a patient is currently asymptomatic, it is less likely to find an increase in FEV1 with the use of short-acting bronchodilators like albuterol. This test, when the patient is asymptomatic, may be falsely negative. When the patient is asymptomatic, the most accurate test of reactive airway disease is a 20% decrease in FEV1 with the use of methacholine or histamine. Chest CT, like an x-ray, shows either nothing or hyperinflation. The ABG and PEF are useful during an acute exacerbation. Flow-volume loops are best for fixed obstructions such as tracheal lesions or COPD.

Pulmonary Function Testing in Asthma

Pulmonary function tests (PFTs) in asthma show:

- Decreased FEV1 and decreased FVC with a decreased ratio of FEV1/FVC
- Increase in FEV1 of more than 12% with the use of albuterol
- Decrease in FEV1 of more than 20% with the use of methacholine or histamine
- Increase in the diffusion capacity of the lung for carbon monoxide (DLCO)

Acetylcholine and histamine provoke bronchoconstriction and an increase in bronchial secretions. **Methacholine** is an artificial form of acetylcholine used in diagnostic testing.

Additional testing options include:

- **CBC** may show an **increased eosinophil count**.
- **Skin testing** is used to identify specific allergens that provoke broncho-constriction.
- Increased **IgE levels** suggest an allergic etiology. IgE levels may also help guide therapy such as the use of the anti-IgE medication omalizumab. Increased IgE levels are also associated with allergic bronchopulmonary aspergillosis.

TREATMENT

Asthma is managed in a stepwise fashion of progressively adding more types of treatment if there is no response.

Step 1. Always start the treatment of asthma with an **inhaled short-acting beta agonist** (SABA) as needed. Examples of SABA are:

- **Albuterol**
- Pirbuterol
- Levalbuterol

Step 2. Add a long-term control agent to a SABA. **Low-dose inhaled cortico-steroids** (ICS) are the best initial long-term control agent.

Example of ICS are:

- Beclomethasone, budesonide, flunisolide, fluticasone, mometasone, triamcinolone

Alternate long-term control agents include:

- Cromolyn and nedocromil to inhibit mast cell mediator release and eosin-ophil recruitment
- Theophylline
- Leukotriene modifiers: montelukast, zafirleukast, or zileuton (best with atopic patients)

> **Adverse effects** of inhaled steroids are **dysphonia** and **oral candidiasis**.

> **Zafirleukast** is hepatotoxic and has been **associated with Churg–Strauss syndrome**.

Step 3. Add a long-acting beta agonist (LABA) to a SABA and ICS, **or** increase the dose of the ICS.

LABA medications are salmeterol or formoterol.

Step 4. Increase the dose of the ICS to maximum **in addition** to the LABA and SABA.

Step 5. Omalizumab may be added to the SABA, LABA, and ICS in those who have an increased IgE level.

Step 6. Oral corticosteroids such as prednisone are added when all the other therapies are not sufficient to control symptoms.

Adverse Effects of Systemic Corticosteroids

They should be used as a last resort because of very harsh adverse effects such as:

- Osteoporosis
- Cataracts
- Adrenal suppression and fat redistribution
- Hyperlipidemia, hyperglycemia, acne, and hirsutism (particularly in women)
- Thinning of skin, striae, and easy bruising

> High-dose inhaled steroids rarely lead to the adverse effects associated with prednisone.

Anticholinergics

The role of ipratropium and tiotropium in asthma management is not clear. Anticholinergic agents will dilate bronchi and decrease secretions. **They are very effective in COPD.**

> Influenza and pneumococcal vaccine are given in all asthma patients.

Acute Asthma Exacerbation

A 47-year-old man with a history of asthma comes to the emergency department with several days of increasing shortness of breath, cough, and sputum production. On physical examination his respiratory rate is 34 per minute. He has diffuse expiratory wheezing and a prolonged expiratory phase.

Which of the following would you use as the best indication of the severity of his asthma?

a. Respiratory rate
b. Use of accessory muscles
c. Pulse oximetry
d. Pulmonary function testing
e. Pulse rate

Answer: The correct answer is (A). A normal respiratory rate is 10 to 16 per minute. By itself, a respiratory rate of 34 indicates severe shortness of breath. Accessory muscle use is hard to assess and is subjective. Pulse oximetry will not show hypoxia until the patient is nearly at the point of imminent respiratory failure. Oxygen saturation can be maintained above 90% by hyperventilating. Pulmonary function testing cannot be done when a patient is acutely short of breath.

DIAGNOSTIC TESTS

The **severity of an asthma exacerbation** is quantified by:

- Decreased **PEF**
- **ABG** with an increased A-a gradient

The PEF is an approximation of the FVC. There is no precise "normal" value. It is **based predominantly on height** and age, not on weight. The PEF is used in acute assessment by seeing how much difference there is from the patient's usual PEF when the patient is stable.

Chest x-ray is used to see if there is an infection leading to the exacerbation. In addition, asthma predisposes to pneumothorax.

TREATMENT

- Oxygen
- Albuterol
- Steroids —???

The best initial therapy is oxygen combined with inhaled beta agonists such as albuterol and a bolus of steroids. Corticosteroids need 4 to 6 hours to begin to work, so give them right away. **Epinephrine injections are no more effective than albuterol** and have more adverse systemic effects. Ipratropium should be used, but does not work as rapidly as albuterol.

Epinephrine is **rarely used** and only as a **drug of last resort**. Magnesium has some modest effect in bronchodilation. **Magnesium** is **not as effective as albuterol**, ipratropium, or steroids, but it does help.

> Magnesium helps bronchospasm. Magnesium is used only in an acute, severe asthma exacerbation not responsive to several rounds of albuterol while waiting for steroids to take effect.

The following are not effective in acute exacerbations:

- Theophylline
- Cromolyn and nedocromil (best with extrinsic allergies like hay fever)
- Leukotriene modifiers
- Omalizumab
- Salmeterol

If the patient does not respond to oxygen, albuterol, and steroids or develops respiratory acidosis (increased pCO_2), the patient **may have to undergo endotracheal intubation** for mechanical ventilation. **These patients should be placed in the intensive care unit.**

CHRONIC OBSTRUCTIVE PULMONARY DISEASE

DEFINITION

COPD is the presence of shortness of breath from lung destruction decreasing the elastic recoil of the lungs. Most of the ability to exhale is from elastin fibers in the lungs passively allowing exhalation. This is lost in COPD, resulting in a decrease in FEV1 and FVC with an increase in the total lung capacity (TLC). COPD is not always associated with reactive airway disease such as asthma.

ETIOLOGY

Tobacco smoking leads to almost all COPD. Tobacco destroys elastin fibers.

PRESENTATION

- **Shortness of breath** worsened by exertion
- Intermittent exacerbations with increased cough, sputum, and shortness of breath often brought on by infection
- **"Barrel chest"** from increased air trapping
- Muscle wasting and cachexia

> If the case describes a patient who is **young** and a **nonsmoker**, you should answer **alpha-1 antitrypsin deficiency** as the most likely cause.

DIAGNOSTIC TESTS

The best initial test is **chest x-ray**:

- **Increased anterior-posterior (AP) diameter**
- Air trapping and **flattened diaphragms**

The most accurate diagnostic test is **PFT**:

- Decreased FEV1, decreased FVC, decreased FEV1/FVC ratio (under 70%)
- **Increased TLC** because of an **increase in residual volume**
- Decreased DLCO
- Incomplete improvement with albuterol
- Little or no worsening with methacholine

Reversibility with Inhaled Bronchodilators

Patients with COPD have a broad range of response to inhaled bronchodilators such as albuterol. This ranges from **no reversibility** to **complete reversibility**. About 50% will have **some degree** of response.

> Full reversibility in response to bronchodilators is defined as greater than 12% increase and 200 mL increase in FEV_1.

Plethysmography will show an increase in residual volume.

Arterial blood gas (ABG): Acute exacerbations of COPD are associated with increased pCO_2 and hypoxia. Respiratory acidosis may be present if there is insufficient metabolic compensation and the bicarbonate level will be elevated to compensate. In between exacerbation, not all those with COPD will retain CO_2.

CBC: May have an increase in hematocrit from chronic hypoxia

EKG:

- Right atrial hypertrophy and right ventricular hypertrophy
- Atrial fibrillation or multifocal atrial tachycardia (MAT)

Echocardiography:

- Right atrial and right ventricular hypertrophy
- Pulmonary hypertension

TREATMENT

Improves Mortality and Delays Progression of Disease

- Smoking cessation
- Oxygen therapy for those with hypoxia; mortality benefit from oxygen is directly proportional to the number of hours that the oxygen is used.
- Influenza and pneumococcal vaccinations

Definitely Improves Symptoms (But Does Not Decrease Disease Progression)

- Short-acting beta agonists (eg, albuterol)
- **Anticholinergic agents: tiotropium, ipratropium**
- Inhaled steroids
- Long-acting beta agonists (eg, salmeterol)
- Pulmonary rehabilitation

Inhaled **anticholinergic agents** are most effective in **COPD**.

▶ **TIP**

Asthmatics not controlled with albuterol → **inhaled steroid**

COPD not controlled with albuterol → **anticholinergic (eg, tiotropium)** → inhaled steroid

Possibly Improves Symptoms

- Theophylline
- Lung volume reduction surgery

When all medical therapy is insufficient, the answer is "refer for transplantation."

No Benefit

- Cromolyn
- Leukotriene modifiers (eg, montelukast)

Treatment of Acute Exacerbations of Chronic Bronchitis

The management of acute episodes of increased shortness of breath is similar to the treatment of acute asthma exacerbations. The use of bronchodilators and corticosteroid therapy is combined with antibiotics.

Antibiotics are generally used in acute exacerbations of chronic bronchitis (AECB) because infection is by far the most commonly identified cause.

> AECB treatment is identical to asthma treatment, just with less proven benefit.

Most Effective

Although viruses cause 20% to 50% of episodes, coverage should be provided against *Streptococcus pneumoniae*, *H. influenzae*, and *Moraxella catarrhalis*.

- Macrolides: azithromycin, clarithromycin
- Cephalosporins: cefuroxime, cefixime, cefaclor, ceftibuten
- Amoxicillin/clavulanic acid
- Quinolones: levofloxacin, moxifloxacin, gemifloxacin

Second-line Agents

- Doxycycline
- Trimethoprim/sulfamethoxazole

Criteria for Oxygen Use in COPD

Oxygen decreases mortality. Criteria are:

- **pO_2 below 55** mm Hg or oxygen **saturation below 88%**

OR

If there are **signs of right-sided heart disease**/failure or an elevated hematocrit:

- **pO_2 less than 60** mm Hg or oxygen **saturation below 90%**

Although the "hypoxic drive elimination" concept is not correct, you would still avoid reflexively placing a patient with COPD on a very high-flow 100% nonrebreather mask. Use only as much oxygen as is necessary to raise the pO_2 above 90% saturation.

> The idea of "eliminating hypoxic drive" is not accurate. Dyspneic, hypoxic patients with COPD must get oxygen.

BRONCHIECTASIS

DEFINITION

Bronchiectasis is an uncommon disease from chronic dilation of the large bronchi. This is a **permanent anatomic abnormality** that cannot be reversed or cured. Bronchiectasis is uncommon because of better control of infections of the lung which lead to the weakening of the bronchial walls.

ETIOLOGY

The single most common cause of bronchiectasis is **cystic fibrosis**, which accounts for **half** of cases. Other causes are:

- Infections: tuberculosis, pneumonia, abscess
- Panhypogammaglobulinemia and immune deficiency
- Foreign body or tumors
- Allergic bronchopulmonary aspergillosis (ABPA)
- Collagen-vascular disease such as rheumatoid arthritis

PRESENTATION/"WHAT IS THE MOST LIKELY DIAGNOSIS?"

Recurrent episodes of very high volume purulent sputum production is the key to the suggestion of the diagnosis. Hemoptysis can occur. Dyspnea and wheezing are present in 75% of cases. Other findings are:

- Weight loss
- Anemia of chronic disease
- Crackles on lung exam
- Clubbing is uncommon

DIAGNOSTIC TESTS

The best initial test is a chest x-ray that shows dilated, thickened bronchi, sometimes with "tram-tracks," which is the thickening of the bronchi.

The most accurate test is a high-resolution CT scan.

> It is impossible to diagnose bronchiectasis without an imaging study of the lungs such as a CT scan.

Figure 5.1: Bronchiectasis with widening of the bronchi in multiple areas. *Source: Leyla Medinasab, MD.*

Sputum culture is the only way to determine the specific bacterial etiology of the recurrent episodes of infection.

TREATMENT

1. Chest physiotherapy ("cupping and clapping") and postural drainage are essential for dislodging plugged-up bronchi.
2. Treat each episode of infection as it arises. Use the same antibiotics as for exacerbations of COPD. The only difference is that inhaled antibiotics seem to have some efficacy and a specific microbiologic diagnosis is preferred since *Mycobacterium avium intracellulare* (MAI) can be found.
3. Surgical resection of focal lesions may be indicated.

ALLERGIC BRONCHOPULMONARY ASPERGILLOSIS (ABPA)

DEFINITION/ETIOLOGY

ABPA is hypersensitivity of the lungs to fungal antigens that colonize the bronchial tree. ABPA occurs almost exclusively in patients with asthma and a history of atopic disorders.

"WHAT IS THE MOST LIKELY DIAGNOSIS?"

Look for an asthmatic patient with recurrent episodes of brown-flecked sputum and transient infiltrates on chest x-ray.

Cough, wheezing, hemoptysis, and sometimes bronchiectasis occur.

Brown-flecked sputum

DIAGNOSTIC TESTS

- Peripheral eosinophilia
- Skin test reactivity to aspergillus antigens
- Precipitating antibodies to aspergillus on blood test
- Elevated serum IgE levels
- Pulmonary infiltrates on chest x-ray or CT

TREATMENT

1. Oral steroids (prednisone) for severe cases; **inhaled steroids are not effective for ABPA**
2. Itraconazole orally for recurrent episodes

> An inhaler cannot deliver a high enough dose of steroids to be effective in ABPA.

CYSTIC FIBROSIS

ETIOLOGY

Cystic fibrosis (CF) is an **autosomal recessive** disorder caused by a mutation in the genes that code for chloride transport. This is known as the **cystic fibrosis transmembrane conductance regulator (CFTR)**. Mutations in the CFTR gene damage chloride and water transport across the apical surface of epithelial cells in exocrine glands throughout the body. This leads to abnormally thick mucus in the lungs, as well as damage to the pancreas, liver, sinuses, intestines, and genitourinary tract. They all clog up.

Damaged mucus clearance decreases the ability to get rid of inhaled bacteria.

> Neutrophils in CF dump tons of DNA into airway secretions, clogging them up.

PRESENTATION

Over one-third of CF patients are adults. Look for a young adult with **chronic lung disease** (cough, sputum, hemoptysis, bronchiectasis, wheezing, and dyspnea) and recurrent episodes of infection. Sinus pain and **polyps** are common.

> Lung disease accounts for 95% of deaths in CF.

Gastrointestinal Involvement

- **Meconium ileus** in infants with abdominal distention
- **Pancreatic insufficiency** (in 90%) with steatorrhea and vitamin A, D, E, and K malabsorption
- **Recurrent pancreatitis**
- Distal **intestinal obstruction**
- Biliary **cirrhosis**

> Islets are spared. Beta cell function is **normal** until much later in life.

Genitourinary Involvement

Men are often infertile; 95% have **azoospermia**, with the **vas deferens missing** in 20%. Women are infertile because chronic lung disease alters the menstrual cycle and thick cervical mucus blocks sperm entry.

DIAGNOSTIC TESTS

The most accurate test is an **increased sweat chloride test**. Pilocarpine increases acetylcholine levels which increases sweat production. Chloride levels in sweat above 60 meq/L on repeated testing establishes the diagnosis.

- **Genotyping is not as accurate** as finding an increased sweat chloride level. This is because there are so many different types of mutations leading to CF.

Additional Diagnostic Tests

Chest x-ray and CT: There is no single abnormality on imaging of the chest to confirm a diagnosis of CF. Findings include:

- Bronchiectasis
- Pneumothorax
- Scarring
- Atelectasis
- Hyperinflation

Arterial blood gas may show hypoxemia and, in advanced disease, a respiratory acidosis.

PFTs show mixed obstructive and restrictive patterns; decrease in FVC and total lung capacity; and decreased diffusing capacity for carbon monoxide.

Sputum Culture:

- Nontypable *Haemophilus influenzae*
- *Pseudomonas aeruginosa*
- *Staphylococcus aureus*
- *Burkholderia cepacia*

TREATMENT

1. **Antibiotics are routine**. See the choices listed for bronchiectasis. Eliminating colonization is difficult and sputum culture is essential to guide therapy. Inhaled aminoglycosides as a treatment method are almost exclusively limited to CF.
2. Inhaled **recombinant human deoxyribonuclease** (rhDNase). This breaks down the massive amounts of DNA in respiratory mucus that clogs up the airways.
3. Inhaled **bronchodilators** such as albuterol
4. Pneumococcal and influenza **vaccinations**
5. **Lung transplantation** is used only in advanced disease not responsive to the therapy previously listed.

6. CHEST PHYSIOTHERAPY

PNEUMONIA

Community-Acquired Pneumonia

DEFINITION

Community-acquired pneumonia (CAP) is defined as pneumonia occurring before hospitalization or within 48 hours of hospital admission. CAP is the most common infectious cause of death in the United States, and is the only infectious disease that is among the top 10 causes of death nationwide.

ETIOLOGY

Streptococcus pneumoniae is the most common cause of CAP. Neither the environmental reservoir of *S. pneumoniae* nor its method of acquisition is known.

NEWBORNS	GBS	E. Coli	LISTERIA	CT		AMP & GENT (VANC)
1-4 mos	RSV	CT	PARAFLU		MACROLIDES +/- CEF
4 mos - 4yrs	VIRAL	S. pneumo	myco		AMOX / AMP
4yrs - 15yrs	S pneumo	myco	VIRAL		AMOX + clarithromycin

Common Pathogens in CAP and Their Associations	
Pathogen	**Association**
Haemophilus influenzae	COPD
Staphylococcus aureus	Recent viral infection (influenza)
Klebsiella pneumoniae	Alcoholism, diabetes
Anaerobes	Poor dentition, aspiration
Mycoplasma pneumoniae	Young, healthy patients
Chlamydophila pneumoniae	Hoarseness
Legionella	Contaminated water sources, air conditioning, ventilation systems
Chlamydia psittaci	Birds
Coxiella burnetii	Animals at the time of giving birth, veterinarians, farmers *PLACENTA*

PRESENTATION

All forms of pneumonia present with **fever** and **cough**. Severe infection is associated with **dyspnea**. *SEVERE* Cough, from any etiology, may be associated with hemoptysis. **Dullness to percussion** is found if there is an effusion. "Bronchial" breath sounds and egophony occur from consolidation of air spaces. Severe infections are distinguished by abnormalities of vital signs (**tachycardia**, **hypotension**, **tachypnea**) or mental status. Rales, rhonchi, and crepitations are auscultory findings from virtually any form of lung infection. Abdominal pain or diarrhea can occur with infection in the lower lobes irritating the intestines through the diaphragm. Chills or **"rigors" are a sign of bacteremia** often with bacterial pathogens. Chest pain occurs from inflammation of the pleura. Hypothermia is just as bad as a fever in terms of pathologic significance.

> Chest pain from pneumonia is often pleuritic, changing with respiration.

▶ **TIP**

USMLE Step 2 CK may play abnormal breath sounds as part of multimedia and ask you to recognize them.

> Dyspnea, high fever, and an abnormal chest x-ray are the main ways to distinguish pneumonia from bronchitis.

Organism-specific Associations on Presentation	
Pathogen	**Association**
Klebsiella pneumoniae	Hemoptysis from necrotizing disease, "currant jelly" sputum
Anaerobes	Foul-smelling sputum, "rotten eggs"
Mycoplasma pneumoniae	Dry cough, rarely severe, bullous myringitis
Legionella	Gastrointestinal symptoms (abdominal pain, diarrhea) or CNS symptoms such as headache and confusion
Pneumocystis	AIDS with <200 CD4 cells

Infections often with a "dry" or non-productive cough

- *Mycoplasma*
- Viruses
- *Coxiella*
- *Pneumocystis*
- *Chlamydia*

These infections preferentially involve the interstitial space and more often leave the air spaces of the alveoli empty. That is why there is less sputum production.

> Specific sputum colors are useless in determining an etiology.

DIAGNOSTIC TESTS

The best initial test for all respiratory infections is a chest x-ray. The x-ray, however, cannot determine a specific etiology. Sputum Gram stain and sputum culture are the best ways to first try to determine a specific microbial etiology. Unfortunately, many organisms will not be detected on a sputum stain or culture. The term **atypical pneumonia** refers to an organism not visible on Gram stain and not culturable on standard blood agar. The use of sputum stain and culture is somewhat controversial because of their low sensitivity. Even after thorough sputum examination, no etiology is found in at least 50% of cases. This is because *Mycoplasma, Chlamydophila, Legionella, Coxiella,* and viruses are not visible on Gram stain, and these agents account for 30% to 50% of cases of CAP.

Leukocytosis (elevated white blood cell count) is often present, but is a nonspecific marker of infection.

Figure 5.2: Right middle lobe infiltrate characteristic of bacterial pneumonia. *Source: Nirav Thakar, MD.*

Chest x-ray: Bilateral interstitial infiltrates are seen with:

- *Mycoplasma*
- Viruses
- *Coxiella*
- *Pneumocystis*
- *Chlamydia*

These are the same organisms that typically present with a nonproductive cough. X-rays lag behind clinical findings.

Figure 5.3: Interstitial infiltrates leave the air space empty. This chest x-ray can be consistent with PCP, *Mycoplasma*, viruses, and *Chlamydia*. Source: Craig Thurm, MD.

Chest CT and MRI show greater definition of abnormalities found on a chest x-ray but will still not be able to determine a specific microbiologic etiology.

▶ **TIP**

In infectious diseases, the radiologic test is never the most accurate test.

Blood Cultures are positive in 5% to 15% of cases of CAP, particularly with *S. pneumoniae*.

Tests Done in Severe Disease with an Unclear Etiology, or Those Not Responding to Treatment

Thoracentesis: Analysis of a pleural effusion can sometimes be useful to determine the presence of an empyema if the diagnosis is unclear. Any new large effusion should be analyzed. Empyema is an infected pleural effusion. Empyema acts like an abscess and will improve more rapidly if it is drained with a chest tube.

Empyema: Look for LDH above 60% of serum level and protein above 50% of serum level. A white cell count above 1000/µl is suggestive of infection.

Bronchoscopy: This is rarely needed in CAP. Bronchoscopy is used if there is severe disease such as someone needing placement in an intensive care unit (ICU) when initial testing such as sputum stain and culture and blood

> The first chest x-ray can be falsely negative in at least 10% to 20% of cases.

> Sputum Gram stain is "adequate" if there are more than 25 white blood cells and fewer than 10 epithelial cells.

> It is **impossible** to make specific diagnosis of the cause of pneumonia from history and physical.

> New, large effusions secondary to pneumonia should be tapped.

cultures do not yield an organism and the patient's condition is worsening despite empiric therapy. An exception is pneumocystis pneumonia in which noninvasive testing rarely reveals a diagnosis, and precise confirmation of the etiology is critical to guide therapy.

Specific Diagnostic Tests by Organism	
Organism	**Diagnostic test**
Mycoplasma pneumoniae	PCR, cold agglutins, serology, special culture media
Chlamydophila pneumoniae	Rising serologic titers
Legionella	Urine antigen, culture on charcoal-yeast extract
Chlamydia psittaci	Rising serologic titers
Coxiella burnetii	Rising serologic titers
Pneumocystis jiroveci (PCP)	Bronchoalveolar lavage (BAL)

Mycoplasma and *Chlamydophila* are rarely confirmed because they are simply treated empirically.

It is **the severity of disease, not the etiology,** that drives initial therapy.

TREATMENT

It is rare to have a specific organism identified at the time treatment is initiated. If the case presented describes an organism on Gram stain, then treatment is directed towards that organism. Usually, the most important step in the initial management of pneumonia is determining the severity of disease in order to determine the location in which to place the patient.

Outpatient Versus Inpatient Treatment

Outpatient Treatment

Previously healthy or no antibiotics in the past 3 months and mild symptoms → **macrolide** (azithromycin or clarithromycin)

or

doxycycline

Comorbidities or antibiotics in the past 3 months → **respiratory fluoroquinolone** (levofloxacin or moxifloxacin)

Inpatient Treatment

Respiratory fluoroquinolone: levofloxacin or moxifloxacin

or

Ceftriaxone and azithromycin

▶ TIP

Almost all infectious diseases are initially treated empirically—that is, without a specific etiology.

Reasons to *Hospitalize*

In 80% of cases, patients with pneumonia can be safely treated as outpatients with oral antibiotics. Severe disease is defined as a **combination** of:

- Hypotension (systolic below 90 mm Hg)
- Respiratory rate above 30 per minute or pO_2 less than 60 mm Hg, pH below 7.35
- Elevated BUN above 30 mg/dL, sodium less than 130 mmol/L, glucose above 250 mg/dL
- Pulse above 125 per minute
- Confusion
- Temperature above 104°F
- Age 65 or older, or comorbidities such as cancer, COPD, CHF, renal failure, or liver disease

> Hypoxia and hypotension as single factors are a reason to hospitalize a patient.

> Notice that the chest **x-ray** **does not guide admission.** X-ray cannot tell severity of hypoxia.

A 65-year-old woman is admitted to the hospital with CAP. Sputum Gram stain shows Gram-positive diplococci but the sputum culture does not grow a specific organism. Chest x-ray shows a lobar infiltrate and a large effusion. She is placed on ceftriaxone and azithromycin. Thoracentesis reveals a marked elevated LDH and protein level with 17,000 white blood cells per µl. Blood cultures grow Streptococcus pneumoniae *with a minimal inhibitory concentration (MIC) to penicillin less than 0.1 µg/mL. Her oxygen saturation is 96% on room air. Blood pressure is 110/70, temperature is 102°F, and pulse is 112 per minute.*

What is the most appropriate next step in the management of this patient?

a. Repeated thoracentesis
b. Placement of chest tube for suction
c. Add ampicillin to treatment
d. Place patient in intensive care unit
e. Consult pulmonary

*Answer: The correct answer is **(B)**. Infected pleural effusion or empyema will respond most rapidly to drainage by chest tube or thoracostomy. A large effusion acts like an abscess and is hard to sterilize. Each side of the chest can accommodate 2 to 3 liters of fluid. There is no benefit of adding ampicillin to ceftriaxone. A low MIC to penicillin automatically means that the organism is sensitive to ceftriaxone and, in fact, all cephalosporins. There is no need to be in the ICU just because of an effusion or for chest tube drainage. The patient is not unstable and, despite the effusion, has no evidence of instability because her pulse is only mildly abnormal and the blood pressure and pulse oximeter are normal. Pulmonary consultation will not add anything, although it may be commonly done in practice.*

Figure 5.4: Pleural effusion with a large meniscus sign. Only a fluid sample from thoracentesis can determine the specific cause. *Source: Craig Thurm, MD.*

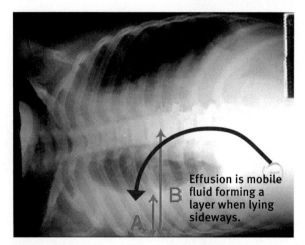

Effusion is mobile fluid forming a layer when lying sideways.

Figure 5.5: Effusion should be freely mobile and form a layer when the patient lies on her side. *Source: Nishith Patel.*

Air ("Pneumo")

Fluid ("Hydro")

Figure 5.6: Hydropneumothorax is both abnormal air and fluid (effusion) in the pleural space. Chest tube drainage is the most effective way to remove this condition. *Source: Albert Takem, MD.*

> Consultation is almost never the right answer on USMLE Step 2 CK.

Pneumococcal Vaccination

Everyone above the age of 65 should receive vaccination with the 23 polyvalent vaccine. In addition, those with chronic heart, liver, kidney, or lung disease (including asthma) should also be vaccinated as soon as their underlying disease is apparent, regardless of age. Other reasons to vaccinate are:

- Functional or anatomic asplenia (eg, sickle cell disease)

- Hematologic malignancy (leukemia, lymphoma)
- Immunosuppression: diabetes mellitus, alcoholics, corticosteroid users, AIDS or HIV positive
- CSF leak and cochlear implantation recipients

Those who are **generally healthy should receive a single dose at the age of 65**. If the first vaccination was given before age 65 or with the other conditions previously described, a second dose should also be given 5 years after the first dose.

> Healthcare workers do **not** need pneumococcal vaccine.

Healthcare-Associated Pneumonia or Hospital-Acquired Pneumonia

Hospital-acquired pneumonia (HAP) is defined as a pneumonia developing more than 48 hours after admission. These patients have a much higher incidence of Gram-negative bacilli such as *E. coli* or *Pseudomonas* as the cause of their infection. The main difference in management is that **macrolides (azithromycin or clarithromycin) are not acceptable** as empiric therapy. Instead, treatment of HAP is centered around therapy for Gram-negative bacilli such as:

Antipseudomonal cephalosporins: cefepime or ceftazidime

or

Antipseudomonal penicillin: piperacillin/tazobactam

or

Carbapenems: imipenem, meropenem, or doripenem

> Piperacillin and ticarcillin are always used in combination with a beta-lactamase inhibitor such as tazobactam or clavulanic acid.

Ventilator-Associated Pneumonia

DEFINITION

Mechanical ventilation interferes with normal mucociliary clearance of the respiratory tract such as the ability to cough. Positive pressure is tremendously damaging to the normal ability to clear colonization. Ventilator-associated pneumonia (VAP) has an incidence as high as 5% per day in the first few days on a ventilator.

"WHAT IS THE MOST LIKELY DIAGNOSIS?"

Because of multiple countercurrent illnesses such as CHF, even a diagnosis of VAP can be hard to establish. Look for:

- **Fever** and/or rising white blood cell count
- **New infiltrate** on chest x-ray
- **Purulent secretions** coming from the endotracheal tube

DIAGNOSTIC TESTS

Because of colonization of the endotracheal tube (ET), sputum culture is nearly worthless. The diagnosis of a specific etiology is extremely difficult on a ventilator. The following tests are given in order from the least accurate but easiest to do, to the most accurate but most dangerous:

- **Tracheal aspirate:** A suction catheter is placed into the ET and aspirates the contents below the trachea when the catheter is past the end of the ET tube.

- **Bronchoalveolar lavage (BAL):** A bronchoscope is placed deeper into the lungs where there are not supposed to be any organisms. Can be contaminated when passed through the nasopharynx.

- **Protected brush specimen:** The tip of the bronchoscope is covered when passed through the nasopharynx, then uncovered only inside the lungs. Much more specific because of decreased contamination.

- **Video-assisted thoracoscopy (VAT):** A scope is placed through the chest wall, and a sample of the lung is biopsied. This allows a large piece of lung to be taken without the need for cutting the chest open (thoracotomy). It is like sigmoidoscopy of the chest.

- **Open lung biopsy:** The most accurate diagnostic test of VAP, but with much greater morbidity and potential complication of the procedure because of the need for thoracotomy.

Figure 5.7: Subcutaneous emphysema is air abnormally leaking into the soft tissue of the chest wall. Chest tube placement may cause air to leak into soft tissues of the chest wall. *Source: Birju Shah, MD.*

> Culturing an endotracheal tube is like culturing urine with a Foley catheter in place: It will always grow something because of colonization.

TREATMENT

Combine **3** different drugs

1. Antipseudomonal beta-lactam

  - Cephalosporin (ceftazidime or cefepime)

    or

- Penicillin (piperacillin/tazobactam)

or

- Carbapenem (imipenem, meropenem, or doripenem)

plus

2. Second antipseudomonal agent
   - Aminoglycoside (gentamicin or tobramycin or amikacin)

or

   - Fluoroquinolone (ciprofloxacin or levofloxacin)

plus

3. Methicillin-resistant antistaphylococcal agent
   - Vancomycin

or

   - Linezolid

> Change the initial therapy for VAP if a specific etiology is identified.

A patient is admitted to the hospital for head trauma and a subdural hematoma. The patient is intubated for hyperventilation and a subsequent craniotomy. Several days after admission, the patient starts to vomit blood and is found to have stress ulcers of the stomach. Lansoprazole is started. VAP develops and the patient is placed on imipenem, linezolid, and gentamicin. Phenytoin is started prophylactically. Three days later, the creatinine rises. The patient then starts having seizures. A repeat head CT shows no changes.

What is the most appropriate next step in the management of this patient?

a. Switch phenytoin to carbamazepine
b. Stop lansoprazole
c. Stop imipenem
d. Stop linezolid
e. Perform an electroencephalogram

*Answer: The correct answer is **(C)**. Imipenem can cause seizures. Imipenem is excreted through the kidneys. The renal failure has caused a rise in imipenem levels leading to toxicity. This is much more likely than a failure of phenytoin. Carbamazepine is no more effective than phenytoin at stopping seizures.*

Lung Abscess

ETIOLOGY

Lung abscesses are rare because of prompt treatment of aspiration pneumonia. A lung abscess occurs only in a patient with a large-volume aspiration of oral/pharyngeal contents, usually with poor dentition, who is not adequately treated. Large-volume aspiration occurs from:

> Aspiration pneumonia happens in the **upper** lobe **when lying flat**.

- Stroke with loss of gag reflex
- Seizures
- Intoxication
- Endotracheal intubation

"WHAT IS THE MOST LIKELY DIAGNOSIS?"

Look for a person with one of these risk factors presenting a chronic infection developing over several weeks with large-volume **sputum that is foul smelling** because of anaerobes. Weight loss is common.

DIAGNOSTIC TEST/TREATMENT

Chest x-ray is the best initial test and will show a cavity, possibly with an air-fluid level. Chest CT is more accurate than a chest x-ray, but only a **lung biopsy** can establish the specific microbiologic etiology. Clindamycin or penicillin are best to cover a lung abscess.

> Sputum culture is the **wrong answer** for diagnosing a lung abscess. Everyone's sputum has anaerobes from mouth flora.

Figures 5.8, 5.9: Cavity consistent with an abscess with a thick wall and an air-fluid level. *Source: Alejandro de la Cruz, MD.*

Pneumocystis Pneumonia

ETIOLOGY

The agent causing pneumocystis pneumonia (PCP) has been renamed *P. jiroveci* instead of *P. carinii*. PCP occurs almost exclusively in patients with AIDS whose CD4 cell count has dropped below 200/μl and who are not on prophylactic therapy.

"WHAT IS THE MOST LIKELY DIAGNOSIS?"

Look for a patient with AIDS presenting with dyspnea on exertion, dry cough, and fever. The question will often suggest or directly state that the CD4 count is low (below 200/μl) and that the patient is not on prophylaxis.

DIAGNOSTIC TESTS

The best initial test can be either a chest x-ray showing bilateral interstitial infiltrates or an arterial blood gas looking for hypoxia or an increased A-a gradient. LDH levels are always elevated. The most accurate test is a bronchoalveolar lavage. Sputum stain for pneumocystis is quite specific if it is positive. If the stain is stated to be positive, there is no need to do further testing.

A negative sputum stain means you should answer bronchoscopy as "the best diagnostic test."

▶ **TIP**

A normal LDH means you should not answer PCP as "the most likely diagnosis."

▶ **TIP**

Remember that the questions on USMLE Step 2 CK ask what is "the **most likely** diagnosis," not what is "the **for sure** diagnosis."

> You cannot distinguish PCP from *Mycoplasma, Chlamydophila,* or viruses by x-ray alone. However, in HIV, PCP is "most likely" with interstitial infiltrates.

TREATMENT

Trimethoprim/sulfamethoxazole (TMP/SMX) is unquestionably the best initial therapy both for treatment and for prophylaxis. Add steroids to decrease mortality if the PCP is severe. Severe PCP is defined as a pO_2 below 70 or an A-a gradient above 35. Atovoquone can also be used as an alternative to TMP/SMX if the PCP is mild, meaning there is only mild hypoxia.

If there is toxicity from TMP/SMX, switch treatment to either:

- Clindamycin and primaquine

or

- Pentamidine

An HIV-positive African American man is admitted with dyspnea, dry cough, high LDH, and a pO_2 of 63 mm Hg. He is started on TMP/SMX and prednisone. On the third hospital day he develops severe neutropenia and a rash. He has anemia and there are bite cells visible on his smear.

What is the most appropriate next step in the management of this patient?

a. Stop TMP/SMX
b. Begin antiretroviral medications
c. Switch TMP/SMX to intravenous pentamidine
d. Switch TMP/SMX to aerosol pentamidine
e. Switch TMP/SMX to clindamycin and primaquine

*Answer: The correct answer is (**C**). Rash is the most common adverse effect of TMP/SMX and bone marrow suppression is the second most common adverse effect. Although clindamycin and primaquine may have more efficacy than pentamidine, the patient seems to have glucose 6 phosphate dehydrogenase (G6PD) deficiency and primaquine is contraindicated in G6PD deficiency. He is an African American man and there are bite cells suggestive of G6PD deficiency on his smear. For active disease, intravenous pentamidine is used, not aerosol. Starting antiretroviral medications should be done eventually, but they will not help an acute opportunistic infection. In addition, antiretrovirals are relatively contraindicated in acute opportunistic infections because of the possibility of immune reconstitution syndrome.*

▶ **TIP**

Often students will see 2 correct treatments and think there is a mistake in the question. If there are 2 correct treatments, look for a contraindication to one of them.

PCP Prophylaxis

Start treatment to prevent PCP in those with AIDS whose **CD4 count is below 200/μl**.

1. TMP/SMX

If there is a rash or neutropenia from TMP/SMX, use:

2. Atovoquone or dapsone

Aerosol pentamidine is not used as second-line therapy for prophylaxis because it has less efficacy than either atovoquone or dapsone.

▶ **TIP**

Always choose therapy based first on efficacy, not adverse effects.

> Dapsone is contraindicated in those with glucose 6 phosphate dehydrogenase deficiency.

An HIV-positive woman with 22 CD4 cells/μl is admitted with PCP and is treated successfully with TMP/SMX. Prophylactic TMP/SMX and azithromycin are started. She is then started on antiretroviral medication and her CD4 rises to 420 cells for the last 6 months.

What is the most appropriate next step in the management of this patient?

a. Stop TMP/SMX.
b. Stop both TMP/SMX and azithromycin
c. Stop all medications and observe
d. Stop all medications if the PCR-RNA viral load is undetectable
e. Continue all the medications
f. Stop the azithromycin

Answer: The correct answer is (B). If the CD4 count is maintained above 200/μl for several months, prophylactic TMP/SMX can be stopped. Azithromycin is used as prophylaxis for atypical mycobacteria and is used when the CD4 count drops below 50/μl. You cannot stop the antiretroviral medications because her CD4 count will drop. It is the antiretroviral medications that are maintaining her CD4 count. If the CD4 rises and is maintained high, there is no need for prophylactic medications. These cells are fully functional and they will prevent opportunistic infections. The use of prophylactic medications is based on the CD4 count, not the viral load.

TUBERCULOSIS

ETIOLOGY

Tuberculosis (TB) continues to diminish in the United States. Two-thirds of domestic TB cases occur in those who are recent immigrants from countries with poor control, including those who have been previously vaccinated with bacille Calmette-Guérin (BCG). This is why **previous BCG vaccine has no impact or effect on recommendations for treatment of latent tuberculosis infection** (positive test for purified protein derivative of tuberculin, or PPD). Almost all patients with TB have one or more established risk factors such as:

- Recent immigrants (in the past 5 years)
- Prisoners
- HIV positive
- Healthcare workers
- Close contacts of someone with TB
- Steroid use
- Hematologic malignancy
- Alcoholics
- Diabetes mellitus

PRESENTATION/"WHAT IS THE MOST LIKELY DIAGNOSIS?"

Look for a person with one of the previously listed risk factors presenting with fever, cough, sputum, weight loss, hemoptysis, and night sweats.

DIAGNOSTIC TESTS

The best initial test is a chest x-ray as with all respiratory infections. Sputum stain and culture specifically for acid-fast bacilli (mycobacteria) must be done 3 times to fully exclude TB. Pleural biopsy is the single most accurate diagnostic test.

> You cannot answer TB as the diagnosis without a clear risk factor, a cavity on chest x-ray, or a positive smear.

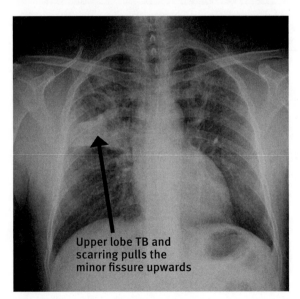

Upper lobe TB and scarring pulls the minor fissure upwards

Figure 5.10: Chest x-ray with upper lobe disease consistent with tuberculosis. *Source: Craig Thurm, MD.*

▶ **TIP**

PPD skin testing is never the best test for TB in a symptomatic patient.

TREATMENT

When the smear is positive, begin therapy with 4 drugs: **r**ifampin, **i**soniazid, **p**yrazinamide, and **e**thambutol (RIPE). You do not need the ethambutol if it is known at the beginning of therapy that the organism is sensitive to all TB medications. Ethambutol is given as part of 4-drug empiric therapy prior to knowing the sensitivity of the organism. After using RIPE for the first 2 months, stop ethambutol and pyrazinamide and continue rifampin and isoniazid for the next 4 months. The standard of care is 6 months total of therapy.

Treatment is extended to 9 months for:

- Osteomyelitis
- Miliary tuberculosis
- Meningitis
- Pregnancy or any other time pyrazinamide is not used

Toxicity of Therapy

All of the TB medications cause hepatoxicity, but do not stop them unless the transaminases rise to 3 to 5 times the **upper** limit of normal.

Adverse Effects of Antituberculosis Therapy		
Drug	**Toxicity**	**Management**
Rifampin	Red color to body secretions	None, benign finding
Isoniazid	Peripheral neuropathy	Use pyridoxine to prevent
Pyrazinamide	Hyperuricemia	No treatment unless symptomatic
Ethambutol	Optic neuritis/color vision	Decrease dose in renal failure

Use of Steroids

Glucocorticoids decrease the risk of constrictive pericarditis in those with pericardial involvement. They also decrease neurologic complication in TB meningitis.

Pregnant patients should not receive pyrazinamide or streptomycin.

Latent Tuberculosis (PPD Testing and Treatment)
Indications for PPD Testing

The PPD is not a general screening test for the whole population. Only those in the risk groups previously described should be screened. PPD testing is not useful in those who are symptomatic or those with abnormal chest x-rays. These patients should have sputum acid fast testing done.

What Is Considered a Positive Test?

Only induration is counted towards a positive test. Erythema is irrelevant.

Induration larger than 5 millimeters:

- HIV-positive patients
- Glucocorticoid users
- Close contacts of those with active TB
- Abnormal calcifications on chest x-ray
- Organ transplant recipients

Induration larger than 10 millimeters

- Recent immigrants (past 5 years)
- Prisoners
- Healthcare workers
- Close contacts of someone with TB
- Hematologic malignancy, alcoholics, diabetes mellitus

Induration larger than 15 millimeters

- Those with no risk factors

Two-Stage Testing

If the patient has never had a PPD skin test before, a second test is indicated within 1 to 2 weeks if the first test is negative. This is because the first test may be falsely negative. If the second test is negative, it means the patient is truly negative. If the second test is positive, it means the first test was a false negative.

Treatment for a Positive PPD

After active tuberculosis has been excluded with a chest x-ray, patients should receive 9 months of isoniazid. A positive PPD confers a 10% lifetime risk of active tuberculosis. Isoniazid results in a 90% reduction in this risk; after isoniazid, the lifetime risk of TB goes from 10% to 1%. The PPD test should not be repeated once it is positive.

Those at high risk, such as healthcare workers, should have a PPD done every year to screen for conversion. Most of the risk of developing active TB lies within the first 2 years after conversion.

▶ TIP

PPD testing is one of the hardest and most misunderstood tests on USMLE Step 2 CK. Reread the preceding section and forget what you have learned in the past.

> Everyone with a reactive PPD test should have a chest x-ray to exclude active disease.

> If the first test is positive, a second test is not necessary.

> Once the PPD is positive, it will always be positive in the future.

> Previous BCG has no effect on these recommendations. If the PPD is positive, the patient must take isoniazid for 9 months even if he or she had BCG.

Solitary Pulmonary Nodule

The key issue for this question is: "When do you answer a biopsy?"

Qualities of Benign and Malignant Pulmonary Nodules	
Benign	**Malignant**
<30 years old	>40 years old
No change in size	Enlarging
Nonsmoker	Smoker
Smooth border	Spiculated (spikes)
Small, <1 cm	Large, >2 cm
Normal lung	Atelectasis
No adenopathy	Yes adenopathy
Dense, central calcification	Sparse, eccentric calcification
Normal PET scan	Abnormal PET scan

▶ **TIP**

The best initial step in all lung lesions is to compare the size with old x-rays.

> Biopsy all enlarging lung lesions, particularly if they are rapidly enlarging.

Management of High-Probability Lesions

When many of the features described under "malignant" in the previous table are present, the answer is to resect (remove) the lesion. When many features of malignancy are present, sputum cytology, needle biopsy, and PET scanning should not be done because a negative test is likely a false negative. If "resection" is one of the choices, then that is the answer.

Management of Intermediate-Probability Lesions

You may notice that there are some "gray" or inconclusive aspects of the solitary pulmonary nodule in the previous table, such at the gap in age ranges (under 30 or over 40) or size (under 1 cm or over 2 cm). This is the definition of "intermediate probability."

Sputum cytology: If the question says cytology is positive, this is highly specific and the "most appropriate next step in management" is resection of the lesion. A negative cytology does not exclude malignancy.

Bronchoscopy or transthoracic needle biopsy: These are "the most appropriate next step" in most patients with intermediate probability of malignancy. Use bronchoscopy for central lesions and transthoracic biopsy for peripheral lesions.

▶ **TIP**

Relax about the diagnostic test question in intermediate lesions; a clear answer must be present. For instance, the choice of test may not be clear, but the adverse effects are always clear. The most common adverse effect of a transthoracic biopsy is pneumothorax.

Positron emission tomography (PET scan): This is a way of telling whether the content of the lesion is malignant without a biopsy. Malignancy has increased uptake of tagged glucose. The sensitivity of PET scan is 85% to 95%. A negative scan points away from malignancy.

Video-assisted thoracic surgery (VATS): VATS is both more sensitive and more specific than all the other forms of testing. Frozen section in the operating room allows for immediate conversion to an open thoracoscopy and lobectomy if malignancy is found.

INTERSTITIAL LUNG DISEASE

DEFINITION

Pulmonary fibrosis is thickening of the interstitial septum of the lung between the arteriolar space and the alveolus. Fibrosis interferes with gas exchange in both directions.

ETIOLOGY

Fibrosis can be idiopathic or secondary to a large number of inflammatory conditions, radiation, drugs, or from inhalation of toxins. All of them thicken the septum. Only some have white cell infiltrates with lymphocytes or neutrophils. Chronic conditions lead to fibrosis and thickening. It is also known as **idiopathic fibrosing interstitial pneumonia**.

Specific Causes of Pulmonary Fibrosis
- Idiopathic; interstitial pulmonary fibrosis
- Radiation
- Drugs: bleomycin, busulfan, amiodarone, methylsergide, nitrofurantoin, cyclophosphamide

Types of Pneumoconioses	
Exposure	**Disease**
Coal	Coal worker's pneumoconiosis
Sandblasting, rock mining, tunneling	Silicosis ↑ TB RISK
Shipyard workers, pipe fitting, insulators	Asbestosis BRONCHOGENIC Ca / MESOTHELIOMA
Cotton	Byssinosis
Electronic manufacture	Berylliosis
Moldy sugar cane	Bagassosis

> Inflammatory infiltration with white cells is reversible (treatable), whereas fibrosis is irreversible.

PRESENTATION

All forms of pulmonary fibrosis, regardless of etiology, present with:

- Dyspnea, worsening on exertion
- Fine rales or "crackles" on examination
- Loud P_2 heart sound
- Clubbing of the fingers

DIAGNOSTIC TESTS

The best initial test is always a chest x-ray. **High resolution CT scan is more accurate than a chest x-ray, but the most accurate test is a lung biopsy.** Echocardiography will often show pulmonary hypertension and possibly right ventricular hypertrophy.

Figure 5.11: Severe, long-standing interstitial fibrosis produces thick walls between alveoli that give the appearance of "honeycombing." *Source: Craig Thurm, MD.*

> Biopsy shows granulomas in berylliosis.

PFTs: Restrictive lung disease with decrease of everything proportionately. The FEV_1, FVC, TLC, and residual volume will all be decreased, but since everything is decreased, the **FEV_1/FVC ratio will be normal**. The **DLCO is decreased** in proportion to the severity of the thickening of the alveolar septum.

TREATMENT

Most types of interstitial lung diseases are untreatable.

If the biopsy shows white cell or inflammatory infiltrate, prednisone should be used. Of all the causes of pneumoconioses, berylliosis is the most likely to respond to treatment with steroids. This is due to the presence of granulomas, which are a sign of inflammation.

SARCOIDOSIS

DEFINITION/ETIOLOGY

Sarcoidosis is more common in African American women. It is an idiopathic inflammatory disorder predominantly of the lungs but can affect most of the body.

PRESENTATION/"WHAT IS THE MOST LIKELY DIAGNOSIS?"

Look for a young African American woman with shortness of breath on exertion and occasional fine rales on lung exam, but without the wheezing of asthma. Erythema nodosum and lymphadenopathy, either on examination or especially on chest x-ray, will hand you the diagnosis question.

Sarcoidosis also presents with:

- Parotid gland enlargement
- Facial palsy
- Heart block and restrictive cardiomyopathy
- CNS involvement
- Iritis and uveitis

> Although liver and kidney granulomas are very common on autopsy, they are rarely symptomatic.

▶ **TIP**

Answer sarcoidosis when a chest x-ray or CT shows hilar adenopathy in a generally healthy African American woman.

DIAGNOSTIC TESTS

Chest x-ray is the best initial test. Hilar adenopathy is present in more than 95% of patients with sarcoidosis. Parenchymal involvement is also present in combination with lymphadenopathy.

Lymph node biopsy is the most accurate test. The granulomas are noncaseating.

Elevated ACE level: 60%

Hypercalciuria: 20%

Hypercalcemia: 5% (granulomas in sarcoidosis make vitamin D)

PFTs: restrictive lung disease (decreased FEV_1, FVC, and TLC with a normal FEV_1/FVC ratio)

> Bronchoalveolar lavage shows an elevated level of helper cells.

TREATMENT

Prednisone is the clear drug of choice. Few patients fail to respond.

Asymptomatic hilar adenopathy does not need to be treated.

THROMBOEMBOLIC DISEASE

DEFINITION

Pulmonary emboli (PE) and deep venous thrombosis (DVT) are essentially treated as a spectrum of the same disease. PE derives from DVT of the large vessels of the **legs in 70%** and **pelvic veins in 30%**, but since the risks and treatment are the same they can be discussed at the same time.

ETIOLOGY

DVTs arise because of **stasis** from **immobility, surgery, trauma, joint replacement**, or thrombophilia such as **factor V Leiden mutation. Malignancy** of any kind leads to DVT.

PRESENTATION/"WHAT IS THE MOST LIKELY DIAGNOSIS?"

Look for the sudden onset of shortness of breath with clear lungs on examination and a normal chest x-ray.

Other findings in PE are:

- Tachypnea, tachycardia, cough, and hemoptysis
- Leg pain from DVT
- Pleuritic chest pain from lung infarction
- Fever can arise from any cause of clot or hematoma
- Extremely severe emboli will produce hypotension

▶ **TIP**

Most questions about PE concern diagnostic testing and treatment.

DIAGNOSTIC TESTS

There is no single, uncomplicated diagnostic test for a PE. Chest x-ray, EKG, and ABG are the best initial tests. Angiography is the most accurate test, but can be fatal in 0.5% of cases.

▶ **TIP**

In PE, the main issue is to know "What is the most common finding?" and "What is the most common abnormality when there is an abnormality?"

Chest x-ray: Usually normal in PE. The most common abnormality is atelectasis. Wedge-shaped infarction, pleural-based lesion (Hampton hump), and oligemia of one lobe (Westermark sign) are much less common than simple atelectasis.

CXR → CAN SEE ATELECTASIS IN PE

EKG: Usually shows sinus tachycardia. The most common abnormality is nonspecific ST-T wave changes. Only 5% will show right axis deviation, RV hypertrophy or right bundle branch block.

ABG: Hypoxia and respiratory alkalosis (high pH and low p CO_2) with a normal chest x-ray is extremely suggestive of PE.

> The most common **wrong** answer is to choose S1, Q3, T3 as the most common abnormality that will be found on EKG.

↳ REALLY NON SPECIFIC ST-T WAVE CHANGES

A 65-year-old woman who recently underwent hip replacement comes to the emergency department with the acute onset of shortness of breath and tachycardia. The chest x-ray is normal, with hypoxia on ABG, an increased A-a gradient, and an EKG with sinus tachycardia.

What is the most appropriate next step in management?

a. Intravenous unfractionated heparin
b. Thrombolytics
c. Inferior vena cava filter
d. Embolectomy
e. Spiral CT scan
f. Ventilation/perfusion (V/Q) scan
g. Lower-extremity Doppler studies
h. D-dimer

Answer: The correct answer is (A). When the history and initial labs are suggestive of PE, it is far more important to start therapy than to wait for the results of confirmatory testing such as the spiral CT or V/Q scan. D-dimer is a poor choice when the presentation is clear because its specificity is poor. Embolectomy is rarely done and is performed only if heparin is ineffective and there is persistent hypotension, hypoxia, and tachycardia.

Spiral CT scan: Also called a CT angiogram, the spiral CT has become the standard of care in terms of diagnostic testing to confirm the presence of a PE after the x-ray, EKG, and ABG are done. The specificity is excellent (over 95%). However, with a sensitivity of 85%, it can miss 15% of clots.

Ventilation/Perfusion (V/Q) scan: High probability scans have no clot (false positive) in 15%. Low-probability scans have a clot (false negative) in 15%. A completely normal scan essentially excludes a clot.

Figure 5.12: V/Q or ventilation/perfusion scanning is still very useful in evaluating pulmonary emboli. A positive test is an area that is ventilated with decreased perfusion. *Source: Nishith Patel.*

D-dimer: This test is **very sensitive** (better than 97% negative predictive value), but the **specificity is poor** since any cause of clot or increased bleeding can elevate the d-dimer level. A **negative test excludes a clot, but a positive test doesn't mean anything**.

> The chest x-ray must be normal for the V/Q scan to have any degree of accuracy. Do a spiral CT if the chest x-ray is abnormal.

▶ **TIP**

D-dimer is the answer when the pretest **probability of PE is low** and you need a simple, noninvasive test to exclude thromboembolic disease.

Lower extremity (LE) Doppler study: If the LE Doppler is positive, no further testing is needed. Only 70% of PEs originate in the legs, so it will miss 30% of cases. You do not need a spiral CT or V/Q scan to confirm a PE if there is a clot in the legs because they will not change therapy. The patient will still need heparin and 6 months of warfarin.

Spiral CT negative → V/Q or LE Doppler → negative → withhold therapy with heparin

> LE Dopplers are a good test if the V/Q and spiral CT do not give a clear diagnosis.

Angiography: The most accurate test with nearly 100% specificity and a false negative rate under 1%. Unfortunately, there is a 0.5% mortality, which is high if you consider the tens of thousands of tests a year that would need to be done to exclude PE in all cases.

> When testing for PE, angiography is rarely done.

▶ **TIP**

What to do is not always clear. However, the adverse effects of angiography (allergy, renal toxicity, and death) is a very clear question.

TREATMENT

Heparin is the best initial therapy. Warfarin should be started at the same time as the heparin in order to achieve a therapeutic INR of 2 to 3 times normal as quickly as possible.

When is an **inferior vena cava** (IVC) filter the right answer?

- **Contraindication to the use of anticoagulants** (eg, melena, CNS bleeding)
- **Recurrent emboli** while on heparin or fully therapeutic warfarin (INR of 2–3)
- **Right ventricular (RV) dysfunction** with an enlarged RV on echo. In this case, disease is so severe that an IVC filter is placed because the next embolus, even if seemingly small, could be potentially fatal.

> There is no specific time limit in which to use thrombolytics as there is in stroke or MI.

When are thrombolytics the right answer?

- Hemodynamically unstable patients (eg, hypotension and tachycardia) *SADDLE EMBOLUS*
- Acute RV dysfunction

When are direct-acting thrombin inhibitors (argatroban, lepirudin) the answer?

- Heparin-induced thrombocytopenia   HIT

When is aspirin the answer?

- Never

PULMONARY HYPERTENSION

DEFINITION

The lung, or pulmonary, circulation normally is extremely low pressure (systolic 25 mm Hg, diastolic 8 mm Hg), so any chronic lung disease leads to back pressure into the pulmonary artery, obstructing flow out of the right side of the heart.

ETIOLOGY

Primary pulmonary hypertension is by definition idiopathic. Any form of chronic lung disease such as COPD or fibrosis elevates the pulmonary artery pressure. Hypoxemia causes vasoconstriction of the pulmonary circulation as a normal reflex in the lungs to shunt blood away from areas of the lung it considers to have poor oxygenation. This is why hypoxia leads to pulmonary hypertension, and pulmonary hypertension results in more hypoxemia.

PRESENTATION

- Dyspnea and fatigue
- Syncope
- Chest pain
- Narrow splitting of S2 with a loud P2 or tricuspid and pulmonary valve insufficiency

> It is impossible to know that pulmonary hypertension is causing the dyspnea without tests.

DIAGNOSTIC TESTS

Chest x-ray and CT: best initial tests showing dilation of the proximal pulmonary arteries with narrowing or "pruning" of distal vessels

Right heart or Swan-Ganz catheter: most accurate test and the most precise method to measure pressures

EKG: right axis deviation, right atrial and ventricular hypertrophy

Echocardiography: RA and RV hypertrophy; Doppler estimates pulmonary artery (PA) pressure

V/Q scanning identifies chronic PE as the cause of pulmonary hypertension. CBC shows polycythemia from chronic hypoxia.

TREATMENT

1. Correct the underlying cause when one is clear.
2. Idiopathic disease is treated with:

   - Prostacyclin analogues (PA vasodilators): epoprostenol, treprostinil, iloprost, beraprost
   - Endothelin antagonists: bosentan
   - Phosphodiesterase inhibitors: sildenafil

These are **all better** than calcium channel blockers, hydralazine, and nitroglycerin.

3. Oxygen slows progression, particularly with COPD.

> Only **lung transplantation is curative** for idiopathic pulmonary hypertension.

OBSTRUCTIVE SLEEP APNEA

Obesity is the most commonly identified cause of obstructive sleep apnea. Patients present with daytime somnolence and a history of loud snoring.

Other symptoms include:

- Headache
- Impaired memory and judgement
- Depression
- Hypertension
- Erectile dysfunction
- "Bull neck"

The **most accurate test is polysomnography** (sleep study) which shows multiple episodes of apnea. Arrythmias and erythrocytosis are common.

TREATMENT

1. **Weight loss and** avoidance of alcohol
2. Nasal continuous positive airway pressure (nasal **CPAP**)
3. Surgical widening of the airway (uvuloplatopharyngoplasty) if this fails
4. Avoid use of sedatives

ACUTE RESPIRATORY DISTRESS SYNDROME

DEFINITION

Acute respiratory distress syndrome (ARDS) is respiratory failure from overwhelming lung injury or systemic disease leading to severe hypoxia with a chest x-ray suggestive of congestive failure but normal cardiac hemodynamic measurements. ARDS decreases surfactant and makes the lung cells "leaky" so that the alveoli fill up with fluid.

ETIOLOGY

ARDS is idiopathic. A large number of illnesses and injuries are associated with alveolar epithelial cell and capillary endothelial cell damage.

Examples of illnesses and injuries associated with developing ARDS include:

- Sepsis or aspiration
- Lung contusion/trauma
- Near-drowning
- Burns or pancreatitis

DIAGNOSTIC TESTS

The chest x-ray shows bilateral infiltrates that quickly become confluent ("white out"). Air bronchograms are common.

Figure 5.13: Air bronchograms are a sign of dense consolidation of the lung air space. This is a case of pneumococcal pneumonia that left only the air space in the larger bronchi open or air bronchograms. *Source: Omid Edrissian, MD.*

ARDS is defined as having a pO_2/FIO_2 ratio below 200. The FIO_2 is expressed as a decimal, so room air with 21% oxygen would be 0.21. If the pO_2 is 105 on room air (21% oxygen or 0.21), then the ratio of pO_2/FIO_2 is 500 (105/.21). If the pO_2 (as measured on an ABG) is 70 while breathing 50% oxygen, the ratio is 70/0.5 or 140.

By definition, ARDS is associated with normal findings on right heart catheterization. The **wedge pressure is normal**.

TREATMENT   5-8 m/kg

> No treatment is proven to reverse ARDS. Don't forget to treat the underlying cause.

Low tidal-volume mechanical ventilation is the best support while waiting to see if the lungs will recover. Use **6 mL per kg of tidal volume. Steroids are not clearly beneficial** in most cases. They may help in late-stage disease in which pulmonary fibrosis develops.

Positive end-expiratory pressure (PEEP) is used when the patient is undergoing mechanical ventilation to try to decrease the FIO_2. Levels of FIO_2 above 50% are toxic to the lungs. Maintain the **plateau pressure of less than 30 cm of water.** This is measured on the ventilator.

No STEROIDS

PLATEAU PRESSURE < 30 cm H_2O

THORACENTESIS

TRANSUDATE	EXUDATE

TRANS - CHF | CIRRHOSIS | PE | NEPHROTIC SYN | ATELECTASIS

EXUDATE - INF | MALIG | COLLAGEN

PLEURAL PROTEIN:
SERUM PROTEIN   > 0.5

P LDH :
S LDH   > 0.6

P LDH > $\frac{2}{3}$ NML S LDH

RHEUMATOLOGY

6

OSTEOARTHRITIS

DEFINITION

Osteoarthritis, or degenerative joint disease (DJD), is a **chronic**, slowly progressive, erosive damage to joint surfaces; this **loss of articular cartilage** causes increasing pain with minimal or **absent inflammation**.

ETIOLOGY

The incidence of DJD is directly proportional to **increasing age and trauma** to the joint. Modest recreational running does not cause DJD, but playing contact sports with trauma does. Obesity increases DJD.

> DJD is, by far, the most common cause of joint disease.

PRESENTATION

DJD is most commonly symptomatic in **weight-bearing joints** (knee, hip, ankle). The hand is affected, but is not as great a cause of disability. Distal interphalangeal (DIP) joints are more commonly affected in the hand compared to the proximal interphalangeal joints (PIP) and metacarpophalangeal joints (MCP). **Crepitations** of the involved joints are common. Effusion is rare. Stiffness is of short duration (under 15 minutes).

DIP enlargement: Heberden nodes

PIP enlargement: Bouchard nodes

DIAGNOSTIC TESTS

Laboratory tests are **normal:**

- Erythrocyte sedimentation rate (ESR)
- Complete blood count (CBC)
- Antinuclear antibody (ANA)
- Rheumatoid factor

The most accurate test is radiography of the affected joint. X-rays show:

- Joint space narrowing
- Osteophytes
- Dense subchondral bone
- Bone cysts

> Absence of inflammation, normal lab tests, and short duration of stiffness distinguishes DJD from rheumatoid arthritis.

TREATMENT

1. **Weight loss** and **moderate exercise** (hydrotherapy [swimming], tai chi, yoga)
2. **Acetaminophen:** best initial analgesic
3. **NSAIDs:** used if symptoms are not controlled with acetaminophen; second because of toxicity, particularly GI bleeding
4. Capsaicin cream
5. **Intraarticular steroids** if other medical therapy does not control pain
6. Joint **replacement** if disease is severe

> Glucosamine and chondroitin sulfate are no more effective than placebo.

GOUT

DEFINITION/ETIOLOGY

Gouty arthritis is a defect in urate metabolism with **90% of cases in men**. This can be from overproduction or underexcretion.

Overproduction:

- Idiopathic
- **Increased turnover of cells** (cancer, hemolysis, psoriasis, chemotherapy)
- **Enzyme deficiency** (Lesch-Nyhan syndrome, glycogen storage disease)

Underexcretion:

- Renal insufficiency
- Ketoacidosis or lactic acidosis
- Thiazides and aspirin

PRESENTATION/"WHAT IS THE MOST LIKELY DIAGNOSIS?"

Look for a **man** who develops **sudden, excruciating pain, redness**, and **tenderness** of the **big toe** at night after binge drinking with beer. **Fever** is common, and it can be hard to distinguish the initial gouty attack from infection without arthrocentesis.

Although the metatarsal phalangeal (MTP) joint of the great toe is the most frequently affected site, gout can also be symptomatic in the ankle, feet, and knees.

Chronic Gout

- **Tophi**: tissue deposits of urate crystals with foreign body reaction. Most often tophi occur in cartilage, subcutaneous tissues, bone, and kidney. They often take years to develop.
- **Uric acid kidney stones** occur in 5% to 10% of patients.
- **Long asymptomatic periods** between attacks are common.

> Tophi can occur anywhere in the body.

DIAGNOSTIC TESTS

The most accurate test is **aspiration of the joint showing needle-shaped crystals** with **negative birefringence** on polarized light microscopy. The white cell count on joint fluid is elevated between 2000 and 50,000/µl and are predominantly neutrophils. Because gout can look like an infected joint with redness, warmth, and tenderness, **it is essential to tap the joint to exclude infection**.

▶ TIP

Protein and glucose levels in synovial fluid don't help answer the "most likely diagnosis" question.

Uric acid levels: elevated at some point in 95% of patients. A single level during an acute gouty attack is normal in 25%.

Acute attacks are associated with an **elevated ESR** and **leukocytosis**.

X-rays: normal in early disease. Erosions of cortical bone happen later.

TREATMENT

Acute Attack

1. **NSAIDs are superior to colchicine** as the best initial therapy of acute, painful gouty arthritis.
2. **Corticosteroids** by injection in a single joint or orally for multiple joints are extremely effective. Steroids (eg, triamcinolone) is the answer when:
   - No response to NSAIDs
   - Contraindication to NSAIDs such as renal insufficiency

▶ TIP

Contraindication questions are always clear.

> Colchicine gives diarrhea and bone marrow suppression (neutropenia).

Chronic Management

Management between attacks prevents recurrences.

1. **Diet**:
   - Decrease consumption of alcohol, particularly beer.
   - Lose weight.
   - Decrease high-purine foods such as meat and seafood.

Probenecid, NSAIDs, and sulfinpyrazone are contraindicated in renal insufficiency. Allopurinol is safe with renal injury.

2. **Stop thiazides,** aspirin, and niacin.

3. **Colchicine** is effective at preventing a second attack of gout. Colchicine is also effective at preventing attacks brought on by sudden fluctuations in uric acid levels due to probenecid or allopurinol.

4. Probenecid and sulfinpyrazone increase the excretion of uric acid in the kidney (uricosuric).

5. Allopurinol decreases production of uric acid.

Do not start uricosuric agents or allopurinol during acute attacks of gout. If the patient is already on allopurinol, you can safely continue it.

Adverse Effects of Chronic Treatment

- Hypersensitivity (rash, hemolysis, allergic interstitial nephritis) occurs with uricosuric agents and allopurinol.

- Colchicine can suppress white cell production.

- Toxic epidermal necrolysis or Stevens-Johnson syndrome may occur from allopurinol.

CALCIUM PYROPHOSPHATE DEPOSITION DISEASE OR "PSEUDOGOUT"

DEFINITION/ETIOLOGY

Calcium pyrophosphate deposition disease (CPPD) is from calcium-containing salts depositing in the articular cartilage. The most common **risk factors are hemochromatosis** and **hyperparathyroidism**. CPPD is also associated with diabetes, hypothyroidism, and Wilson disease.

PRESENTATION

CPPD differs from gout in that large joints such as the knee and wrist are affected, but not particularly the first MCP of the foot. It differs from DJD in that **the DIP and PIP are not affected.**

DIAGNOSTIC TESTS

You cannot confirm a diagnosis of CPPD without aspiration of the joint.

Uric acid levels are normal. X-ray shows calcification of the cartilaginous structures of the joint and DJD. The most accurate test is arthrocentesis, which reveals positively birefringent rhomboid-shaped crystals. Synovial fluid will show an elevated level of white blood cells between 2000 and 50,000/μl, but this will not distinguish CPPD from gout or other inflammatory disorders of the joint such as rheumatoid arthritis (RA).

Disease	DJD	Gout	CPPD	Rheumatoid arthritis	Septic arthritis
Characteristic History	Older, slow, worse with use	Men, acute, binge drinking	Hemochromatosis Hyperparathyroidism	Young, female, morning stiffness better with use	High fever, very acute
Physical Findings	DIP, PIP, hip, and knees	1st big toe	Wrists and knees	Multiple joints of hands and feet	Single hot joint
Synovial Fluid Analysis	<200 WBCs, osteophytes and joint space narrowing	2,000–50,000 WBCs, negatively birefringent needles	2,000–50,000 WBCs, positively birefringent rhomboids	Anti-cyclic citrulinated peptide (anti-CCP)	>50,000 neutrophils, culture of fluid

TREATMENT

The best **initial therapy** is **NSAIDs**. If there is severe disease not responsive to NSAIDs, give **intraarticular steroids** such as triamcinolone. **Colchicine helps prevent subsequent attacks** as prophylaxis between attacks.

LOW BACK PAIN

ETIOLOGY

Low back pain is so common over a lifetime (80% of population) that the most important issue is to identify those few patients that have serious pathology that will require radiologic testing and possible surgical treatment.

DJD on x-ray or MRI of the spine is nearly universal in those above 50 years of age and has no meaning when it is found.

▶ TIP

The most frequently tested issue is who **not** to get an imaging study on.

"WHAT IS THE MOST LIKELY DIAGNOSIS?"

If all of the diseases described in the following are excluded, the patient has simple low back pain from "lumbosacral strain" or is simply idiopathic. These patients require no imaging studies and **no treatment beyond NSAIDs**.

Compression of the Spinal Cord

Malignancy or infection compressing the spinal cord is a neurological emergency that needs urgent identification and treatment. Look for a **history of cancer** with the sudden onset of **focal neurological deficits** such as a **sensory level**. For instance, compression at the level of the fourth thoracic vertebra would result in a loss of sensation below the nipples. Compression at the 10th thoracic vertebra leads to sensory loss below the umbilicus. **Point tenderness** at the spine with percussion of the vertebra is **highly suggestive** of cord compression. **Hyperreflexia** is found below the level of compression. Epidural abscess is most often from *Staphylococcus aureus*. Epidural abscess presents in the same way as cord compression from cancer, but there is a high fever and markedly elevated ESR.

Disk Herniation (Sciatica)

Herniations at the L4/5 and L5/S1 level account for 95% of all disk herniations. **The straight leg raise (SLR) test is pain going into the buttock and below the knee when the leg is raised above 60 degrees.** Although only 50% of those with a positive SLR actually have a herniated disk, the sensitivity is excellent. A **negative SLR excludes herniation with 95% sensitivity.**

Nerve Root Innervation			
Nerve root	**Motor deficit**	**Reflex affected (lost)**	**Sensory area affected**
L4	Dorsiflexion of foot	Knee jerk	Inner calf
L5	Dorsiflexion of toe	None	Inner forefoot
S1	Eversion of foot	Ankle jerk	Outer foot

DIAGNOSTIC TESTS

Imaging is required for cord compression, epidural abscess, ankylosing spondylitis, and cauda equina syndrome.

The best initial test for cancer with compression, infection, and fractures is a plain x-ray. The **most accurate test is an MRI**. CT scan is used as the most accurate test if there is a contraindication to MRI such as a pacemaker. If CT scan is used, intrathecal contrast must be given to increase accuracy (CT myelogram).

Imaging in disk herniation is somewhat controversial because it is not clear that it changes management. **We recommend you answer "no MRI" for just low back pain and a positive SLR alone.** If severe or progressive neurological deficits (paralysis, weakness) are described, then an MRI should be done.

Figure 6.1: MRI is the most accurate test of cord compression. Using glucocorticoids to relieve compression is more important than waiting for test results. *Source: Nirav Thakur, MD.*

Classification of Back Pain				
Cord compression	**Epidural abscess**	**Cauda equina**	**Ankylosing spondylitis**	**Disk herniation**
History of cancer	Fever, high ESR	Bowel and bladder incontinence, erectile dysfunction	Under age 40, pain worsens with rest and improves with activity	Pain/numbness of medial calf or foot
Vertebral tenderness, sensory level, hyperreflexia	Same as cord compression	Bilateral leg weakness, saddle area anesthesia	Decreased chest mobility	Loss of knee and ankle reflexes, positive straight leg raise

Diagnosis	**Cord compression**	**Epidural abscess**	**Cauda equina**	**Ankylosing spondylitis**	**Disk herniation**
History to answer "Most Likely Diagnosis"	History of cancer	Fever, high ESR	Bowel and bladder incontinence, erectile dysfunction	Under age 40, pain worsens with rest and improves with activity	Pain/numbness of medial calf or foot
Physical Findings	Vertebral tenderness, sensory level, hyperreflexia	Same as cord compression	Bilateral leg weakness, saddle area anesthesia	Decreased chest mobility	Loss of knee and ankle reflexes, positive straight leg raise

TREATMENT

Cord compression: systemic **glucocorticoids**, chemotherapy for lymphoma, radiation for many solid tumors. Surgical decompression if steroids and radiation are not effective.

Epidural abscess: Steroids are used to control acute neurological deficits. Use **antistaphylococcal antibiotics** such as **vancomycin** or **linezolid** until the sensitivity of the organism is known. If a **sensitive staphylococcus** is found, switch to beta-lactam antibiotics such as **oxacillin**, **nafcillin**, or **cefazolin**. Beta-lactam antibiotics have greater efficacy when the organism is sensitive. Gentamicin is added for synergy with *staphylococcus* as is done for endocarditis. Surgical drainage is needed for larger collections of infected material.

> Think of **epidural abscess like endocarditis.** Use vancomycin as initial empiric therapy. Switch to oxacillin if it is sensitive. Drain it if the infection is large enough to produce neurological deficits or it does not respond to antibiotics alone.

Cauda equina syndrome: surgical decompression

Disk herniation (sciatica): NSAIDs with continuation of ordinary activities (conservative management) is superior to bed rest. Yoga is just as effective as a more regimented or supposedly specific formal back exercise program. **Steroid injection** into the epidural space achieves **rapid and dramatic benefit** for those with sciatica who do not improve with conservative management. Surgery is rarely needed; it is the answer only if focal neurological deficits develop or progress.

The most common **wrong** answer for sciatica is **bed rest.**

A man with a history of prostate cancer comes to the emergency department with severe back pain and leg weakness. He has tenderness of the spine, hyperreflexia, and decreased sensation below his umbilicus.

What is the most appropriate next step in the management of this patient?

a. Dexamethasone
b. MRI
c. X-ray
d. Radiation
e. Flutamide
f. Ketoconazole
g. Finasteride
h. Leuprolide (GnRH agonist)
i. Biopsy
j. Orchiectomy

Answer: The correct answer is *(A)*. When there is obvious cord compression, the most important step is to begin steroids urgently in order to decrease the pressure on the cord. Radiation is necessary in those with metastatic cancer to the cord, but it does not work as fast as giving steroids. X-ray may show vertebral damage, and **MRI is the most accurate imaging study**, but **preventing permanent paralysis with steroids is more important to do first**. Leuprolide is actually dangerous without first blocking the peripheral receptors to testosterone with flutamide. GnRH agonists will give a transient burst up in testosterone levels. Finasteride is a 5-alpha reductase inhibitor that is not helpful for prostate cancer. Finasteride is used for benign prostatic hypertrophy and male pattern hair loss. Ketoconazole is a second-line agent in inhibiting androgens. The fastest way to lower androgen levels is with orchiectomy, but this step is rarely necessary. Biopsy is done if the etiology is not clear. The key issue in this question is timing: What decompresses the spine fastest? The answer is glucocorticoids like dexamethasone.

▶ **TIP**

Most commonly tested point: Do not do imaging studies in those patients **without focal neurological abnormalities** or with simple lumbosacral strain.

LUMBAR SPINAL STENOSIS

DEFINITION/ETIOLOGY

Narrowing of the spinal canal leading to pressure on the cord is idiopathic. Pain occurs when the back is in extension and the cord presses backwards against the ligamentum flavum.

> Exertion with leaning back leads to worse pain because of pressure on the cord.

PRESENTATION/"WHAT IS THE MOST LIKELY DIAGNOSIS?"

Look for a person over age 60 with back pain while walking, radiating into the buttocks and thighs bilaterally. The pain is described as **worse when walking downhill**, and better when sitting, but the pedal pulses and **ankle/brachial index are normal**. Unsteady gait and leg weakness when walking also occur. About a quarter have diminished lower extremity reflexes. **Pain** is much **less** with activities that have the **patient leaning forward** such as cycling.

> Spinal stenosis can simulate peripheral arterial disease, but the vascular studies are normal.

DIAGNOSTIC TEST/TREATMENT

The only test is **MRI**. Weight loss and steroid injections into the lumbar epidural space improve 25% to 50% of cases. **Surgical correction** to dilate the spinal canal is needed in 75% of patients.

PAGET'S DISEASE
- HAS DOESN'T FIT / BONE PAIN
    - ↑ ALK PHOS   NML Ca²⁺/PHOS
- OSTEOLYTIC LESIONS / MOSAIC BONE
- BISPHOSPHONATES

OSTEOPETROSIS
- HAS DOESN'T FIT
- IMPAIRED OSTEOCLASTS
- DEAFNESS
- ↓ H ↑ H   ↑ CREATINE KINASE
- TRANSFUSIONS
- ACTIVITY RESTRICTIONS

FIBROMYALGIA

"WHAT IS THE MOST LIKELY DIAGNOSIS?"

Look for a **young woman** with chronic musculoskeletal pain and **tenderness with trigger points** of focal tenderness at the trapezius, medial fat pad of the knee, and lateral epicondyle. The cause of fibromyalgia is unknown. **Pain occurs at many sites** (neck, shoulders, back, and hips) and is associated with:

- Stiffness, numbness, and fatigue
- Headaches
- Sleep disorder

DIAGNOSTIC TESTS/TREATMENT

There is **no test to confirm fibromyalgia**. It is based on a complex of symptoms with trigger points at predictable points. **All lab tests are normal** such as ESR, C-reactive protein, rheumatoid factor (RF), and CPK levels.

The best initial therapy is **amitriptyline**. Other treatments are **milnacipran** and **pregabalin**. Milnacipran is an inhibitor of the reuptake of serotonin and norepinephrine and is approved specifically for the management of fibromyalgia. **Trigger point injections** with local anesthetic are also sometimes used.

> Steroids are the wrong answer for fibromyalgia.

CARPAL TUNNEL SYNDROME

DEFINITION

Carpal tunnel syndrome is a peripheral neuropathy from the compression of the median nerve as it passes under the flexor retinaculum. Pressure on the nerve interferes with both sensory and motor function of the nerve.

ETIOLOGY

Carpal tunnel syndrome is most often of unclear etiology, but it is associated with overuse of the hand and wrist as well as:

- Pregnancy
- Diabetes
- Rheumatoid arthritis
- Acromegaly
- Amyloidosis
- Hypothyroidism

"WHAT IS THE MOST LIKELY DIAGNOSIS?"

Look for a person with **pain** in the **hand** affecting the palm, thumb, index finger, and the radial half of the ring finger with muscle **atrophy of the thenar eminence.** The pain is **worse at night** and is more frequent in those whose work involves prolonged use of the hands such as typing.

- **Tinel sign:** reproduction of the pain and tingling with **tapping or percussion** of the median nerve
- **Phalen sign:** reproduction of symptoms with **flexion of the wrists to 90 degrees**

DIAGNOSTIC TESTS/TREATMENT

Carpal tunnel is usually obvious from the symptoms. Besides the Tinel and Phalen signs, simple compression of the nerve by squeezing it helps confirm the diagnosis. The **most accurate diagnostic tests** are **electromyography** and **nerve conduction testing.**

The **best initial therapy** is with **wrist splints** to immobilize the hand in a position to relieve pressure. Patients should **avoid manual activity. Steroid injection** is used if splints and NSAIDs do not control symptoms. **Surgery can be curative** by mechanically decompressing the tunnel such as with cutting open the flexor retinaculum.

> Sensory symptoms happen before motor symptoms.

DUPUYTREN CONTRACTURE

This is the **hyperplasia of the palmar fascia** leading to nodule formation and **contracture of the fourth and fifth fingers.** There is a genetic predisposition and an association with alcoholism and cirrhosis. Patients lose the ability to extend their fingers, which is more often a cosmetic embarrassment than a functional impairment. **Triamcinolone injection may help.** Surgical release is performed when function is impaired.

SPORTS MEDICINE

Rotator Cuff Injury

Damage to the rotator cuff of muscles, tendons, and the bursae around the shoulder leads to the inability to flex or abduct the shoulder. It presents with pain in the shoulder that is worse at night when lying on the affected shoulder. There can be **severe tenderness at the insertion of the supraspinatus.**

MRI is the most accurate test.

Treat with **NSAIDs, rest, and physical therapy.** If these are ineffective, steroid injection relieves pain. **Surgery is used with complete tears** and those not responding to NSAIDs, steroids, and physical therapy.

Patellofemoral Syndrome

This is a cause of anterior **knee pain** secondary to **trauma**, imbalance of quadriceps strength, or **meniscal tear**. The pain is in front of the knee or underneath the patella. The pain is particularly bad when walking up or down stairs. **Symptoms are worse just after starting to walk after having been seated for a prolonged period**. It improves after walking. Examination reveals crepitus, joint locking, and instability. **X-rays are normal**.

GELLING

Most cases respond to **physical therapy** and strength training with cycling. Knee braces don't help. There is **nothing to fix surgically**.

Plantar Fasciitis

Plantar fasciitis presents with **very severe pain in the bottom of the foot near the calcaneus** where the fascia inserts. It is of unclear etiology. The pain is **worst in the morning** and **improves with walking a few steps**. There is **point tenderness** at the bottom of the foot where the fascia inserts at the calcaneus. You can distinguish this from tarsal tunnel syndrome because the pain of that disorder worsens with use, and **plantar fasciitis clearly improves with use**. Treatment consists of stretching exercises, arch supports, and NSAIDs. **Steroid injection** is performed if these don't solve the problem. Surgical release of the plantar fascia is rarely necessary.

> **X-ray** of the foot is **not useful** in plantar fasciitis. There is no correlation with the presence of heel spurs.

RHEUMATOID ARTHRITIS

DEFINITION/ETIOLOGY

RA is an autoimmune disorder predominantly of the joints but with many systemic manifestations of chronic inflammation. The cause is unknown although there is an association with specific HLA types. As with most autoimmune diseases, RA is more common in women. Chronic synovitis leads to overgrowth, or pannus formation, which damages all the structures surrounding the joint (bone, ligaments, tendons, and cartilage).

> **Morning stiffness** of multiple small, inflamed joints is the key to the diagnosis.

PRESENTATION

- Bilateral, **symmetrical joint involvement:** PIP joints of the fingers, MCP joints of the hands, and involvement of the wrists, knees, and ankles
- **Morning stiffness** lasting at least 30 minutes, but often much longer
- Rheumatoid **nodules** (20%), most often over bony prominences
- **Ocular** symptoms: episcleritis
- **Lung involvement:** pleural effusion and nodules of lung parenchyma
- Vasculitis: skin, bowel, and peripheral nerves
- **Cervical joint** involvement, particularly at **C1 and C2**, which can lead to subluxation

- Baker cyst may rupture and mimic a DVT
- Pericarditis and pleural disease
- Carpal tunnel syndrome

> **DIP is spared** in RA. DIP involvement happens in DJD.

Figure 6.2: Boutonnière and swan neck are classic deformities of the hands in rheumatoid arthritis. *Source: Nirav Thakur, MD.*

DIAGNOSTIC TESTS

- Rheumatoid factor **(RF) in 70% to 80%**. RF is rather nonspecific and can be associated with many autoimmune and chronic infectious diseases.
- **Anti-cyclic citrulinated peptide (anti-CCP)** is more than 80% sensitive and more than **95% specific**.
- Radiographs:
  - Erosion of joints
  - Osteopenia
- Elevated ESR and C-reactive protein
- **Anemia:** Normocytic
- Arthrocentesis is useful on initial presentation to exclude crystal disease and infection if the diagnosis is not clear. Will find modest elevation in lymphocytes.
- Abnormal x-rays are no longer needed to establish a diagnosis of RA. Instead, diagnostic criteria are assessed on a point system. A total of 6 or more points = RA.
  - Joint involvement (up to 5 points)
  - ESR or CRP (1 point)
  - Duration for longer than 6 weeks (1 point)
  - RF or anti-CCP (1 point)

> Sicca syndrome: dry eyes, mouth, and other mucous membranes.

Felty syndrome:

I FELT THE LIVER OF THAT R.A. PATIENT

- RA
- Splenomegaly
- Neutropenia

Caplan syndrome:

- RA
- Pneumoconiosis
- Lung nodules

> The most common cause of death in RA is coronary artery disease.

▶ **TIP**

The most important issue in RA is stopping the progression of the disease. **Any patient with erosive disease or x-ray abnormalities needs at least methotrexate to slow disease progression.**

TREATMENT

Disease Modifying Antirheumatic Drugs

Neither **NSAIDs nor steroids stop RA from progressing**. Any patient with erosive RA needs a disease modifying antirheumatic drug (DMARD) as part of initial therapy.

A patient with long-standing RA is to have coronary bypass surgery. Which of the following is most important prior to surgery?

a. Cervical spine x-ray
b. Rheumatoid factor
c. Extra dose of methotrexate
d. ESR
e. Pneumococcal vaccination

Answer: The correct answer is (A). RA is associated with C1/C2 subluxation. Cervical spine imaging to detect possible instability of the vertebra is essential prior to the hyperextension of the neck that typically occurs with endotracheal intubation. Methotrexate does not work acutely and additional doses are not useful. Although pneumococcal vaccination is useful in any immunocompromised person, there is no particular indication for vaccination surrounding surgical procedures.

"Erosive" disease means:

- Joint space narrowing
- Physical deformity of joints
- X-ray abnormalities

Methotrexate

Methotrexate is the best initial DMARD. Adverse effects are:

- Liver toxicity
- Bone marrow suppression
- Pulmonary toxicity

Tumor Necrosis Factor Inhibitors (infliximab, adalimumab, etanercept)

Tumor necrosis factor (TNF) inhibitors are the first line as DMARDS for those not responding to methotrexate or intolerant of methotrexate. They are often used initially in combination with methotrexate to prevent disease progression.

Toxicity of anti-TNF drugs:

- **Reactivation of TB: screen with a PPD prior to their use**
- Infection

Rituximab

This agent, originally developed for non-Hodgkin lymphoma, is effective in RA as a DMARD by **removing CD20 positive lymphocytes** from circulation. This leads to excellent long-term control of RA. Rituximab is used in combination with methotrexate in those not responding to anti-TNF medications.

Hydroxychloroquine

This agent can be used as monotherapy as a **DMARD in cases of mild disease** in which we wish to avoid the toxicity of methotrexate. More often hydroxychloroquine is used in combination with methotrexate as a DMARD. Hydroxychloroquine is toxic to the retina.

> Hydroxychloroquine leads to retinal toxicity. Do a dilated eye exam.

Sulfasalazine, Leflunomide, and Abatacept

These agents are alternative DMARDs to add to methotrexate if anti-TNF agents do not control disease. **Sulfasalazine** causes:

- Bone marrow toxicity
- Hemolysis with G6 PD deficiency
- Rash

Symptomatic Control of RA

NSAIDs are the best initial therapy for the pain of RA. They work immediately to improve inflammation, but do nothing to prevent the progression of disease.

Steroids also work in a matter of hours to control the pain of RA secondary to inflammation. Steroids are used:

- When NSAIDs do not control symptoms immediately
- As a bridge when waiting for DMARDs to take effect; DMARDs are much slower in onset of action than steroids

> Steroids do not prevent the progression of RA.

▶ **TIP**

It would be difficult to test you on which agent to use as a DMARD with methotrexate or after methotrexate fails, because the answer is not clear. **However, adverse effects are mandatory for you to know,** since the answers to that question would be very clear.

Adverse Effects of RA Medications	
Drug	**Adverse effect**
Anti-TNF	Reactivation of <u>tuberculosis</u>
Hydroxychloroquine	Ocular
Sulfasalazine	Rash, hemolysis, oligospermia
Rituximab	Infection
Gold salts	Nephrotic syndrome
Methotrexate	Liver, lung, marrow , MACROCYTIC ANEMIA

JUVENILE RHEUMATOID ARTHRITIS OR ADULT STILL DISEASE

DEFINITION/ETIOLOGY

Juvenile rheumatoid arthritis (JRA) is very difficult to define and there is no known etiology. This does not stop it, however, from appearing on virtually every USMLE exam as either the correct answer or one of the distracters.

PRESENTATION/"WHAT IS THE MOST LIKELY DIAGNOSIS?"

This is unquestionably the single most important, and nearly the only, fact you need to know about JRA. The <u>most important</u> feature of **JRA** is the presence of high, spiking **fever** (often above <u>104°F</u>) in a **young person** that has no clearly identified etiology but is associated with a **rash**.

HIGH FEVER SALMON RASH

Features of JRA rash: *SALMON TRUNK RASH*

- Often only with fever spikes
- "Salmon" colored
- On chest and abdomen

Other features of JRA:

- Splenomegaly
- Pericardial effusion
- Mild **joint** symptoms

Laboratory Abnormalities

There is **no clear diagnostic test**; however, anemia and leukocytosis are often present. ANA is normal.

Treatment

Half of cases improve with aspirin or NSAIDs. If there is no response, then use steroids.

Systemic Lupus Erythematosus

Definition/Etiology

Systemic lupus erythematosus (SLE) is an autoimmune disorder with a number of autoantibodies (ANA, double-stranded DNA). It causes inflammation diffusely through the body (skin, brain, kidneys, joints) and the blood. SLE has numerous abnormal blood tests associated with it (anemia, anti-Sm, antiphospholipid antibodies), but this is not the same thing as knowing what causes SLE. Its cause is a mystery.

Drug Induced
- Hydralazine
- Procainamide
- Isoniazid

Presentation

The diagnosis of SLE is based on the presence of at least 4 of 11 known manifestations of the disease.

Skin: Four of the manifestations of SLE are of the skin:

1. Malar rash
2. Discoid rash
3. Photosensitivity
4. Oral ulcers

> Alopecia is common in SLE but is not one of the "official" diagnostic criteria.

Joint: Arthritis is present in 90% of those with SLE and is often the first symptom that brings patients to seek medical attention. SLE gives joint pain without deformation or erosion. That is why the **x-ray is normal**.

Serositis: Inflammation of the pleura and pericardium gives **chest pain** potentially with both pericardial and pleural effusion.

Renal: Any degree of abnormality can occur, from mild proteinuria to end-stage renal disease requiring dialysis. The **most common glomerulonephritis is membranous**. Red cell casts and hematuria occur.

Neurologic: Symptoms include psychosis, seizures, or stroke from vasculitis.

> Pneumonia, alveolar hemorrhage, and restrictive lung disease happen in SLE but are not criteria for the diagnosis of the disease.

Ocular findings are not part of formal diagnostic criteria:

- Photophobia
- Retinal lesions (cotton wool spots)
- Blindness

Hematologic: Hemolytic anemia is part of the diagnostic criteria, but the anemia of chronic disease is more commonly found. Lymphopenia, leukopenia, and thrombocytopenia are also seen.

Immunologic (laboratory) abnormalities: Criteria include positive ANA, or **any** one of the following:

- **Anti-double-stranded DNA**
- **Anti-Sm**™
- False positive test for syphilis
- Positive LE cell preparation

Additional findings:

- Mesenteric vasculitis
- Raynaud phenomenon
- Antiphospholipid syndromes

− ANA = No LUPUS (handwritten)

Do not treat an asymptomatic ANA.

+ DS DNA/sm = LUPUS (handwritten)

DIAGNOSTIC TESTS

ANA: found in 95% to 99% of cases. A negative ANA is extremely sensitive for lupus, but a positive ANA has little specificity. Many rheumatologic diseases are associated with a positive ANA.

Anti-double-stranded (DS) DNA (60%) and anti-Sm (30%): These are found only in SLE. They are extremely specific for SLE.

Decreased complement levels: They can correlate with disease activity. They can **drop further with acute disease exacerbations**.

Anti-SSA and anti-SSB: Found in 10% to 20% of cases. They add little to the diagnosis. These tests are most often found in Sjögren syndrome (65% of cases).

A 34-year-old woman with a history of SLE is admitted with pneumonia and confusion. As you are wrestling with the decision over a bolus of high-dose steroids in a person with an infection, you need to determine if this is a flare of lupus, or simply an infection with sepsis causing confusion.

Which of the following will help you the most?

a. Rise in anti-Sm

b. Rise in ANA

c. Decrease in complement

d. Decrease in complement and rise in anti-DS DNA

e. MRI of the brain

f. Response to steroids

*Answer: The correct answer is **(D)**. Although anti-Sm is specific for SLE, the level does not change in an acute flare. ANA levels do not tell severity of disease. MRI of the brain is most often normal in lupus cerebritis unless there has been a stroke. **In an acute lupus flare, complement levels drop and anti-DS DNA levels rise.***

[handwritten: FLARE UP — ↓ COMPLEMENT — ↑ ANTI-DS DNA]

TREATMENT

Acute lupus **flare** is treated with high-dose **boluses of steroids**. Hydroxychloroquine can control mildly chronic disease limited to skin and joint manifestations.

Lupus nephritis may need steroids either alone or in combination with cyclophosphamide or mycophenolate. The only way to determine the severity of lupus nephritis is with a kidney biopsy. The urinalysis is insufficient to tell the severity of lupus nephritis. Biopsy is the only way to tell if there is simple glomerulo**sclerosis**, or scarring of the kidney, which will not respond to therapy.

[handwritten: STEROIDS + HYDROXYCHLOROQUINE]

> **Young** patients most commonly **die of infection**. In **older patients**, accelerated atherosclerosis makes myocardial infarction the most common cause of death.

ANTIPHOSPHOLIPID SYNDROME

DEFINITION

Antiphospholipid (APL) syndrome is best treated as a separate topic because the majority of cases are not associated with SLE. APL syndrome is an idiopathic disorder with IgG or IgM antibodies made against negatively charged phospholipids.

The 2 main types are:

- Lupus anticoagulant
- Anticardiolipin antibodies

PRESENTATION/DIAGNOSTIC TESTS

APL syndrome presents with thromboses of both arteries and veins as well as recurrent spontaneous abortions. Unlike the other causes of thrombophilia, APL syndrome is often associated with an **elevation of the aPTT** with a normal prothrombin time (PT) and normal INR. **False positive VDRL or RPR** with a normal FTA occurs because the antibody reacts with the reagent in the lab which is a cardiolipin. Anticardiolipin antibodies more often give spontaneous abortion, and the lupus anticoagulant is more often associated with an elevated aPTT.

> APL = clotting + **elevated aPTT** and normal PT

185

The **best initial test is the mixing study**, in which the patient's plasma is mixed with an equal amount of normal plasma. If the elevation in aPTT is from a clotting factor deficiency, the aPTT will come down to normal. If the APL syndrome antibody is present in plasma, the aPTT will remain elevated.

The **most specific test** for the lupus anticoagulant is the **Russell viper venom test** (RVVT). The RVVT is prolonged with APL antibodies and does not correct on mixing with normal plasma.

TREATMENT

An asymptomatic APL antibody does not need to be treated.

Thromboses (DVT or PE) are treated with heparin and warfarin as you would any other form of thrombosis with an INR of 2 to 3. The duration of treatment with warfarin is controversial. It is not clear if lifelong warfarin, instead of the usual 6 months of treatment, is indicated after a single thrombotic episode. Recurrent thrombotic episodes are treated lifelong.

▶ **TIP**

USMLE Step 2 CK questions have to be unequivocally clear. If an area is controversial, USMLE will avoid it, and ask only what is clear. The exam will not trick you.

Spontaneous Abortion

There is no treatment for a spontaneous abortion that is in the process of occurring. It is too late. The most commonly asked questions are:

- What should be investigated for anticardiolipin antibody as a cause of spontaneous abortion?
  - Answer: Two or more first-trimester events or a single second-trimester event
- What is the treatment to prevent a recurrence?
  - Answer: heparin and aspirin

▶ **TIP**

Warfarin or steroids are wrong answers for preventing spontaneous abortion. Steroids are not effective.

> Warfarin is contraindicated in pregnancy secondary to teratogenicity.

SCLERODERMA (SYSTEMIC SCLEROSIS)

The cause of scleroderma is unknown. Scleroderma is diffuse in 20% of cases and limited in 80%. Limited scleroderma is also known as CREST syndrome (**c**alcinosis, **R**aynaud, **e**sophageal dysmotility, **s**clerodactyly, **t**elangiectasia).

"WHAT IS THE MOST LIKELY DIAGNOSIS?"

Look for a young (20s to 40s) woman (3 times more likely than men) with fibrosis of the skin and internal organs such as the lung, kidney, and GI tract.

PRESENTATION

Raynaud syndrome: increased vascular reactivity of the fingers beginning with pain and pallor (white) or cyanosis (blue) followed by reactive hyperemia (red). Raynaud is precipitated by cold and emotional stress. Some cases lead to ulceration and gangrene.

Skin manifestations: fibrosis of the hands, face, neck, and extremities; telangiectasia and abnormalities of pigmentation occur

Gastrointestinal: esophageal dysmotility with GERD, large-mouthed diverticuli of small and large bowel

Renal: sudden **hypertensive crisis**

Lung: fibrosis leading to **restrictive lung disease** and **pulmonary hypertension**

Cardiac: myocardial fibrosis, pericarditis, and heart block; lung disease gives right ventricular hypertrophy

DIAGNOSTIC TESTS

+ CENTROMERE = CREST

ANA: positive in 85% to 90%, but nonspecific

ESR: usually normal

SCL-70: the **most specific test is the SCL-70** (anti-topoisomerase), but present in only 30% of those with diffuse disease and 20% of those with limited disease

Anticentromere: present in half of those with CREST syndrome

> Anticentromere antibodies are extremely specific for CREST syndrome.

TREATMENT

No treatment stops the underlying disease process of scleroderma. **Penicillamine is not effective.**

Renal crisis: ACE inhibitors (use even if the creatinine is elevated)

Esophageal dysmotility: PPIs for GERD

Raynaud: calcium channel blockers

Pulmonary fibrosis: Cyclophosphamide improves dyspnea and PFTs. Pulmonary hypertension is treated like primary pulmonary hypertension with bosentan (endothelin antagonist).

Polymyositis and Dermatomyositis

Presentation

Inflammatory myopathies present with **proximal muscle weakness** leading to difficulty getting up from a seated position or walking up stairs. They do not affect facial or ocular muscles as occurs in myasthenia gravis. The proximal muscles are weak, but only a quarter have pain and tenderness. Dysphagia occurs from involvement of the striated muscles of the pharynx, making it difficult to initiate swallowing. Cardiac muscle involvement is rare, even though the CK-MB level may be elevated.

Dermatomyositis presents with:

- Malar involvement
- **Shawl sign:** erythema of the face, neck, shoulders, upper chest, and back
- **Heliotrope rash:** edema and purplish discoloration of the eyelids
- **Gottron papules:** scaly patches over the back of the hands, particularly the PIP and MCP joints

> **Dermatomyositis is associated with cancer in 25% of cases. Common sites are:**
> - Ovary
> - Lung
> - Gastrointestinal
> - Lymphoma

Diagnostic Tests

The best initial test is **CPK** and **aldolase**. The most accurate test is a **muscle biopsy**.

CPK & Aldolase → Biopsy

ANA is frequently positive, but nonspecific. **Anti-Jo antibodies are associated with lung fibrosis**. MRI detects patchy muscle involvement. Electromyography is often abnormal.

Other labs that are occasionally abnormal are the ESR, C-reactive protein, and rheumatoid factor. Like the occasional presence of anemia, none of these tests will help establish the diagnosis.

Treatment

Steroids are usually sufficient.

When patient is unresponsive or intolerant of steroids, use:

- Methotrexate
- Azathioprine

- Intravenous immunoglobulin
- Mycophenolate

Hydroxychloroquine helps the skin lesions.

SJÖGREN SYNDROME

DEFINITION/ETIOLOGY

Sjögren syndrome is an idiopathic autoimmune disorder secondary to **antibodies predominantly against lacrimal and salivary glands**; 90% of those affected are women. Sjögren syndrome is associated with:

- Rheumatoid arthritis
- SLE
- Primary biliary cirrhosis
- Polymyositis
- Hashimoto thyroiditis

PRESENTATION

Sjögren presents with **dryness of the mouth and eyes**. Ocular abnormalities give the feeling of "sand in the eyes" as well as burning and itching. This is called **keratoconjunctivitis sicca**.

Dryness of the mouth gives a patient presenting with **the need to constantly drink water** and difficulty swallowing, especially dry foods. Loss of saliva leads to **rampant dental caries** and loss of teeth. The main function of saliva is to neutralize acid on teeth and physically wash food off teeth.

> Loss of vaginal secretions leads to **dyspareunia**.

Less common manifestations are:

- Vasculitis
- Lung disease
- Pancreatitis
- Renal tubular acidosis (20%)

▶ TIP

When asked what is the most **"dangerous"** complication of Sjögren, answer **lymphoma.**

DIAGNOSTIC TESTS

The best initial test is called a **Schirmer test** in which a piece of **filter paper is placed against the eye** and then observed for the amount of tears produced by the amount of wetness on the filter paper.

The **most accurate test is a lip or parotid gland biopsy**. These reveal lymphoid infiltration in the salivary glands.

Best initial test on blood: SS-A and SS-B. These are also called "Ro" and "La" and are each present in about 65% of patients. SLE is associated with SS-A and SS-B in 10% to 20% of cases.

Other abnormalities that are present, but are nonspecific: ANA, RF, anemia, leukopenia, and eosinophilia.

TREATMENT

The best **initial therapy is to water the mouth**. Use frequent sips of water, sugar-free gum, and **fluoride** treatments. Use **artificial tears** to avoid corneal ulcers.

Pilocarpine and **cevimeline increase acetylcholine**, the main stimulant to the production of saliva. Cevimeline is a new drug that has the single indication of increasing rates of saliva production.

There is no cure, but lifespan is not shortened. **Evaluate for lymphoma,** which occurs in up to 10% of patients.

VASCULITIS

The cause of vasculitis is unknown. Symptoms develop over weeks to months.

All vasculitides (eg, polyarteritis nodosa, Wegener granulomatosis, Churg-Strauss, giant cell) give:

- Fever
- Malaise/fatigue
- Weight loss
- Arthralgia/myalgia

Polyarteritis Nodosa

DEFINITION

Hep B = PAN

Polyarteritis nodosa (PAN) is a disease of small- and medium-sized arteries leading to a diffuse vasculitis that inexplicably **spares the lungs**. Chronic hepatitis B is associated with PAN.

PRESENTATION

PAN is very difficult to identify because there is no single pathognomonic feature.

Common Features of PAN

Renal: You cannot distinguish from other forms of glomerulonephritis without a biopsy; UA is not enough to confirm it is PAN.

Neurological: Any large peripheral nerve can be involved, but peroneal neuropathy leading to **foot drop** is the most common neurological abnormality. Look for a **stroke in a young person**.

Gastrointestinal: Abdominal pain is worsened by eating from vasculitis of the mesenteric vessels. Bleeding also occurs. Nausea and vomiting are common.

Skin: Lower extremity ulcers are most common; livedo reticularis, purpura, nodules, and rarely gangrene also occur.

Mononeuritis Multiplex

This is a confusing term. How can it be "mono" and "multi" at the same time?

Mononeuritis **multi**plex is **multiple peripheral neuropathies** of **nerves large enough to have a name**. For example, the radial nerve **and** the peroneal nerve or the ulnar nerve **and** the lateral femoral cutaneous.

DIAGNOSTIC TESTS

The most accurate test is a **biopsy of a symptomatic site**.

Angiography of the renal, mesenteric, or hepatic artery shows abnormal dilation or "beading."

Other abnormalities are **anemia**, **leukocytosis**, ESR, and C-reactive protein. **P-ANCA is present in less than 20%**. Urinalysis will show protein and red cells, but has nothing specific to indicate that it is PAN.

TREATMENT

Prednisone and cyclophosphamide. Treat hepatitis B when found.

> Lung is spared in PAN.

> Test all PAN patients for hepatitis B.

Polymyalgia Rheumatica

Polymyalgia rheumatica (PMR) occurs in those **over age 50** with:

- Pain and stiffness in shoulder and pelvic girdle muscles
- Difficulty combing hair and rising from a chair
- **Elevated ESR**
- Normochromic, normocytic anemia

Although there is muscle pain, there are no lab findings of muscle destruction. The **CPK and aldolase are normal**.

PMR has a rapid and enormous response to **steroids even at low doses**.

DRAMATICA - STEROIDS - IMMEDIATE CORE

Giant Cell (Temporal) Arteritis

This disease seems to be on a spectrum with PMR. The difference is the presence of:

- Visual symptoms
- Jaw claudication (pain in jaw when chewing)
- Scalp tenderness

- Headache
- Symptoms in other arteries such as decreased arm pulses, bruits near the clavicles, or aortic regurgitation

ESR and C-reactive protein are elevated. The most accurate test is a biopsy of the affected artery such as the temporal artery. Treat with prednisone. Starting high-dose prednisone quickly is more important than waiting for the biopsy.

> Blindness is not reversible.

Wegener Granulomatosis

"WHAT IS THE MOST LIKELY DIAGNOSIS?"

Look for a combination of **upper and lower respiratory tract findings in association with renal insufficiency**.

Upper Respiratory Tract Involvement
Wegener granulomatosis presents with:

- **Sinusitis**
- **Otitis media**
- Mastoiditis
- Oral and gingival involvement

Wegener is also associated with skin, joint, and eye lesions.

DIAGNOSTIC TESTS

> Wegener: C-ANCA
> Churg-Strauss and microscopic polyangiitis: P-ANCA

The best initial test is antineutrophil cytoplasmic antibody (ANCA). The most accurate test is a biopsy.

Cytoplasmic antibodies are also called "C-ANCA."

C-ANCA = anti-proteinase-3 antibodies

P-ANCA = anti-myeloperoxidase antibodies

▶ **TIP**

When asked about the "best test" for Wegener, **lung biopsy is better than renal biopsy** with **sinus biopsy being the least accurate**. When all 3 are in the choices, choose lung biopsy.

TREATMENT

Treat with prednisone and cyclophosphamide.

▶ **TIP**

The clue to answering the "most likely diagnosis" question is unresolving pneumonia not better with antibiotics. You will not first think of Wegener when presented with the case.

TAKAYASU'S
TIA |STROKE| PULSELETS NESS
MRA STEROIDS

Churg-Strauss Syndrome

A pulmonary-renal syndrome, Churg-Strauss also has:

- **Asthma**

- **Eosinophilia**

As with Wegener granulomatosis, and many vasculitides, there can be fever, weight loss, joint pain, and skin findings, but these will not help you answer "What is the most likely diagnosis?" **Biopsy is the most accurate test**. Treat with prednisone and cyclophosphamide.

Henoch-Schönlein Purpura

A vasculitis more frequently seen in children, Henoch-Schönlein purpura (HSP) is characterized by involvement of:

- **Gastrointestinal tract:** pain, bleeding

- **Skin:** purpura

- **Joint:** arthralgia

- **Renal:** hematuria

HSP is **most often a clinical diagnosis**; however, **biopsy is the most accurate test**.

▶ **TIP**

When the case describes **leukocytoclastic vasculitis** on biopsy, the answer is Henoch-Schönlein purpura.

Figure 6.3: Leukocytoclastic reactions are painless, palpable purpura of the buttocks and legs in Henoch-Schönlein purpura. *Source: Shreya Patel and Nishith Patel.*

Serum IgA levels are the **wrong answer**. They are not reliable when testing for Henoch-Schönlein purpura.

TREATMENT

Most cases resolve spontaneously. **Steroids are the answer when there are severe extrarenal manifestations** associated with progressive renal insufficiency: Steroids do not reverse renal insufficiency.

Cryoglobulinemia

Cryoglobulinemia is most commonly associated with chronic hepatitis C infection. It is also found with endocarditis and other connective tissue disorders such as Sjögren syndrome. **Don't confuse cryoglobulins with cold agglutinins**. Both are IgM antibodies. Neither responds to steroids.

Differences between Cryoglobulins and Cold Agglutinins		
	Cryoglobulins	**Cold agglutinin**
Associated with	Hepatitis C	EBV, *Mycoplasma*, lymphoma
Manifestations	• Joint pain • Glomerulonephritis • Purpuric skin lesions • Neuropathy	• Hemolysis
Treatment	Interferon and ribavirin	• Stay warm • Rituximab, cyclophosphamide, cyclosporine

Lab tests in cryoglobulinemia show a **positive rheumatoid factor** and cold precipitable immune complexes. Steroids have **not** been shown to be effective. Treat the underlying cause, especially hepatitis C, with interferon and ribavirin.

> ▶ **TIP**
>
> Despite the rarity of the condition, the **USMLE loves cryoglobulinemia** questions.

SLE → decreased **C3** or
3 letters (SLE) = C3
Hep C → decreased **C4** or
4 letters (Hep C) = C4

Behçet Syndrome

> ▶ **TIP**
>
> The most common Behçet questions are:
>
> • What is the most likely diagnosis?
> • What is "pathergy"?

Look for an Asian or Middle Eastern person with painful **oral and genital ulcers** in association with erythema nodosum-like lesions of the skin. Also with:

• **Ocular lesions** leading to uveitis and blindness
• Arthritis
• CNS lesions mimicking multiple sclerosis

Pathergy: sterile skin pustules from minor trauma like a needle stick

DIAGNOSTIC TESTS/TREATMENT

There is no characteristic lab abnormality. Patients respond to corticosteroids. To wean patients off of steroids, use:

- Azathioprine
- Cyclophosphamide
- Colchicine
- Thalidomide

SERONEGATIVE SPONDYLOARTHROPATHIES

The 3 types of seronegative spondyloarthropathies are:

- Ankylosing spondylitis
- Psoriatic arthritis
- Reactive arthritis (Reiter syndrome)

These disorders present with joint pain, more often starting in men under the age of 40, with:

- **Involvement of the spine** and large joints
- **Negative rheumatoid factor** (hence the name **seronegative**)
- **Enthesopathy** (inflammation where tendons and ligaments attach to bones)
- **Uveitis**
- **HLA-B27**

Corticosteroids are not a good treatment for seronegative spondyloarthropathy.

▶ **TIP**

Despite the association with HLA-B27, this is never the "best initial" or "most accurate" test for seronegative spondyloarthropathies.

Ankylosing Spondylitis

"WHAT IS THE MOST LIKELY DIAGNOSIS?"

Look for a **young man** with low **backache** and **stiffness** of his back and pain that radiates to the buttocks with **flattening of the normal lumbar curvature** and **decreased chest expansion**. Eventually the spine will not expand in any direction. Enthesopathy occurs at the Achilles tendon.

> Look for back pain **worsened by rest** and relieved by activity.

Other Findings of Ankylosing Spondylitis
- Transient peripheral **arthritis** of knees, hips, and shoulders (50%)
- Cardiac: **atrioventricular block** in 3% to 5%; **aortic insufficiency**
- **Uveitis**

> "Bamboo spine" is a late finding with fusion of vertebral joints.

DIAGNOSTIC TEST

The best initial test is an **x-ray of the sacroiliac (SI) joint**. The most accurate test is an MRI. MRI detects abnormalities years before the x-ray becomes abnormal.

ESR is elevated in 85%.

Narrowing of sacroiliac joint

Figure 6.4: The best initial test for seronegative spondyloarthropathies is an x-ray of the sacroiliac joint. *Source: Conrad Fischer, MD.*

Figure 6.5: Bamboo spine is a late finding of ankylosing spondylitis. The vertebral bodies are fused by bridging syndesmophytes. *Source: Shreya Patel and Nishith Patel.*

▶ **TIP**

HLA B27 is not a confirmatory diagnostic test since 8% of the general population is positive.

TREATMENT

An **exercise program** and **NSAIDs** are the best initial treatment. If NSAIDs are insufficient, use **anti-TNF drugs** such as etanercept, adalimumab, or infliximab.

Psoriatic Arthritis

In patients with psoriatic arthritis, 80% will have preceding psoriasis. It is more common with severe skin disease. Besides SI joint involvement, characteristic findings are:

- **Sausage digits** from enthesopathy
- **Nail pitting**

Figure 6.6: Arthritis with nail pitting accompanies about 10% of those with psoriasis. *Source: Conrad Fischer, MD.*

DIAGNOSTIC TESTS

Although the ESR is elevated in almost all patients, it is nonspecific. The best initial test is an **x-ray of the joint showing a "pencil in a cup" deformity**. There will also be bony erosions and irregular bone destruction. Uric acid level is elevated from increased skin turnover.

TREATMENT

NSAIDs are the best initial therapy. **Methotrexate** is used when the question describes severe disease or no response to NSAIDs.

Anti-TNF agents are the answer when methotrexate does not control disease. Steroids are a wrong choice.

Reactive Arthritis (Reiter Syndrome)

Reactive arthritis occurs secondary to:

- **Inflammatory bowel** disease (equal sex incidence)
- Sexually transmitted infection (far greater in men)
- Gastrointestinal infection (*Yersinia, Salmonella, Campylobacter*)

Keratoderma blennorhagicum is a skin lesion unique to reactive arthritis that looks like pustular psoriasis.

"WHAT IS THE MOST LIKELY DIAGNOSIS?"

Look for the triad of:

- **Joint** pain
- **Ocular** findings (uveitis, conjunctivitis)
- **Genital** abnormalities (urethritis, balanitis)

DIAGNOSTIC TESTS/TREATMENT

There is **no specific test for reactive arthritis**. Hot swollen joints should be tapped to **rule out septic joint**. The diagnosis is based on the triad previously described. **Treat with NSAIDs** and correct the underlying cause. **Sulfasalazine is used when NSAIDs do not control it**.

Antibiotics do not reverse reactive arthritis once joint pain has started.

OSTEOPOROSIS

Look for an older person, more often a woman, with vertebral fractures leading to loss of height or wrist fracture. Many are asymptomatic, and fractures are found on routine screening with bone densitometry, which is recommended for all women above the age of 65.

Osteoporosis gives spontaneous fractures of weight-bearing bones.

DIAGNOSTIC TESTS

The most accurate test is bone densitometry (DEXA) scanning.

The T-score compares bone density with the normal density of a young woman.

Osteopenia: Bone density (T-score) is between 1 and 2.5 standard deviations below normal.

Osteoporosis: T-score more than 2.5 standard deviations below normal.

All blood tests are normal in osteoporosis. Calcium, phosphate, and parathyroid hormone levels are normal.

Bisphosphonates are very rarely associated with **osteonecrosis of the jaw.**

TREATMENT

1. **Vitamin D and calcium** are the best initial therapy.
2. **Bisphosphonates** (alendronate, risendronate, ibandronate) are used when the T-score is more than 2.5 standard deviations below normal.
3. **Estrogen replacement** is especially useful in postmenopausal women.
4. **Raloxifene** is used as a substitute for estrogen in postmenopausal women; it also reduces the risk of breast cancer and decreases LDL levels.
5. **Teriparatide** is an analogue of parathyroid hormone that stimulates new bone matrix formation.
6. Used as a nasal spray, **calcitonin decreases the risk of vertebral fractures.**

Bisphosphonates that have prolonged contact with the esophagus can cause esophagitis (pill esophagitis).

▶ **TIP**

When multiple treatment options are presented, choose **vitamin D, calcium, and bisphosphonates.**

Teriparatide has caused osteosarcoma in rats. It has also caused hypercalcemia.

SEPTIC ARTHRITIS

DEFINITION

Septic arthritis is an infection of any kind finding its way into the joint space.

ETIOLOGY

Because synovial lining has no basement membrane, it is relatively "loose" and both bacteria and antibiotics easily find their way across it. **Septic arthritis is relatively rare in an undamaged joint**. The risk of infection is directly proportional to the degree of joint damage. Osteoarthritis (DJD) provides a slight risk, with rheumatoid arthritis having a greater risk because of greater destruction. The greatest risk is with a prosthetic joint.

Bacteremia can spread into the joint space, which is why endocarditis and injection drug use causes septic arthritis.

Etiology of Septic Arthritis	
Etiology	**Frequency**
Staphylococcus	40%
Streptococcus	30%
Gram-negative rods	20%

PRESENTATION

The joint is **warm**, **red**, and **immobile** and often has a palpable effusion. Chills and fever happen because of bacteremia.

DIAGNOSTIC TESTS

The **best initial and most accurate test is aspiration of the joint** with a needle (arthrocentesis). X-ray, CT, and MRI are not useful and are the wrong answers.

Joint fluid shows:

- **Leukocytosis:** more than 50,000 to 100,000 cells, predominantly neutrophils
- **Gram stain:** positive (50%) Gram-negative bacilli; (75%) with *Staphylococcus*
- **Synovial fluid culture:** 70% to 90% sensitive
- **Blood cultures:** 50% sensitive

TREATMENT

Ceftriaxone and vancomycin are the best initial empiric therapy.

Other Options for Treatment of Septic Arthritis		
Gram-negative bacilli	**Gram-positive cocci (sensitive)**	**Gram-positive cocci (resistant)**
• Quinolones • Aztreonam • Cefotaxime • Piperacillin • Aminoglycosides	• Oxacillin, nafcillin • Cefazolin • Piperacillin with tazobactam	• Linezolid • Daptomycin • Tigecycline

▶ **TIP**

Adjust antibiotics according to culture results.

Prosthetic Joint Infection

Prosthetic joints are placed in over 100,000 people per year in the United States. An infected prosthetic joint gives a **warm, red, immobile, and tender joint**, but without an x-ray or CT scan, it is not possible to tell whether the infection is limited to the joint space or has spread into the bone around the implantation of the joint. MRI is difficult to perform with prosthetic joints because they are made of metal.

If there is lucency around the implantation of the joint on radiologic imaging or **if joint is physically loose, infection is likely present** at the implantation site.

Treatment of Infected Prosthetic Joint

It is much harder to clear or sterilize septic arthritis associated with a prosthetic joint without removing the joint. Hence, the first stage is to **remove the joint, treat with antibiotics for 6 to 8 weeks, and then replace the joint**.

GONOCOCCAL ARTHRITIS (GONORRHEA)

Look for a history of STDs or a sexually active young person. The difference in presentation from septic arthritis is:

- **Polyarticular** involvement
- **Tenosynovitis** (inflammation of the tendon sheaths, making finger movement painful)
- Petechial **rash**

DIAGNOSTIC TESTS

Detecting gonorrhea is much more difficult than detecting the *Staphylococcus*, *Streptococcus*, and Gram-negative bacilli of septic arthritis.

If the *Staphylococcus* is sensitive, vancomycin is associated with a worse outcome than a beta-lactam antibiotic such as oxacillin or cefazolin. Switch drugs if the organism is sensitive.

The most common organism for recently placed artificial joints is *Staphylococcus epidermidis*.

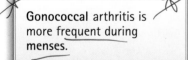

Gonococcal arthritis is more frequent during menses.

Synovial Fluid Analysis for Infectious Arthritis		
Test sensitivity	**Septic arthritis**	**Gonococcal arthritis**
Leukocytosis	>50,000–100,000 cells/μl	30,000–50,000 cells/μl
Gram stain	50–75% sensitive	25% sensitive
Culture	90% sensitive	<50% sensitive
Blood cultures	50% sensitive	<40% sensitive

In order to reach maximum sensitivity, multiple diffuse sites must be cultured for gonorrhea, such as:

- Pharynx
- Rectum
- Urethra
- Cervix

What tells you to culture everywhere?

- Rash
- Tenosynovitis
- Polyarticular involvement

TREATMENT

Ceftrioxone, cefotaxime, or ceftizoxime is the best empiric therapy for disseminated gonorrhea. Fluoroquinolones are **not** the best initial therapy because more than 5% are resistant. Use quinolones only if the organism is confirmed to be sensitive.

▶ **TIP**

If recurrent gonorrhea infection is described, test for terminal complement deficiency—a favorite subject of USMLE Step 2 CK.

OSTEOMYELITIS

DEFINITION/ETIOLOGY

Osteomyelitis is an infection of the bone. Although *Staphylococcus aureus* is the most common cause, any organism can infect the bone. **Children get osteomyelitis through hematogenous spread, but adults get it from a contiguous (nearby) infection**, most often as a result of vascular insufficiency and diabetes.

Salmonella is the most commonly identified organism in patients with sickle cell disease.

PRESENTATION

Look for a **diabetic patient with an ulcer** from peripheral neuropathy or vascular disease with warmth, redness, and swelling in the area. There may also be a draining "purulent sinus tract" in the lesion. Most patients are afebrile.

DIAGNOSTIC TESTS

The best initial test is an x-ray. The most accurate test is a biopsy. If the x-ray is normal, the "most appropriate next step in management" is an MRI. CT scan is not very useful.

> Bone scan is the answer only if you want to get an MRI and it is contraindicated (pacemaker).

▶ TIP

When is ESR the answer?

- To follow the response to therapy

▶ TIP

When is "culturing the drainage" the answer?

- Never. You **cannot** reliably **distinguish** superficial **colonization** from whatever organism is inside the bone causing the bone infection.

TREATMENT

Osteomyelitis takes weeks to progress. Obtain a biopsy, and then treat the organism that is found. Without a biopsy, it is impossible to know what organism is present and what it is sensitive to. **Sensitive staphylococci are best treated with oxacillin, cefazolin, nafcillin, or ceftriaxone.** Resistant staphylococci are treated with vancomycin or linezolid. Gram-negative bacilli such as *E. coli* are treated with fluoroquinolones such as ciprofloxacin. **It is essential to confirm the sensitivity of the organism prior to treating with ciprofloxacin.**

> Ciprofloxacin is the only oral therapy for osteomyelitis, but should be used only if the organism is confirmed as a sensitive Gram-negative bacillus.

Toxicity of Quinolones

Fluoroquinolones can cause Achilles tendon rupture from interfering with the growth of chondrocytes. They are also **contraindicated in pregnancy and in children** because they interfere with bone growth.

Hematology

7

Anemia

"What Is the Most Likely Diagnosis?"

All forms of anemia can present with identical symptoms if they have the same hematocrit. Symptoms of anemia are generally based not on the etiology, but on the severity of disease. You cannot answer the "What is the most likely diagnosis?" question simply from symptoms.

Diagnostic Tests

Complete blood count (CBC) is always the best initial test in the evaluation of anemia.

Hematocrit and Symptoms	
Hematocrit	**Expected symptoms**
>30%–35%	None
25%–30%	Dyspnea (worse on exertion), fatigue
20%–25%	Lightheadedness, angina
Under 20%–25%	Syncope, chest pain

Ultimately, cardiac ischemia from anemia proves fatal. Myocytes in the heart cannot distinguish between:

- Anemia
- Hypoxia
- Coronary artery disease
- Carbon monoxide poisoning

All of these conditions result in decreased oxygen delivery to tissues.

Mean Corpuscular Volume

Although CBC establishes the presence of anemia, mean corpuscular volume (MCV) is the first clue to the etiology of anemia.

Microcytosis

Causes of low MCV:

- Iron deficiency   ↓ FERRITIN
- Thalassemia   NORMAL IRON STUDIES
- Sideroblastic anemia   ↑ IRON →LEAD, EtOH, B6, RA, MM
- Anemia of chronic disease   ~~NORMAL IRON STUDIES~~ ↓ TIBC ↑ FERRITIN

Microcytic anemias generally have a **low reticulocyte count.** Most causes of microcytosis are production problems. Production problems are nearly synonymous with low reticulocyte counts. Only alpha thalassemia with 3 genes deleted has an elevated reticulocyte count.

▶ **TIP**

Routine blood smear will **not** be effective in telling the difference between the types of microcytosis. All of them will be hypochromic and all of them potentially give target cells.

Macrocytic Anemia

Causes of high MCV:

- B_{12} and folate deficiency
- Sideroblastic anemia
- Alcoholism
- Antimetabolite medications such as azathioprine, 6-mercaptopurine, or hydroxyurea
- Liver disease or hypothyroidism
- Medications such as zidovudine or phenytoin
- Myelodysplastic syndrome (MDS)

Normocytic Anemia

Acute blood loss or hemolysis can give a drop in hematocrit so rapid that there is no time for the MCV to change. Blood loss ultimately leads to iron deficiency and microcytosis. Eventually, hemolysis will increase the reticulocyte count, and this will raise the MCV since reticulocytes are slightly larger than normal cells.

Sideroblastic anemia can be either **microcytic** or **macrocytic.**

Macrocytic anemias all give a low reticulocyte count.

Blood loss and hemolysis will raise the reticulocyte count.

TREATMENT

If anemia is severe, it is treated with packed red blood cells. Answering the question "At what hematocrit do I transfuse a patient?" depends on the following factors:

1. Is the patient **symptomatic**? Then transfuse.
2. Is the **hematocrit very low** in an **elderly** patient or one with **heart disease**? Then transfuse.

> "Very low" hematocrit means 25 to 30 in the elderly or those with heart disease.

Symptomatic from anemia means:

- Shortness of breath
- Lightheaded, confused, and sometimes syncope
- Hypotension and tachycardia
- Chest pain

▶ **TIP**

Remember, it is **not** necessary to transfuse anemia if the patient is young and **asymptomatic**.

Blood Products

Packed Red Blood Cells

This is a concentrated form of blood. It is a unit of whole blood with about 150 mL of plasma removed. The hematocrit of packed red blood cells (PRBCs) is about 70% to 80%. Because of the removal of plasma, the normal hematocrit in blood of around 40 is nearly doubled.

Each unit of PRBCs should raise the hematocrit by about **3 points per unit**.

Fresh Frozen Plasma

Fresh frozen plasma (FFP) replaces clotting factors in those with an elevated prothrombin time, activated partial thromboplastin time (aPTT), or INR and bleeding. FFP is used as replacement with plasmapheresis.

> FFP is **not** a choice for those with hemophilia A or B or von Willebrand disease.

Cryoprecipitate → DIC | NEVER FIRST LINE

Cryoprecipitate is used to **replace fibrinogen** and has some utility in disseminated intravascular coagulation. Its use provides high amounts of clotting factors in a smaller plasma volume.

> Cryoprecipitate is **never** used **first** for anything.

▶ **TIP**

Whole blood is never correct. Whole blood is divided into either PRBCs or FFP.

MICROCYTIC ANEMIA

DEFINITION/ETIOLOGY

Microcytosis refers specifically to an MCV that is lower than normal, which is usually below 80 fL. The most common causes are:

- **Iron deficiency:** caused by blood loss. The body only needs a very tiny amount of iron, in the range of 1 to 2 mg per day. Menstruating women need a little more, in the range of 2 to 3 mg a day. Pregnant women need as much as 5 to 6 mg a day. The duodenum can absorb only about 4 mg a day. Hence, as little as one teaspoon (5 mL) a day of blood loss will lead to iron deficiency over time.

- **Chronic disease:** includes any form of cancer or chronic infection. The anemia of chronic disease is of unclear etiology. Iron is locked in storage or trapped in macrophages or in ferritin. Hemoglobin synthesis will not occur because the iron just does not move forward. The precise mechanism is clear only in renal failure in which there is a deficiency of erythropoietin. Initially the MCV is normal, and then decreases.

- **Sideroblastic anemia: can be macrocytic** as well when it is associated with myelodysplasia, a preleukemic syndrome. In general, the most common cause is alcohol's suppressive effect on the bone marrow. Less common causes are lead poisoning, isoniazid, and vitamin B_6 deficiency.

- **Thalassemia:** an extremely common cause of microcytosis. Most patients with thalassemia trait alone are asymptomatic.

PRESENTATION/"WHAT IS THE MOST LIKELY DIAGNOSIS?"

You cannot distinguish these forms of anemia based on symptoms. You might have a suggestion from history.

How to Answer "What Is the Most Likely Diagnosis?" for Anemia	
Feature in the history	**What is the most likely diagnosis?**
Blood loss (GI bleeding)	Iron deficiency
Menstruation	Iron deficiency
Cancer or chronic infection	Chronic disease
Rheumatoid arthritis	Chronic disease
Alcoholic	Sideroblastic
Asymptomatic	Thalassemia

DIAGNOSTIC TESTS

The peripheral smear is not useful as all of the causes of microcytic anemia can be hypochromic or associated with target cells. Target cells are **most common** with thalassemia.

Unique findings on iron studies are the best initial test of microcytic anemia.

Iron Studies

Unique Features and Diagnoses of Iron Studies	
Unique feature	**Diagnosis**
Low ferritin ↑ TIBC	Iron deficiency
High iron	Sideroblastic anemia
Normal iron studies	Thalassemia

↑ FERRITIN | ↓ TIBC   CHRONIC DISEASE

- **Iron deficiency:** A low ferritin is extremely specific for iron deficiency anemia. Nearly a **third of patients have a normal or increased ferritin** because ferritin is an acute phase reactant. This means that any counter current infection or inflammation can raise the ferritin level. Both iron deficiency and the anemia of chronic disease are associated with a low serum iron level. However, iron deficiency is associated with an increase in the total iron binding capacity (TIBC). This is a measure of the **unbound** sites on transferrin. When there are a lot of **open** sites on transferrin, the **capacity** or **unbound** sites increase.

- **Chronic disease:** The serum iron is low in circulation, because iron is trapped in storage. That is why the ferritin, or **stored** iron, is elevated or normal. Circulating iron is decreased. However, the major point of difference is that the **TIBC is low**.

- **Sideroblastic anemia:** This is the only form of microcytic anemia in which the **circulating iron level is elevated**.

- **Thalassemia:** This is a genetic disease with **normal iron studies**.

Unique Laboratory Features

- **Iron deficiency:** The red cell distribution of width **(RDW) is increased**. This is because the newer cells are more iron deficient and smaller. As the body runs out of iron, the newer cells have less hemoglobin and get progressively smaller. There is an **elevated platelet count**. The single most accurate test is a bone marrow biopsy for stainable iron which is decreased. This is rarely done, but it is the most accurate test.

- **Sideroblastic anemia: Prussian blue** staining for **ringed sideroblasts** is the most accurate test. Basophilic stippling can occur in any cause of sideroblastic anemia.

- **Thalassemia:** Hemoglobin **electrophoresis** is the most accurate test. For alpha thalassemia, genetic studies are the most accurate test. Only 3-gene deletion alpha thalassemia is associated with hemoglobin H and an increased reticulocyte count. All forms have a normal RDW.

Figure 7.1: Ringed sideroblasts are detected with Prussian blue staining. *Source: Alireza Eghtedar, MD.*

Electrophoresis Findings	
Alpha thalassemia	**Beta thalassemia**
One gene deleted: normal	Increased hemoglobin F and A_2
Two genes deleted: mild anemia, normal electrophoresis	N/A
Three genes deleted: moderate anemia with hemoglobin H, which are beta-4 tetrads; increased reticulocytes	Beta thalassemia intermedia • Normal hemoglobin F • No transfusion dependence
Four genes deleted: gamma-4 tetrads or hemoglobin Bart; CHF causes death in utero	N/A

TREATMENT

- **Iron deficiency:** Replace iron with oral ferrous sulfate. If this is insufficient, occasionally patients are treated with intramuscular iron.
- **Chronic disease:** Correct the underlying disease. Only the anemia associated with end-stage renal failure routinely responds to erythropoietin replacement.
- **Sideroblastic anemia:** Correct the cause. Some patients respond to vitamin B6 or pyridoxine replacement.

Only 3-gene deletion alpha thalassemia has high reticulocytes.

- **Thalassemia:** Trait is not treated. Beta thalassemia major (Cooley anemia) is managed with chronic transfusion lifelong. Iron overload is managed with deferasirox, an oral iron chelator. Deferoxamine is a parenteral version of an iron chelator.

MACROCYTIC ANEMIA

A 73-year-old man comes to the office with fatigue that has become progressively worse over the last several months. He is also short of breath when he walks up one flight of stairs. He drinks 4 vodka martinis a day. He complains of numbness and tingling in his feet. On physical examination he has decreased sensation of his feet. His hematocrit is 28% and his MCV is 114 fL (elevated).

What is the most appropriate next step in management?

a. Vitamin B_{12} level
b. Folate level
c. Peripheral blood smear
d. Schilling test
e. Methylmalonic acid level

Answer: The correct answer is (C). Although a macrocytic anemia could be from B_{12} or folate deficiency, direct alcohol effect on the bone marrow, or liver disease, the first step is a peripheral smear. This is to detect hypersegmented neutrophils. Once hypersegmented neutrophils are seen, then you would get B_{12} and folate levels.

| Megaloblastic anemia is the presence of hypersegmented neutrophils. Many factors raise the MCV, but only B_{12} and folate deficiency and antimetabolite medications cause hypersegmentation. |

ETIOLOGY

Vitamin B_{12} deficiency is caused by:

- Pernicious anemia
- **Pancreatic insufficiency**
- Dietary deficiency (vegan/strict vegetarian)
- Crohn disease damaging terminal ileum
- Blind loop syndrome (gastrectomy or gastric bypass for weight loss)
- Diphyllobothrium latum

Folate deficiency is caused by:

- Dietary deficiency (goat's milk has no folate and provides only limited iron and B_{12})
- Psoriasis and skin loss or turnover
- Drugs: phenytoin, sulfa_ METHOTREXATE

| Celiac disease causes B_{12}, folate, and iron deficiency. |

| Look for methotrexate use in rheumatoid arthritis to suggest folate deficiency. |

PRESENTATION/"WHAT IS THE MOST LIKELY DIAGNOSIS?"

Although alcohol can give a macrocytic anemia and neurological problems, it will not give hypersegmented neutrophils.

► **TIP**

B$_{12}$ deficiency can give **any** neurological abnormality, but peripheral neuropathy is the most common. Dementia is the least common. Posterior column damage to position and vibratory sensation or "subacute combined degeneration" of the cord is classic. Look for ataxia.

DIAGNOSTIC TESTS

Laboratory abnormalities common to both B$_{12}$ and folate deficiency are:

- Megaloblastic anemia
- Increased LDH and increased indirect bilirubin levels
- Decreased reticulocyte count
- Hypercellular bone marrow
- **Macroovalocytes**
- Increased homocysteine levels

B$_{12}$ and folate deficiency are **identical hematologically** and on blood smear.

> Only B$_{12}$ deficiency is associated with an increased methylmalonic acid level.

Figure 7.2: Hypersegmented neutrophils are the best initial test in determining the etiology of macrocytic anemia.
Source: Alireza Eghtedar, MD.

A 73-year-old woman comes with decreased position and vibratory sensation of the lower extremities, a hematocrit of 28%, MCV of 114 fL, and hypersegmented neutrophils. Her B$_{12}$ level is decreased, but near the borderline of normal.

What is the most appropriate next step in the management of this patient?

a. Methylmalonic acid level
b. Anti-intrinsic factor antibodies
c. Anti-parietal cell antibodies
d. Schillings test
e. Folate level
f. Homocysteine level

Answer: The correct answer is (A). USMLE Step 2 CK frequently tests the fact that while both B$_{12}$ and folate deficiency increase homocysteine levels, only B$_{12}$ is associated with an increased MMA. The B$_{12}$ level can be normal in as many as a third of patients with B$_{12}$ deficiency because the carrier protein, transcobalamin, is an acute phase reactant and can be elevated from many forms of stress such as infection, cancer, or trauma. **When the story suggests B$_{12}$ deficiency and the B$_{12}$ level is equivocal, use an increased MMA level to confirm the diagnosis of vitamin B$_{12}$ deficiency.**

▶**TIP**

Tested facts about macrocytic anemia:

- Schilling test is never the right answer.
- Pernicious anemia is confirmed with anti-intrinsic factor and anti-parietal cell antibodies.
- Red cells are destroyed as they leave the marrow, so the reticulocyte count is low.
- B$_{12}$ and folate deficiency can cause pancytopenia as well as macrocytic anemia.
- Pancreatic enzymes are needed to absorb B$_{12}$. They free it from carrier proteins.
- Neurological abnormalities will improve as long as they are **minor** (eg, peripheral) and of **short duration**.

TREATMENT

Replace what is deficient. Folate replacement corrects the hematologic problems of B$_{12}$ deficiency, but not the neurological problems.

> B$_{12}$ can give either neurological or hematological abnormalities alone. You do **not** have to have both.

Which of the following is a complication of B$_{12}$ or folate replacement?

a. Seizures
b. Hemolysis
c. Hypokalemia
d. Hyperkalemia
e. Diarrhea

Answer: The correct answer is (C). Hyperkalemia from massive tissue or cellular breakdown has many causes. Hypokalemia from cell production is rare. When replacing B$_{12}$ and folate, particularly if there is pancytopenia, cells in the marrow are produced so rapidly that the marrow packages up all the potassium, lowering the serum level. Observe and replace.

> Pancreatic enzymes are needed to remove B$_{12}$ from the R-protein so it can bind with intrinsic factor.

HEMOLYTIC ANEMIA

All forms of hemolysis can lead to:

- Sudden decrease in hematocrit
- Increased levels of LDH, indirect bilirubin, and reticulocytes
- Decreased haptoglobin level

Chronic hemolysis is associated with bilirubin gallstones.

- Slight increase in MCV because reticulocytes are larger than normal cells
- Hyperkalemia from cell breakdown
- Folate deficiency from increased cell production using it up; folate stores are limited

Sickle Cell Disease

DEFINITION/ETIOLOGY

Sickle cell is caused by a point mutation at position 6 of the beta globin chain: Valine replaces glutamic acid.

Sickle cell is a chronic, usually well-compensated hemolytic anemia with a reticulocyte count that is always high. Acute painful vasoocclusive crisis is caused by:

- Hypoxia
- Dehydration
- Infection
- Cold temperatures

"WHAT IS THE MOST LIKELY DIAGNOSIS?"

Look for an African American patient with sudden, severe pain in the chest, back, and thighs that may be accompanied by fever. It is rare for an adult to present with an acute crisis without a clear history of sickle cell disease.

Other Common Manifestations of Sickle Cell Disease

These include:

- **Bilirubin gallstones** from chronically elevated bilirubin levels
- Increased **infection** from autosplenectomy, particularly encapsulated organisms
- **Osteomyelitis**, most commonly from *Salmonella*
- **Retinopathy**
- **Stroke**
- Enlarged heart with hyperdynamic features and a systolic murmur
- Lower extremity **skin ulcers**
- **Avascular necrosis** of the femoral head

Children present with dactylitis (inflammation of fingers).

DIAGNOSTIC TESTS

Papillary necrosis of the kidney happens from chronic kidney damage.

The best **initial** test is a **peripheral smear**. Sickle cell trait (AS disease) does **not** give sickled cells. The most **accurate** test is the hemoglobin **electrophoresis**.

Figure 7.3: Target cells can occur with many hematological diseases, including sickle cell disease. *Source: Abhay Vakil, MD.*

Which of the following can be found on smear in sickle cell disease?

a. *Basophilic stippling*
b. *Howell-Jolly bodies*
c. *Bite cells*
d. *Schistocytes*
e. *Morulae*

*Answer: The correct answer is (B). These are precipitated remnants of nuclear material seen inside the red cells of a patient who does not have a spleen. There is no change in therapy or management based on the presence of Howell-Jolly bodies. **Basophilic stippling** is associated with a number of causes of **sideroblastic** anemia, especially lead poisoning. Bite cells are seen in glucose 6 phosphate dehydrogenase deficiency. Schistocytes are fragmented red cells seen with intravascular hemolysis. Morulae are seen inside neutrophils in **Ehrlichia** infections.*

> Nucleated red blood cells are found with premature release of precursor blood cells.

TREATMENT

1. Begin with oxygen/hydration/analgesia.
2. If fever or a white cell count higher than usual is present, then antibiotics are given. Use ceftriaxone, levofloxacin, or moxifloxacin.
3. Folic acid replacement is necessary on a chronic basis.
4. Give pneumococcal vaccination because of autosplenectomy.
5. Hydroxyurea prevents recurrences of sickle cell crises by increasing hemoglobin F.

> Do not wait for results of testing to start antibiotics if there is a fever. The absence of a functional spleen leads to overwhelming infection.

> **Exchange transfusion is used if there is severe vasoocclusive crisis presenting with:**
>
> - Acute chest syndrome
> - Priapism
> - Stroke
> - Visual disturbance from retinal infarction

Aplastic Crisis

A 43-year-old man with sickle cell disease is admitted with an acute pain crisis. His only routine medication is folic acid. His hematocrit on admission is 34%. On the third hospital day, the hematocrit drops to 22%.

What is the best initial test?

a. Reticulocyte count
b. Peripheral smear
c. Folate level
d. Parvovirus B-19 IgM level
e. Bone marrow

> The most accurate test for parvovirus B-19 is a PCR for DNA. This is more accurate than the IgM level. Intravenous immunoglobulin is the best initial therapy.

*Answer: The correct answer is (A). Patients with sickle cell disease usually have very high reticulocyte counts because of the chronic compensated hemolysis. Parvovirus B-19 causes an aplastic crisis which freezes the growth of the marrow. Nothing will be visible on blood smear. Although the **bone marrow will show giant pronormoblasts**, this would not be done routinely, and certainly never as the initial test. The first clue to parvovirus is a sudden drop in reticulocyte level.*

Sickle Cell Trait

Sickle cell trait means the patient is **heterozygous** for the sickle gene (AS). The only manifestation of sickle cell trait is a **defect in the ability to concentrate the urine** or "isosthenuria." They are clinically asymptomatic and have both a normal CBC level and a normal smear result. **Hematuria** may sometimes occur. There is **no treatment** for sickle cell trait.

Hereditary Spherocytosis

ETIOLOGY

This is a defect in the cytoskeleton of the red cell leading to an abnormal round shape and loss of the normal flexibility characteristic of the biconcave disc that allows red cells to bend in the spleen.

"WHAT IS THE MOST LIKELY DIAGNOSIS?"

- Recurrent episodes of hemolysis
- Intermittent jaundice
- Splenomegaly

- Family history of anemia or hemolysis
- Bilirubin gallstones

DIAGNOSTIC TESTS

- Low MCV
- Increased mean corpuscular hemoglobin concentration (MCHC)
- Negative Coombs test

The most accurate test is osmotic fragility. When cells are placed in a slightly hypotonic solution, the increased swelling of the cells leads to hemolysis.

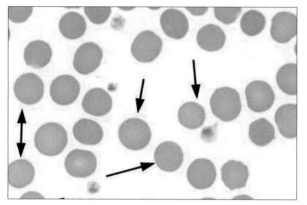

Figure 7.4: Spherocytes lose the central pallor of normal red cells. The MCHC is elevated. *Source: Alireza Eghtedar, MD.*

TREATMENT

1. Chronic **folic acid** replacement supports red cell production.
2. **Splenectomy** stops the hemolysis but does not eliminate the spherocytes.

Autoimmune (Warm or IgG) Hemolysis

ETIOLOGY

Fifty percent of cases have no identified etiology. Clear causes are:

- Chronic lymphocytic leukemia (CLL)
- Lymphoma
- Systemic lupus erythematosus (SLE)
- Drugs: penicillin, alpha-methyldopa, rifampin, phenytoin

DIAGNOSTIC TESTS

The most accurate diagnostic test is the **Coombs test**, which detects IgG antibody on the surface of the red cells. The direct and indirect Coombs tests tell basically the same thing, but the indirect test is associated with a greater amount of antibody.

Autoantibodies remove small amounts of red cell membrane and lead to a smaller membrane, forcing the cell to become round. Biconcave discs need a

> Autoimmune hemolysis is also associated with spherocytes.

greater surface area than a sphere. Autoimmune hemolysis is associated with microspherocytes.

▶ **TIP**

The smear does not show fragmented cells in autoimmune hemolysis because the red cell destruction occurs inside the spleen or liver, not in the blood vessel.

TREATMENT

1. **Glucocorticoids** such as prednisone are the "best initial therapy."
2. Recurrent episodes respond to **splenectomy**.
3. Severe, acute hemolysis not responding to prednisone is controlled with intravenous immunoglobulin (**IVIG**).
4. **Rituximab** is used when splenectomy does not control the hemolysis.

[Handwritten margin note: GLUCOCORTICOIDS ↓ IVIG ↓ SPLENECTOMY ↓ RITUXIMAB]

Alternate treatments to diminish the need for steroids in general are:

- Cyclophosphamide
- Cyclosporine
- Azathioprine
- Mycophenolate mofetil

Cold Agglutinin Disease

DEFINITION/ETIOLOGY

Cold agglutinins are IgM antibodies against the red cell developing in association with Epstein-Barr virus, Waldenström macroglobulinemia, or *Mycoplasma pneumoniae.*

PRESENTATION

Symptoms occur in colder parts of the body such as numbness or mottling of the nose, ears, fingers, and toes. Symptoms resolve on warming up the body part.

DIAGNOSTIC TESTS

The direct Coombs test is positive only for complement. The smear is normal, or may show only spherocytes.

TREATMENT

1. Stay warm.
2. Administer **rituximab.**
3. Cyclophosphamide, cyclosporine, or other immunosuppressive agents stop the production of the antibody.

[Handwritten note: No STEROIDS]

▶ **TIP**

Steroids and splenectomy do not work in cold agglutinin disease. **Prednisone is the most common wrong answer.**

Cryoglobulins are often mixed up with cold agglutinins. Although both are IgM and do not respond to steroids, cryoglobulins are associated with:

- Hepatitis C
- Joint pain
- Glomerulonephritis

Glucose 6 Phosphate Dehydrogenase Deficiency

ETIOLOGY

Glucose 6 phosphate dehydrogenase (G6PD) deficiency is an X-linked recessive disorder leading to an inability to generate glutathione reductase and protect the red cells from oxidant stress. The most common oxidant stress is **infection**. Other causes are dapsone, quinidine, sulfa drugs, primaquine, nitrofurantoin, and fava beans.

> Because G6PD deficiency is X-linked recessive, it manifests almost exclusively in **men**.

"WHAT IS THE MOST LIKELY DIAGNOSIS?"

Look for African American or Mediterranean **men** with **sudden anemia** and jaundice who have a normal-sized spleen with an infection or are using one of the drugs previously listed.

DIAGNOSTIC TESTS

The best initial test is for Heinz bodies and bite cells. The G6PD level will be **normal** after a hemolytic event. The most accurate test is the G6PD level after waiting 1 to 2 months after an acute episode of hemolysis.

Figure 7.5: Bite cells. *Source: Alireza Eghtedar, MD.*

Treatment

Nothing reverses the hemolysis. Avoid oxidant stress.

Hemolytic Uremic Syndrome and Thrombotic Thrombocytopenic Purpura

Hemolytic uremic syndrome (HUS) and thrombotic thrombocytopenic purpura (TTP) are different versions of the same basic disease. HUS is associated with *E. coli* 0157:H7 and is more frequent in children. TTP is associated with ticlopidine, clopidogrel, cyclosporine, and AIDS.

Both disorders are characterized by:

- Intravascular hemolysis with fragmented red cells (schistocytes)
- Thrombocytopenia
- Renal insufficiency

> If there is a delay to plasmapheresis, infuse FFP.

TTP is also associated with neurological disorders and fever and is more common in adults. Neurological symptoms include confusion and seizures. There is no one specific test to diagnose either disorder. HUS and TTP both have normal PT/aPTT and negative Coombs test. Severe cases are treated with plasmapheresis or plasma exchange. STEROIDS

> Do not transfuse platelets into patients with HUS or TTP. Platelet transfusion worsens the disease.

Paroxysmal Nocturnal Hemoglobinuria

Etiology

Paroxysmal nocturnal hemoglobinuria (PNH) is a clonal stem cell defect with increased sensitivity of red cells to complement in acidosis. This is from deficiency of the complement regulatory proteins CD 55 and 59 also known as **decay accelerating factor**. The gene for phosphatidylinositol class A (PIG-A) is defective. This leads to overactivation of the complement system. During sleep, the relative hypoventilation leads to a mild increase in pCO_2 and acidosis. This does nothing to an unaffected person, but in PNH it leads to hemolysis and thrombosis.

> PNH is a stem cell defect that may cause aplastic anemia, **myelodysplasia**, or **acute leukemia**.

Presentation/"What Is the Most Likely Diagnosis?"

- **Episodic dark urine** with the first urination of the day from hemoglobin
- **Pancytopenia** and iron deficiency anemia

▶ **TIP**

Thrombosis is the most common cause of death.

Diagnostic Tests

CD55/59 LEVELS

CBC often shows pancytopenia in addition to anemia. The most accurate test is a decreased level of **CD55** and **CD59**. The Ham test and the sucrose hemolysis test are in vitro methods of activating the complement pathway. If CD55 and

CD59 are in the answer, Ham test and sucrose hemolysis are **never** the correct answer. Flow cytometry is another way of saying CD55/CD59 testing.

TREATMENT

1. **Prednisone** is the best initial therapy for hemolysis. The mechanism is not clear.
2. Allogeneic **bone marrow transplant** is the only method of **cure**.
3. **Eculizumab** inactivates C5 in the complement pathway and decreases red cell destruction. Complement overactivation is the mechanism of PNH. Eculizumab is, essentially, a complement inhibitor.
4. Give supportive care such as folic acid replacement and transfusions as needed.

Large vessel thrombosis of the mesenteric and hepatic veins is the most common site of thrombosis.

APLASTIC ANEMIA

DEFINITION/ETIOLOGY

PNH & Aplastic Anemia = Bone Marrow Transplant

Aplastic anemia is **pancytopenia** of unclear etiology. Any infection or cancer can invade the bone marrow, causing decreased production or hypoplasia. Other causes of pancytopenia are:

- Radiation and toxins such as toluene, insecticides (DDT), and benzene
- Drug effect: sulfa, phenytoin, carbamazepine, chloramphenicol, alcohol, chemotherapy
- SLE
- PNH
- Infection: HIV, hepatitis, CMV, EBV
- B_{12} and folate deficiency
- Thyroid-inhibiting medications such as propylthiouracil (PTU) and methimazole

PRESENTATION/DIAGNOSTIC TESTS

FATTY BONE MARROW

Patients present with the **fatigue** of anemia, **infections** from low white cell counts, and **bleeding** from thrombocytopenia. Aplastic anemia is confirmed by excluding all the causes of pancytopenia. The most accurate test is a bone marrow biopsy.

TREATMENT

Besides supportive therapy such as blood transfusion for anemia, antibiotics for infection, and platelets for bleeding, you should treat any underlying cause that is identified. A true aplastic anemia is treated with **allogeneic bone marrow transplantation (BMT)** if the patient is young enough and there is a matched donor.

Aplastic anemia acts as an autoimmune disorder in which the T cells attack the patient's own marrow. Treatment is based on medications like cyclosporine that inhibit T cells. This brings the marrow back to life.

When the patient is too old for BMT (above age 50) or there is no matched donor, the treatment is **antithymocyte globulin** (ATG) and **cyclosporine**. **Tacrolimus** is an alternative to cyclosporine.

POLYCYTHEMIA VERA

DEFINITION

Polycythemia vera (p. vera) is the unregulated overproduction of all 3 cell lines, but red cell overproduction is the most prominent. There is a mutation in the JAK2 protein which regulates marrow production. The **red cells grow wildly despite a low erythropoietin level**.

"WHAT IS THE MOST LIKELY DIAGNOSIS?"

Patients present with symptoms of hyperviscosity from the increased red blood cell mass such as:

- Headache, blurred vision, and tinnitus
- **Hypertension**
- Fatigue
- **Splenomegaly**
- **Bleeding** from engorged blood vessels
- **Thrombosis** from hyperviscosity

[handwritten: TRIAD — Thrombosis — Burning of Hands/Feet — Pruritus]

> Pruritus often follows warm showers because of histamine release from increased numbers of basophils.

DIAGNOSTIC TESTS

The hematocrit is markedly elevated above 60% and the platelets and white cell count are often up as well. You must exclude hypoxia as a cause of the erythrocytosis. The total red cell mass is elevated. **Oxygen levels are normal** and **erythropoietin levels are low**.

Vitamin B$_{12}$ levels are elevated for unclear reasons. Iron levels are low because it has all been used up to make red cells. The **most accurate test is the JAK2 mutation**, found in 95% of patients. Increased numbers of basophils are present, as occurs in all forms of myeloproliferative disorders. A small number of patients can convert to AML.

> Renal cell cancer is associated with an elevated hematocrit, but the erythropoietin level is elevated with kidney cancer.

> The MCV is low in p. vera.

TREATMENT

1. Phlebotomy
2. Hydroxyurea, which helps lower the cell count

> Platelet counts elevate temporarily after spleen removal.

[handwritten: Too much stuff → Hydroxyurea]

ESSENTIAL THROMBOCYTOSIS

This is a markedly elevated platelet count above one million leading to both thrombosis and bleeding. Essential thrombocytosis (ET) can be very difficult to distinguish from an elevated platelet count as a reaction to another stress such as infection, cancer, or iron deficiency.

TREATMENT

If the patient is under age 60 and is asymptomatic with a platelet count under 1.5 million, no treatment is necessary. If the patient is above 60 and there are thromboses or the platelet count is above 1.5 million, begin treatment. **The best initial therapy is hydroxyurea.** Anagrelide is used when there is red cell suppression from hydroxyurea. **Aspirin is used for erythromelalgia.**

> JAK2 mutation is found in 50% of ET cases.

> Erythromelalgia = painful, red hands in ET. Treat with aspirin.

MYELOFIBROSIS

Myelofibrosis is a disease of older persons with a pancytopenia associated with a bone marrow showing marked fibrosis. Blood production shifts to the spleen and liver, which become markedly enlarged. Look for **teardrop-shaped cells** and nucleated red blood cells on blood smear. **Thalidomide** and **lenalidomide** are tumor necrosis factor inhibitors that increase bone marrow production. In the occasional patient presenting under age 50 to 55, allogeneic bone marrow transplantation is attempted.

< 10% BLASTS = CHRONIC

> 30% BLASTS = ACUTE

ACUTE LEUKEMIA   *AML / ALL*

Patients present with signs of **pancytopenia** (fatigue, infection, bleeding) even though the white blood cell count is normal or increased in many patients. Despite an increase in white cell count, **infection** is a common presentation because leukemic cells (blasts) do not function normally in controlling infection.

lymphoblast *OR* *ALL*

myeloblast *AML*

The most frequently tested type of acute leukemia is M3 or acute promyelocytic leukemia. This is because promyelocytic leukemia is associated with disseminated intravascular coagulation (DIC). There is no distinct clinical presentation between the 3 subtypes of acute lymphocytic leukemia (ALL), so for the USMLE Step 2 CK, there is no point in learning the differences between them.

The **best initial test is a blood smear showing blasts.**

The most accurate test is flow cytometry, which will distinguish the different subtypes of acute leukemia. Flow cytometry is the method of detecting the specific CD subtypes associated with each type of leukemia. **Myeloperoxidase is characteristic of acute myelocytic leukemia (AML).**

> Look for a history of myelodysplastic syndrome to suggest acute leukemia.

> M3 is associated with translocation between chromosomes 15 and 17.

> Auer rods are eosinophilic inclusions associated with AML. M3 or acute promyelocytic leukemia is most commonly associated with Auer rods.

M3 = DIC

M3 AML = t(15,17) | AUER RODS | DIC | ALL-TRANS VIT A

Figure 7.6: Auer rods are characteristic of AML.
Source: Shreya Patel, Nishith Patel.

TREATMENT

Both AML and ALL are treated initially with chemotherapy to remove blasts from the peripheral blood smear. This is known as inducing remission. The question is whether to proceed directly to BMT after remission or only give more chemotherapy. If prognosis is poor, then go straight to BMT; if prognosis is good, give more chemotherapy.

The **best indicator of prognosis in acute leukemia is cytogenetics** or assessing the specific chromosomal characteristics found in each patient.

> Good cytogenetics = less chance of relapse = more chemotherapy

> Bad cytogenetics = more chance of relapse = immediate BMT

1. Add all-trans-retinoic acid (ATRA) to those with M3 (promyelocytic leukemia).
2. Add intrathecal chemotherapy such as methotrexate to ALL treatment. This prevents relapse of ALL in the CNS.

▶ **TIP**

The most tested facts for acute leukemia are:

- M3 (promyelocytic leukemia) gives DIC.
- Add ATRA to M3.
- Auer rods = AML.
- Add intrathecal methotrexate to ALL.

[Handwritten margin notes: ALL = INTRATHECAL CHEMO; M3 = DIC; ATRA TO M3; AUER RODS = AML; INTRATHECAL CHEMO = ALL]

CHRONIC MYELOGENOUS LEUKEMIA

"WHAT IS THE MOST LIKELY DIAGNOSIS?"

Look for a patient with a persistently high WBC count that is all neutrophils. → MYELO

- **Pruritus** is common after hot baths/showers from histamine release from basophils.
- **Splenomegaly** presents with early satiety, abdominal fullness, and left upper quadrant pain.
- Chronic myelogenous leukemia (CML) can present with vague symptoms of fatigue, night sweats, and fever from hypermetabolic syndrome.
- CML can present with **high WBC on routine exam**.

DIAGNOSTIC TESTS

After the high neutrophil count is found, you must determine if it is a reaction to another infection or stress (leukemoid reaction), or genuinely represents a leukemia.

If the leukocyte alkaline phosphatase score (LAP) **is** a choice, then this is first. Leukemic cells do **not** have normal amounts of alkaline phosphatase and the LAP score is low in CML. → JUST NOT AS MUCH STUFF IN A RUSH B/C THEY ARE

If LAP score is **not** a choice, or the question is "What is the most accurate test?" then answer "BCR-ABL," which can be done by PCR on peripheral blood.

In CML, you may find small numbers of blasts, but it should be under 5%. Basophils are increased.

> "BCR-ABL" = 9:22 translocation = Philadelphia chromosome

TREATMENT

→ BLOCKS TYROSINE KINASE

Tyrosine kinase inhibitors such as imatinib (Gleevec; Novartis, East Hanover, New Jersey), dasatinib, or nilotinib are the **best initial therapy**.

Only a **BMT** can cure CML, but this should **never be the first therapy**. BMT is, however, the answer to the question "Which of the following is the most effective cure for the disease?"

CML = IMITINAB & BM TRANSPLANT

> CML has the greatest likelihood of all myeloproliferative disorders **to transform into acute leukemia (blast crisis)**. If CML is untreated, this will happen in 20% of patients a year.

CML = IMATINIB

LEUKOSTASIS REACTION

A 54-year-old man comes to the emergency department for shortness of breath, blurry vision, confusion, and priapism. His WBC count is found to be 225,000/µL. The cells are predominantly neutrophils with about 4% blasts.

What is the most appropriate next step in the management of this case?

a. Leukapheresis
b. BCR-ABL testing
c. Bone marrow biopsy
d. Bone marrow transplant

e. Consult hematology/oncology

f. Flow cytometry

g. Hydroxyurea

Answer: The correct answer is (A). In acute leukostasis reaction, it is more important to remove the excessive white cells from the blood than to establish a specific diagnosis. Specific testing is not as important as treatment. No matter what the etiology, you still have to take the cells off. The symptoms are caused by blocking the delivery of oxygen to tissues because the red cells simply cannot get to the tissues. Afterward, you can establish a specific diagnosis. Hydroxyurea will lower the cell count, but not as rapidly as leukapheresis.

MYELODYSPLASTIC SYNDROME

DEFINITION

MDS is a preleukemic disorder presenting in older patients (over 60) with a pancytopenia despite a hypercellular bone marrow. Most patients never develop acute myelogenous leukemia because **complications of infection and bleeding lead to death before leukemia occurs**.

> 5q deletion is the characteristic abnormality of MDS. Patients with 5q have a better prognosis than do those without it.

PRESENTATION

Many patients present with an **asymptomatic pancytopenia on routine CBC**. Symptoms that do occur are:

- Fatigue and weight loss
- Infection
- Bleeding
- Sometimes splenomegaly

There is no single pathognomonic finding in the history or physical examination.

DIAGNOSTIC TESTS

- CBC: anemia with an **increased MCV**, **nucleated red cells,** and a small number of blasts
- Marrow: hypercellular
- Prussian blue stain shows **ringed sideroblasts**
- **Severity is based on the percentage of blasts**

> Pelger-Huet cells are the most distinct lab abnormality in MDS.

Bilobed nucleus
of Pelger-Huet cell

Figure 7.7: Pelger-Huet cells are found in myelodysplastic syndrome. *Source: Alireza Eghtedar, MD.*

$\overline{EPO} = \uparrow HTN$

TREATMENT

1. **Transfusion**; support with blood products as needed.
2. **Erythropoietin** gives about 20% response.
3. **Lenalidomide** for those with the 5q deletion can decrease transfusion dependence.

LENALIDOMIDE

Azacitidine decreases transfusion dependence but does not increase survival.

CHRONIC LYMPHOCYTIC LEUKEMIA

PRESENTATION

Chronic lymphocytic leukemia (CLL) is a clonal proliferation of normal, mature-appearing B lymphocytes that function abnormally. CLL occurs over the age of 50 in 90% of those affected. Many are asymptomatic at presentation with only a markedly elevated white cell count. The **most common symptom is fatigue**. Other symptoms include:

- **Lymphadenopathy** (80%)
- **Spleen or liver enlargement** (50%)
- **Infection** from poor lymphocyte function

CLL has no unique physical findings.

Richter phenomenon, the conversion of CLL into high-grade lymphoma, happens in 5% of patients.

DIAGNOSTIC TESTS

The WBC count is usually at least above 20,000/µL with 80% to 98% lymphocytes. Half of patients are hypogammaglobulinemic.

Anemia and thrombocytopenia can occur from marrow infiltration or autoimmune warm IgG antibodies. CLL is paradoxical. When the body needs a useful antibody for an infection, it is often not made; on the other hand, the CLL cells attack normal red cells and platelets.

A smudge cell is a lab artifact in which the fragile nucleus is crushed by the cover slip.

TREATMENT

For stage 0 (elevated WBC) and stage I (lymphadenopathy), there is no treatment.

Stage II (hepatosplenomegaly), stage III (anemia), and stage IV (thrombocytopenia) are treated with **fludarabine.**

If there is a choice that lists fludarabine **and** rituximab, then this is the best initial therapy for advanced-stage disease (II, III, IV) or any patient who is symptomatic (severe fatigue, painful nodes).

> **PCP prophylaxis is indicated in CLL.**

> *CLL = FLUDARABINE*

To get a 99 on Step 2 CK, know:

- Refractory cases: **cyclophosphamide** (more efficacy, but more toxic)
- Mild cases: **chlorambucil**
- Severe infection: intravenous immunoglobulins
- Autoimmune thrombocytopenia or hemolysis: **prednisone**

▶ **TIP**

Which is less dangerous? Thrombocytopenia and anemia from autoimmune effect, or from marrow infiltration with CLL cells? The answer is autoimmune effect. This is treated with prednisone, and is not the same as stage III and IV disease.

HAIRY CELL LEUKEMIA

Hairy cell leukemia (HCL) presents in middle-aged men with:

- Pancytopenia
- Massive splenomegaly
- Monocytopenia
- Inaspirable "dry" tap despite hypercellularity of the marrow

> **Hairy cell leukemia is from B-cells with filamentous projections on smear.**

The most accurate test is tartrate resistant acid phosphatase (TRAP) or CD11c. **Treat with cladribine.**

NON-HODGKIN LYMPHOMA

DEFINITION

> *DIFFUSE LARGE B-CELL IS M.C.*

Non-Hodgkin lymphoma (NHL) is a proliferation of lymphocytes in the lymph nodes and spleen. NHL is most often widespread at presentation and can affect any lymph node or organ that has lymphoid tissue. NHL and CLL are extremely similar, but NHL is a solid mass and CLL is "liquid" or circulating.

PRESENTATION/"WHAT IS THE MOST LIKELY DIAGNOSIS?"

- **Painless lymphadenopathy** (NOT CERVICAL)
- May involve pelvic, retroperitoneal, or mesenteric structures
- Nodes **not warm, red, or tender**
- "B" symptoms: fever, weight loss, drenching night sweats

> Infection, not NHL, gives nodes that are warm, red, and tender.

DIAGNOSTIC TESTS

The best initial test is an **excisional biopsy. The CBC is normal in most cases.** High LDH levels correlate with worse severity. Staging determines the intensity of therapy. Staging NHL does not often change treatment because in most cases, disease is widespread (stage III and IV). Typical staging procedures are:

↑ LDH = WORSE DZ

- CT scan of the chest, abdomen, and pelvis
- Bone marrow biopsy

▶ **TIP**

The most common **wrong answer** is to do a **needle aspiration** of the lymph node. Aspiration is not enough because the individual lymphocytes appear normal.

Staging
- Stage I: 1 lymph node group
- Stage II: 2 or more lymph node groups on the same side of the diaphragm
- Stage III: both sides of the diaphragm
- Stage IV: widespread disease

TREATMENT

Local disease (stage Ia and IIa): local radiation

Advanced disease (stage III and IV, any "B" symptoms): combination chemotherapy with CHOP and rituximab, an antibody against CD20

C = cyclophosphamide

H = adriamycin (doxorubicin or "hydroxydaunorubicin")

O = vincristine (oncovin)

P = prednisone

> NHL presents in advanced stages in 80% to 90% of cases.

Mucosal Associated Lymphoid Tissue

This is lymphoma of the stomach in association with *Helicobacter pylori*. Treat the *Helicobacter* with clarithromycin and amoxicillin.

HODGKIN DISEASE

The definition, presentation, diagnostic tests, "B" symptoms, and staging of Hodgkin disease (HD) are the same as NHL. HD has Reed-Sternberg cells on pathology.

NODULAR SCLEROIS - MC.

* PAINLESS CERVICAL LYMPHADENOPATH

Differences between HD and NHL	
Hodgkin disease	**Non-Hodgkin lymphoma**
Local, stage I, and stage II in 80%–90%	Stage III and stage IV in 80%–90%
Centers around cervical area	Disseminated
Reed-Sternberg cells on pathology	No Reed-Sternberg cells
Pathologic classification: Lymphocyte predominant has the best prognosis. Lymphocyte depleted has the worst prognosis.	Pathologic classification: Burkitt and immunoblastic have the worst prognosis.

TREATMENT

Stage Ia and IIa: local radiation

Stage III and IV or anyone with "B" symptoms: ABVD

A = adriamycin (doxorubicin)

B = bleomycin

V = vinblastine

D = dacarbazine

> Relapses after radiation therapy are treated with chemotherapy. Relapses after chemotherapy are treated with extra high dose chemotherapy and bone marrow transplantation.

Complications of Radiation and Chemotherapy

Radiation increases the risk of **solid tumors** such as **breast cancer** or **lung cancer**. Screening for breast cancer is recommended 8 years or more after treatment. **Radiation also increases the chance of premature coronary artery disease**. The risk of acute leukemia, MDS, and NHL as a complication of chemotherapy is about 1% per year.

Which of the following is the most useful to determine dosing of chemotherapy in HD?

a. Echocardiogram

b. Bone marrow biopsy

c. Gender

d. MUGA or nuclear ventriculogram

e. Hematocrit

f. Symptoms

*Answer: The correct answer is **(D)**. Adriamycin (or doxorubicin) is cardiotoxic. The nuclear ventriculogram is the most accurate method of assessing left ventricular ejection fraction. Use the MUGA scan to determine whether cardiac toxicity has occurred prior to the development of symptoms.*

Adverse Effects of Chemotherapy	
Chemotherapeutic agent	**Toxicity**
Doxorubicin	Cardiomyopathy
Vincristine	Neuropathy
Bleomycin	Lung fibrosis
Cyclophosphamide	Hemorrhagic cystitis
Cisplatin	Renal and ototoxicity

MULTIPLE MYELOMA

> 10% PLASMA CELLS

DEFINITION

Myeloma is an abnormal proliferation of plasma cells. These plasma cells are unregulated in their production of useless immunoglobulin that is usually IgG or IgA. IgM is a separate disease called **Waldenström macroglobulinemia**. These immunoglobulins do not fight infection but clog up the kidney.

"WHAT IS THE MOST LIKELY DIAGNOSIS?"

The most common presentation of myeloma is **bone pain** from pathologic fractures. A pathologic fracture means that the bone breaks under what would be considered normal use. This is from osteoclast activating factor (OAF), which attacks the bone, causing lytic lesions. OAF is also the reason for **hypercalcemia**. Infection is common because the abnormal plasma cells do not make immunoglobulins that are effective against infections.

PRESENTATION

- **Hyperuricemia:** from increased turnover of the nuclear material of plasma cells
- **Anemia:** from infiltration of the marrow with massive numbers of plasma cells
- **Renal failure:** from accumulation of immunoglobulins and Bence-Jones protein in the kidney; hypercalcemia and hyperuricemia also damage the kidney

HYPERCALCEMIA

> Renal failure and infection are the most common causes of death in myeloma.

DIAGNOSTIC TESTS

The first test done is usually an **x-ray** of the affected bone that will **show lytic lesions**.

Myeloma has a decreased anion gap. IgG is cationic. Increased cationic substances will increase chloride and bicarbonate levels. This decreases the anion gap.

Rouleaux form when the IgG paraprotein sticks to the red cells, causing them to adhere to each other in a stack or "roll."

An M-spike on SPEP does **not** mean IgM.

Serum protein electrophoresis **(SPEP)** shows an IgG (60%) or IgA (25%) spike of a single type or "clone." This one clone is called a Monoclonal or "M" spike. Fifteen percent have light chains or Bence-Jones protein only. Additional laboratory abnormalities include:

- **Hypercalcemia**
- **Bence-Jones protein** on urine immunoelectrophoresis (υPEP)
- Beta$_2$ microglobulin levels correspond to severity of disease
- Smear with **rouleaux**
- Elevated BUN and creatinine
- Bone marrow biopsy: **greater than 10% plasma cells defines myeloma**
- Elevated total protein with normal albumin

A 69-year-old woman is admitted with severe back pain that has suddenly worsened. She also feels a "pop" when she coughs followed by tenderness over the ribs. X-ray shows lytic lesions. Her calcium level is 2 points above normal, the hematocrit is 27%, and her creatinine is elevated. Urinalysis shows trace protein, but the 24-hour urine show 5 grams of protein.

What do you expect to find on technetium bone scan?

a. Normal
b. Lytic lesions at the site of the fractures
c. Increased uptake diffusely
d. Decreased uptake

Answer: The correct answer is (A). The radionuclide bone scan will be normal because lytic lesions do not pick up the nuclear isotope. Nuclear bone scan shows increased uptake with osteoblastic activity, which is absent in myeloma.

What is the explanation for the difference between the urinary level of protein on urinalysis and the 24-hour urine?

a. False positive 24-hour urine is common in myeloma.
b. Calcium in urine creates a false negative urinalysis.
c. Uric acid creates a false positive 24-hour urine.
d. Bence-Jones protein is not detected by dipstick.
e. IgG in urine inactivates the urine dipstick.

Answer: The correct answer is (D). Bence-Jones protein is detected by urine immunoelectrophoresis. The urine dipstick will detect only albumin.

What is the single most accurate test for myeloma?

a. Skull x-rays
b. Bone marrow biopsy
c. 24-hour urine
d. SPEP
e. Urine immunoelectrophoresis (Bence-Jones protein)

*Answer: The correct answer is (B). Nothing besides myeloma is associated with **greater than 10% plasma cells on bone marrow biopsy**. The most common wrong answer is SPEP. Of those with an "M-spike" of immunoglobulins, 99% do **not** have myeloma. Most IgG spikes are from monoclonal gammopathy of unknown significance that does not progress or need treatment. Skull x-rays show lytic lesions, but this is not as specific as massive plasma cell levels in the marrow.*

TREATMENT

The best initial therapy is a combination of dexamethasone with lenalidomide, bortezomib, or both.

Melphalan is useful in older, fragile patients who cannot tolerate adverse effects. The most effective therapy in those under age 70 is an autologous bone marrow transplant with stem cell support. This is used after induction chemotherapy with lenalidomide and steroids.

> Myeloma therapy is in a state of rapid flux due to numerous advances.

MONOCLONAL GAMMOPATHY OF UNKNOWN SIGNIFICANCE

IgG or IgA spikes on an SPEP are common in older patients. The main issue is to evaluate with bone marrow biopsy to exclude myeloma. Monoclonal gammopathy of unknown significance (MGUS) has small numbers of plasma cells. There is **no therapy for MGUS**, although about **1% a year transform into myeloma**. The quantity or amount of immunoglobulin in the spike is the main correlate of risk for myeloma: more MGUS, more myeloma.

WALDENSTRÖM MACROGLOBULINEMIA

This is the overproduction of IgM from malignant B cells leading to hyperviscosity. It presents with:

- Lethargy
- Blurry vision and vertigo
- **Engorged blood vessels in the eye**
- **Mucosal bleeding**
- Raynaud phenomenon

Anemia is common, but an IgM spike on SPEP results in hyperviscosity. There are no bone lesions. **Plasmapheresis is the best initial therapy** to remove the IgM and decrease viscosity. Long-term treatment is with chlorambucil or fludarabine and prednisone. Control the cells that make the abnormal immunoglobulins. Decrease the means of production.

[Handwritten notes in left margin:]

PLATELET PLUG
↓
FIBRIN PLUG

HEPARIN MONITORED w/ PTT

LMWH IS NOT MONITORED
↳ ANTI FACTOR XA IF WANT TO CHECK

WARFARIN INHIBITS
II, VII, IX, X, C, S

ASPIRIN — COX INHIBITOR   ACS POST-MI STROKE

CLOPIDIGREL — ADP BLOCK   IF CAN'T GIVE ASPIRIN

ABCICIXIMAB — GP IIb/IIIa BLOCK   POST MI

DIPYRIMADOLE — ADENOSINE lambe BLOCK

HEPARIN — BINDS ANTI-THROMBIN TO INCREASE ACTIVITY

LMWH — BINDS XA
(ENOXIPARIN)

WARFARIN — STOPS II,VII,IX,X PRODUCTION

DISCO STARTED IN 1972

BLEEDING DISORDERS

The first step in the evaluation of bleeding is determining if the bleeding seems related to platelets or clotting factors.

	Types of Bleeding	
1ST		**2ND**
Platelet bleeding	**Factor bleeding**
Superficial	Deep
Epistaxis, gingival, petechiae, purpura, mucosal surfaces such as the gums, vaginal bleeding	Joints and muscles

Idiopathic Thrombocytopenic Purpura

"WHAT IS THE MOST LIKELY DIAGNOSIS?"

Look for:

- Isolated thrombocytopenia (normal hematocrit, normal WBC count)
- **Normal-sized spleen**

[Handwritten:] ANTI PLATELET Abs

A 23-year-old woman comes to the emergency department with markedly increased menstrual bleeding, gum bleeding when she brushes her teeth, and petechiae on physical examination. Physical examination is otherwise normal. The platelet count is 17,000/µL.

What is the most appropriate next step in therapy?

a. Bone marrow biopsy
b. Intravenous immunoglobulins
c. Prednisone
d. Antiplatelet antibodies
e. Platelet transfusion

*Answer: The correct answer is **(C)**. The bleeding in this case is mild, meaning there is no intracranial bleeding or major GI bleeding, and the platelet is not profoundly low. Prednisone is the best initial therapy. Initiating prednisone is more important than checking for increased megakaryocytes or the presence of antiplatelet antibodies, which is characteristic of ITP.*

DIAGNOSTIC TESTS

Idiopathic thrombocytopenic purpura (ITP) is a diagnosis of exclusion. Occasional diagnostic tests are:

- Antiplatelet antibodies lack specificity, limited benefit.
- Ultrasound or CT scan to exclude hypersplenism
- **Megakaryocytes are elevated** in number.

Treatment	
Presentation	**Management**
No bleeding, count >30,000	No treatment
Mild bleeding, count <30,000	Glucocorticoids
Severe bleeding (GI/CNS), count <10,000	IVIG, Anti-Rho (anti-D) _PLASMAPHERESIS_
Recurrent episodes, steroid dependent	Splenectomy
Splenectomy or steroids not effective	Rituximab, azathioprine, cyclosporine, mycophenolate

TREATMENT

Romiplostim and eltrombopag are therapies for ITP when splenectomy fails. They are never used for acute treatment.

Before splenectomy, give vaccination to:

- *Neisseria meningitidis*
- *Hemophilus influenzae*
- Pneumococcus

Von Willebrand Disease (VWD)

DEFINITION

VWD is the most common inherited bleeding disorder with a decrease in the level or functioning of von Willebrand factor (VWF). It is autosomal dominant.

VWF & FACTOR VIII NOT MADE IN LIVER !!!!

"WHAT IS THE MOST LIKELY DIAGNOSIS?"

Look for bleeding related to platelets (epistaxis, gingival, gums) with a normal platelet count. VWD is markedly worsened after the use of aspirin. The aPTT may be elevated in half of patients.

DIAGNOSTIC TESTS

- **Bleeding time:** increased duration of bleeding
- **VWF (antigen) level may be decreased**
- **Ristocetin cofactor assay**: detects VWF dysfunction

TREATMENT

The **best initial therapy is DDAVP** (desmopressin), which releases subendothelial stores of VWF. If there is no response, use factor VIII replacement or VWF concentrate.

Hemophilia B → "Benign" → B-9 → IX

↑ PTT

DDAVP / specific factor

Hemophilia

Look for delayed joint or muscle bleeding in a male child, since the condition is X-linked recessive. Bleeding is delayed because the primary hemostatic plug is with platelets. The prothrombin time (PT) is normal and the aPTT is prolonged. Mixing studies with normal plasma will correct the aPTT to normal. The most accurate test is a specific assay for factor VIII or IX. Treat mild cases with DDAVP. Severe bleeding with very low levels of factor VIII or IX is treated with replacement of the specific factor.

Factor XI Deficiency

Most of the time, there is no increase in bleeding with factor XI deficiency. With trauma or surgery, there is increased bleeding. Look for a normal PT with a prolonged aPTT. Mixing study will correct the aPTT to normal, as occurs whenever there is a deficiency of clotting factors. Use fresh frozen plasma to stop the bleeding.

Factor XII Deficiency

These patients have an **elevated aPTT** but there is **no bleeding**. There is **no therapy** needed.

Disseminated Intravascular Coagulation

Disseminated intravascular coagulation (DIC) does not occur in otherwise healthy people. Look for a definite risk such as:

- Sepsis
- Burns
- Abruptio placenta or amniotic fluid embolus
- Snake bites
- Trauma resulting in tissue factor release
- Cancer

There is bleeding related to both clotting factor deficiency as well as thrombocytopenia.

DIAGNOSTIC TESTS

Look for:

- Elevation in both the PT and aPTT
- Low platelet count
- Elevated d-dimer and fibrin split products
- Decreased fibrinogen level (it has been consumed)

TREATMENT

Replace platelets if they are under 50,000/μL, as well as clotting factors, by using FFP. Heparin has no definite benefit. Cryoprecipitate may be effective to replace fibrinogen levels if FFP does not control bleeding.

HYPERCOAGUABLE STATES/ THROMBOPHILIA

The most common cause is factor V Leiden mutation. There is no difference in the intensity of anticoagulation. Use warfarin to an INR of 2 to 3 for 6 months.

Heparin Induced Thrombocytopenia

Heparin induced thrombocytopenia (HIT) is more common with the use of unfractionated heparin, but can still occur with low molecular weight heparin. HIT presents 5 to 10 days after the start of heparin with a marked drop in platelet count (more than 30%). Both venous and arterial thromboses can occur, although **venous clots are more common**. HIT rarely leads to bleeding. The platelets just precipitate out.

DIAGNOSTIC TESTS

HIT is confirmed with an ELISA for platelet factor 4 (PF4) antibodies or the serotonin release assay.

TREATMENT

1. Immediately **stop all heparin**-containing products. You cannot just switch unfractionated heparin to low molecular weight heparin.
2. Administer direct thrombin inhibitors: **argatroban, lepirudin,** and **bivalirudin**.
3. Warfarin should not be used first, but after a direct thrombin inhibitor is started, use warfarin.

> Do not transfuse platelets into those with HIT because it may worsen the thrombosis.

Antiphospholipid Syndromes

The 2 main syndromes are the lupus anticoagulant and the anticardiolipin antibody. **Both cause thrombosis.** Anticardiolipin antibodies are associated with multiple spontaneous abortions. The antiphospholipid (APL) syndromes are the only cause of thrombophilia with an abnormality in the aPTT.

The best **initial test is the mixing study**. Because it is a circulating inhibitor, the aPTT will remain elevated even after the mix. The most accurate test for the lupus anticoagulant is the Russell viper venom test.

Treat with heparin and warfarin as you would for any cause of DVT or pulmonary embolus. APL syndrome may require lifelong anticoagulation.

GASTROENTEROLOGY

8

ESOPHAGEAL DISORDERS

Dysphagia is the essential feature of the majority of esophageal disorders. **Dysphagia** means **difficulty** swallowing. **Odynophagia** is the proper term for **pain** while swallowing. Both dysphagia and odynophagia can lead to weight loss. Hence, weight loss cannot be used to answer the "What is the most likely diagnosis?" question.

When severe, some forms of esophageal disorders will also give anemia and heme-positive stool. When any of these **alarm** symptoms are present, **endoscopy should be performed** to exclude cancer.

Alarm symptoms indicating endoscopy include:

- Weight loss
- Blood in stool
- Anemia

Achalasia

DEFINITION/ETIOLOGY

Achalasia is the **inability of the lower esophageal sphincter (LES) to relax** due to a loss of the nerve plexus within the lower esophagus. The etiology is not clear. There is aperistalsis of the esophageal body.

"WHAT IS THE MOST LIKELY DIAGNOSIS?"

Look for:

- **Young** patient (under 50)
- Progressive dysphagia to **both** solids and liquids at the **same time**
- No association with alcohol and tobacco use

DIAGNOSTIC TESTS

- Barium esophagram will show a **"bird's beak"** as the esophagus comes down to a point.
- **Manometry** is the "most accurate test" and will show a failure of the lower esophageal sphincter to relax.
- Chest x-ray may show some abnormal **widening of the esophagus**, but chest x-ray is neither very sensitive nor very specific.
- **Upper endoscopy** shows **normal mucosa** in achalasia; however, endoscopy is useful in some patients to exclude malignancy.

Figure 8.1: Achalasia is from inadequate relaxation of the lower esophageal sphincter. Narrowing is seen at the end of the esophagus on barium study.
Source: Nishith Patel.

> In the esophagus, **only** cancer and Barrett esophagus are diagnosed by biopsy.

▶ **TIP**

In the esophagus, barium studies are acceptable to do first in most patients, although radiologic tests **always** lack the specificity of endoscopic procedures.

TREATMENT

Achalasia cannot exactly be "cured." Nothing can restore the normal function of the missing neurological control of the esophagus. All the treatment is based on simple mechanical dilation of the esophagus.

1. **Pneumatic dilation:** Place an endoscope with the ability to inflate a device that will enlarge the esophagus. Effective in more than 80% to 85% of patients.
2. **Botulinum toxin injection:** This will relax the lower esophageal sphincter, but the effects will wear off in about 3 to 6 months, requiring reinjection.
3. **Surgical sectioning** or **myotomy** can help to alleviate symptoms.

> Pneumatic dilation leads **to perforation** in less than 3% of patients.

Esophageal Cancer

"WHAT IS THE MOST LIKELY DIAGNOSIS?"

Look for:

- Age 50 or older
- Dysphagia **first for solids**, followed **later (progressing) to dysphagia for liquids**
- Association with prolonged alcohol and tobacco use
- More than 5 years of GERD symptoms

DIAGNOSTIC TESTS

1. Endoscopy is indispensible, since **only** a **biopsy can diagnose cancer**.
2. Barium **might** be the "best initial test," but **no** radiologic test can diagnose cancer.
3. CT and MRI scans are **not** enough to diagnose esophageal cancer; they are used to determine the extent of spread into the surrounding tissues.
4. PET scan is used to determine the contents of anatomic lesions if you are not certain whether they contain cancer. PET scan is often used to determine whether a cancer is resectable. Local disease is resectable, and widely metastatic disease is not.

> The single word *progressive* (or "from solids to liquids") is the **most** important clue to the diagnosis of esophageal cancer.

> For cancer, the radiologic test is **never** the "most accurate test."

TREATMENT

1. Surgical resection is **always** the thing to try. No resection (removal) = no cure.
2. Chemotherapy and radiation are used in **addition** to surgical removal.
3. **Stent placement** is used for lesions that cannot be resected surgically just to keep the esophagus open for **palliation** and to improve dysphagia.

Esophageal Spasm

The 2 forms of spastic disorders, diffuse esophageal spasm (DES) and nutcracker esophagus, are clinically indistinguishable. Both present with the **sudden onset of chest pain** that is not related to exertion. Therefore, at first it is impossible to distinguish them from some form of atypical coronary artery spasm or unstable angina. They can be **precipitated by drinking cold liquids**. The case will describe sudden, severe chest pain and the EKG and stress test will be normal.

Esophagram and endoscopy will be normal.

DES and nutcracker esophagus can be distinguished only by the most accurate test: **manometry**, which will show a different pattern of abnormal contraction in each of them.

Figure 8.2: Barium studies can show a corkscrew appearance at the time of the spasm.
Source: Conrad Fischer, MD.

TREATMENT

Esophageal spastic disorders are **treated with calcium channel blockers** and nitrates. This is similar to the treatment of Prinzmetal angina.

Infectious Esophagitis

A 43-year-old man recently diagnosed with AIDS comes to the emergency department with pain on swallowing that has become progressively worse over the last several weeks. There is no pain when not swallowing. His CD4 count is 43 mm³. The patient is not currently taking any medications.

What is the most appropriate next step in management?

a. Esophagram
b. Upper endoscopy
c. Oral nystatin swish and swallow
d. Intravenous amphotericin
e. Oral fluconazole

*Answer: The correct answer is (E). The most commonly asked infectious esophagitis question is esophageal candidiasis in a person with AIDS. Oral candidiasis (thrush) need **not** be present in order to have esophageal candidiasis. One does not automatically follow from the other. Although other infections such as CMV and herpes can also cause esophageal infection, over 90% of esophageal infections in patients with AIDS are caused by Candida. Empiric therapy with fluconazole is the best course of action. If fluconazole does not improve symptoms, then endoscopy is performed. Intravenous amphotericin is used for confirmed candidiasis not responding to fluconazole. Oral nystatin swish and swallow is not sufficient to control esophageal candidiasis. Nystatin treats oral candidiasis.*

Rings and Webs

Schatzki ring and Plummer-Vinson syndrome both give dysphagia. Schatzki ring is often from acid reflux and is associated with hiatal hernia. This is a type of scarring or tightening (also called peptic stricture) of the distal esophagus. Plummer-Vinson syndrome is associated with **iron deficiency anemia** and can rarely transform into **squamous cell cancer**. Plummer-Vinson syndrome is more proximal. Rings are easily detected on barium studies of the esophagus.

Figure 8.3: Schatzki ring is visible as a distal narrowing of the esophagus. This is easily found on barium studies.
Source: Azmeena Laila, MD.

Schatzki ring is associated with **intermittent dysphagia** and is treated with pneumatic dilation in an endoscopic procedure. Plummer-Vinson syndrome is treated with iron replacement at first, which may lead to resolution of the lesion.

> "Steakhouse syndrome" = dysphagia from solid food associated with Schatzki ring

Zenker Diverticulum

Zenker is an outpocketing of the posterior pharyngeal constrictor muscles. There is dysphagia, halitosis, and regurgitation of food particles. Some patients suffer from aspiration pneumonia when the contents of the diverticulum end up in the lung.

> Zenker is associated with **bad smell** and severe halitosis.

DIAGNOSTIC TESTS/TREATMENT

Zenker diverticulum is best **diagnosed with barium studies** and is repaired with surgery. There is **no** medical therapy.

▶ **TIP**

Do **not** answer nasogastric tube placement or upper endoscopy. These are dangerous to people with Zenker diverticulum and may cause perforation.

Scleroderma

These patients present with symptoms of **reflux** and have a clear history of scleroderma, or **progressive systemic sclerosis**. Manometry shows decreased lower esophageal sphincter pressure from an inability to close the LES. The management is with PPIs as it would be for any person with reflux symptoms. The disorder is simply one of mechanical immobility of the esophagus.

▶ **TIP**

Manometry is the answer for:

- Achalasia
- Spasm
- Scleroderma

Mallory-Weiss Tear

Mallory-Weiss tear presents with upper **gastrointestinal bleeding** after prolonged or severe **vomiting or retching**. Repeated retching is followed by hematemesis of bright red blood, or by black stool.

Mallory Weiss does **not** present with dysphagia. There is no specific therapy, and it will resolve spontaneously. Severe cases with persistent bleeding are managed with an injection of epinephrine to stop bleeding or the use of electrocautery.

> Mallory-Weiss is a **nonpenetrating** tear of only the mucosa.

EPIGASTRIC PAIN

DEFINITION

The epigastric area is the part of the abdominal surface just beneath the xiphoid process and in between the 2 sets of ribs. It is above the umbilicus. Pain in the epigastric area is common, occurring in as much as 25% of the population at some point in their lives. Tenderness, which is increased pain on palpation or pressure in the epigastric area, is far less common.

> The presence of **pain**, which is a **complaint** or **sensation** that is stated by the patient, is not the same thing as **tenderness**. Tenderness is a physical finding on examination.

A 44-year-old woman comes to see you because of pain in her epigastric area for the last several months. She denies nausea, vomiting, weight loss, or blood in her stool. On physical examination, you find no abnormalities.

What is the most likely diagnosis?

a. Duodenal ulcer disease
b. Gastric ulcer disease
c. Gastritis
d. Pancreatitis
e. Non-ulcer dyspepsia
f. Pancreatic cancer

*Answer: The correct answer is (E). This is often a **very** hard question for the average medical student. This is because of the selection bias of which cases you, as a student, see admitted to the hospital. Non-ulcer dyspepsia is, by far, the most common cause of epigastric pain and at a minimum accounts for 50% to 90% of all cases of epigastric pain. This is particularly true in patients under the age of 50.*

*In the hospital, you will see far more patients with ulcer disease, pancreatic disorders, or cancer because those are the ones who are admitted. Non-ulcer dyspepsia is virtually **never** a reason to be admitted to hospital.*

| How to Answer "What Is the Most Likely Diagnosis?" about Epigastric Pain ||
If this is in the history:	The most likely diagnosis is:
Pain worse with food	Gastric ulcer
Pain **better** with food	Duodenal ulcer
Weight loss	Cancer, gastric ulcer
Tenderness	Pancreatitis
Bad taste, cough, hoarse	Gastroesophageal reflux
Diabetes, bloating	Gastroparesis
Nothing	Non-ulcer dyspepsia

> Patients hospitalized with epigastric pain are far more likely to have ulcers, biliary disease, pancreatic disease, cancer, and gastritis with bleeding.

> Only endoscopy can **truly** give a precise diagnosis.

DIAGNOSTIC TESTS

Endoscopy is the only way to truly understand the **etiology of epigastric pain from ulcer disease**. Radiologic and barium testing are modest in accuracy at best. You cannot biopsy with radiologic testing.

▶ TIP

In the esophagus, barium studies may be a good place to start with testing, but in the stomach barium is very poor.

TREATMENT

Proton pump inhibitors (PPIs) are always a good place to start in the therapy of epigastric pain. There is no difference in the efficacy of different PPIs.

H2 blockers (ranitidine, nizatidine, cimetidine, famotidine) are **not** as effective, but will work in about 70% of patients.

Liquid antacids have roughly the same efficacy as H2 blockers.

Misoprostol, an artificial prostaglandin analogue, was developed just before the invention of PPIs. Misoprostol was designed to be especially good in preventing and treating NSAID-induced gastric damage. When PPIs arrived, misoprostol became obsolete.

> USMLE Step 2 CK does **not** test dosing.

GASTROESOPHAGEAL REFLUX DISEASE

DEFINITION/ETIOLOGY

Gastroesophageal reflux disease (GERD) is the **inappropriate relaxation of the lower esophageal sphincter**, resulting in the acid contents of the stomach coming up into the esophagus. Symptoms of GERD are worsened by nicotine, alcohol, caffeine, chocolate, peppermint, late-night meals, and obesity.

"WHAT IS THE MOST LIKELY DIAGNOSIS?"

GERD is the answer when you see "**epigastric burning pain** radiating up into the chest."

The patient also complains of **sore throat**, **bad taste** in the mouth (metallic), **hoarseness**, or **cough**.

> There are **no** unique physical findings in GERD. It is a symptom complex.

▶ **TIP**

You do not have to have **all** of these extra symptoms present in order to answer "GERD" as the most likely diagnosis.

A 42-year-old man comes to the office with several weeks of epigastric pain radiating up under his chest which becomes worse after lying flat for an hour. He also has a "brackish" taste in his mouth and a sore throat.

What is the most appropriate next step in the management of this patient?

a. *Ranitidine*
b. *Liquid antacid*
c. *Lansoprazole*
d. *Endoscopy*
e. *Barium swallow*
f. *24-hour pH monitoring*

*Answer: The correct answer is **(C)**. Lansoprazole is a PPI that should be used to control the symptoms of GERD. When the diagnosis is very clear (such as in this case), with epigastric pain **going under the sternum, bad taste**, and **sore throat**, confirmatory testing is not necessary. H2 blockers such as ranitidine are effective in about 70% of patients, but are clearly inferior to PPIs. Endoscopy does not diagnose GERD and is certainly not necessary when the diagnosis is so clear. Barium swallow shows major anatomic abnormalities of the esophagus and is worthless in GERD.*

DIAGNOSTIC TESTS

GERD is a symptom complex that is most often diagnosed based on patient history. In some patients in whom the diagnosis is not clear, 24-hour pH monitoring is done to confirm the etiology.

HIATAL HERNIA

- BARIUM SWALLOW

→ MILD → PPI

→ SURGERY
   ↳ NISSEN
   ↳ GASTROPEXY

Endoscopy is indicated when there is:

- Signs of obstruction such as dysphagia or odynophagia
- Weight loss
- Anemia or heme-positive stools
- More than 5 years of symptoms to exclude Barrett esophagus

GERD may also show redness, erosions, ulcerations, strictures, or Barrett esophagus.

> Endoscopy will show nothing when there is only pyrosis (heartburn).

TREATMENT

All patients should:

- Lose weight if obese.
- Avoid alcohol, nicotine, caffeine, chocolate, and peppermint.
- Avoid eating at night before sleep (within 3 hours of bedtime).
- Elevate head of bed 6 to 8 inches.

Mild or Intermittent Symptoms

Mild or intermittent symptoms may be treated with liquid antacids or H2 blockers.

Persistent Symptoms or Erosive Esophagitis

PPIs. There is no difference in efficacy between different PPIs.

Treatment of Those Not Responsive to Medical Therapy

About 5% of GERD patients do not respond to medical therapies. These patients may require surgical or anatomic correction to tighten the lower esophageal sphincter such as:

- **Nissen fundoplication:** wrapping the stomach around the lower esophageal sphincter
- Endocinch: using a scope to **place a suture around the LES** to tighten it
- Local **heat** or **radiation** of LES: causes scarring

BARRETT ESOPHAGUS

Long-standing GERD leads to histologic changes in the lower esophagus with columnar metaplasia. Columnar metaplasia usually needs at least **5 years** of reflux to develop. There are no unique physical findings or lab tests.

> Only endoscopy can determine the presence of Barrett esophagus.

DIAGNOSTIC TESTS/TREATMENT

Biopsy is the only way to be certain of the presence of Barrett esophagus and/or dysplasia. This is indispensible because the biopsy drives therapy. Columnar metaplasia with intestinal features has the greatest risk of transforming into esophageal cancer.

Each year, about 0.5% of people with **Barrett** esophagus progress to esophageal **cancer**.

Findings and Management

Finding	Management
Barrett alone (metaplasia)	PPIs and rescope every 2–3 years
Low-grade dysplasia	PPIs and rescope every 6–12 months
High-grade dysplasia	Ablation with endoscopy: photodynamic therapy, radiofrequency ablation

GASTRITIS

This is the inflammation or erosion of the gastric lining that is sometimes called **gastropathy**. Gastritis is caused by:

- Alcohol
- NSAIDs
- *Helicobacter pylori*
- Portal hypertension
- Stress such as burns, trauma, sepsis, and multiorgan failure (eg, **uremia**)

Atrophic gastritis is associated with vitamin B12 deficiency.

"WHAT IS THE MOST LIKELY DIAGNOSIS?"

Gastritis often presents with gastrointestinal **bleeding without pain**. Severe, erosive gastritis can present with epigastric pain. NSAIDs or alcoholism in the history is a clue.

> ▶ TIP
>
> You **cannot** answer the "most likely diagnosis" question from the history and physical alone.

There are no unique physical findings for gastritis.

Gastritis can present with almost any degree of bleeding from mild "coffee-ground" emesis, to large-volume vomiting of red blood, to black stool (melena).

Correlation of Manifestations with Volume of Bleeding

Manifestation	Volume of bleeding
Coffee-ground emesis	5–10 mL
Heme (guaiac) positive stool	5–10 mL
Melena	50–100 mL

DIAGNOSTIC TESTS/TREATMENT

Only upper endoscopy can definitively diagnose erosive gastritis. Although anemia may occur, there are no specific blood tests. Radiologic studies such as an upper gastrointestinal (GI) series will **not** be specific enough. **Capsule endoscopy is not appropriate** for upper GI bleeding if endoscopy is one of the choices.

Testing for *Helicobacter pylori* should be performed because this organism should be treated if it is associated with gastritis.

Testing for *Helicobacter pylori*		
The test	**What is good about this test?**	**What is bad about this test?**
Endoscopic biopsy	The most accurate of all the tests	Requires an invasive procedure such as endoscopy
Serology	Inexpensive, easily excludes infection if it is negative; no complications or procedures required	Lacks specificity; a positive test does not easily tell the difference between current and previous infection
Urea C^{13} or C^{14} breath testing	Positive only in active infection; noninvasive	Requires expensive equipment in office
***H. pylori* stool antigen**	Positive only in active infection; noninvasive	Requires stool sample

Treat with PPIs. H2 blockers, sucralfate, and liquid antacids are not as effective as PPIs. Sucralfate is an inert substance (aluminum hydroxide complex) that coats the stomach. If sucralfate is presented as a choice, it is nearly always the wrong answer. Misoprostol is a prostaglandin analogue that has some benefit in preventing NSAID-induced gastritis but is rarely used.

Stress ulcer prophylaxis is indicated in:

- Mechanical ventilation
- Burns
- Head trauma
- Coagulopathy

PEPTIC ULCER DISEASE

DEFINITION

The term *peptic ulcer disease* (PUD) refers to both duodenal ulcer and gastric ulcer disease. They cannot be distinguished definitively **without endoscopy**. The name is a misnomer based on the mistaken belief that they were caused by the protein-digesting enzyme pepsin.

ETIOLOGY

PUD is most commonly caused by *Helicobacter pylori*. NSAIDs are the second most common cause because of their effect in inhibiting the production of the protective mucus barrier in the stomach. NSAIDs inhibit prostaglandins and prostaglandins produce the mucus.

> NSAIDs produce more **bleeding** than pain.

Less common causes of peptic ulcers are:

- Burns
- Head trauma
- Crohn disease
- Gastric cancer
- Gastrinoma (Zollinger-Ellison syndrome)

▶ **TIP**

Alcohol and tobacco do **not** cause ulcers. They delay the healing of ulcers.

PRESENTATION/"WHAT IS THE MOST LIKELY DIAGNOSIS?"

PUD presents with recurrent episodes of epigastric pain that is described as dull, sore, and gnawing. Although the most common cause of upper GI bleeding is PUD, the majority of those with ulcers do not bleed. Tenderness and vomiting are unusual. You cannot answer PUD as the "most likely diagnosis" based on symptoms alone.

> There is no way to diagnose PUD without endoscopy or barium studies.

Duodenal ulcer (**DU**) disease is more often **improved with eating**, whereas gastric ulcer (**GU**) disease is more often **worsened by eating**. Hence, GU is associated with weight loss. You cannot definitively distinguish DU, GU, gastritis, and non-ulcer dyspepsia without endoscopy.

DIAGNOSTIC TESTS

Upper endoscopy is the most accurate test. Radiologic testing such as an upper GI series can detect ulcers, but cannot detect the presence of either cancer or *H. pylori*.

Helicobacter pylori Testing

Please see the table under "Gastritis."

In those who are to undergo endoscopy, there is no point in doing noninvasive testing such as serology, breath testing, or stool antigen detection methods. Biopsy is the answer to "What is the most accurate test?" for *H. pylori*. Endoscopy is the **only** method of detecting gastric cancer. **Cancer is present in 4% of those with GU** but in **none** of those with DU.

TREATMENT

PUD responds to PPIs in over 95% of cases, but will recur unless *H. pylori* is eradicated in those who are infected.

DU is associated with *H. pylori* in more than 80% to 90% of cases, but GU is associated with *H. pylori* in 50% to 70% of cases.

H. pylori is readily eradicated with PPIs in combination with 2 antibiotics. The "best initial therapy" is a PPI combined with clarithromycin and amoxicillin. In those who do not respond to therapy, metronidazole and tetracycline can be used as alternate antibiotics. **Adding bismuth** to a change of antibiotics **may aid in resolution** of treatment-resistant ulcers.

A 56-year-old woman comes to the clinic because her symptoms of epigastric pain from an endoscopically confirmed duodenal ulcer have not responded to several weeks of a PPI, clarithromycin, and amoxicillin.

What is the most appropriate next step in the management of this patient?

a. Refer for surgery
b. Switch the PPI to ranitidine
c. Abdominal CT scan
d. Capsule endoscopy
e. Urea breath testing
f. Vagotomy
g. Add sucralfate

Answer: The correct answer is (E). If there is no response to DU therapy with PPIs, clarithromycin, and amoxicillin, the first thought should be antibiotic resistance of the organism. Persistent H. pylori *infection can be detected with several methods such as urea breath testing, stool antigen detection, or a repeat endoscopy for biopsy. It would be very hard to choose between these, and that is why they are not all given as choices in this question.*

Capsule endoscopy cannot detect H. pylori. *Vagotomy and surgery were done more frequently in the past before we knew that* H. pylori *was the cause of most ulcers and we did not routinely eradicate it. H2 blockers and sucralfate add nothing to a PPI and have less efficacy, not more.*

Treatment of Refractory Ulcers

If the initial therapy does not resolve the DU, then detecting persistent *H. pylori* and switching the antibiotics to metronidazole and tetracycline is appropriate. For those **with GU, a repeat endoscopy is done to exclude cancer** as a reason for not getting better.

Treatment failure most often stems from:

- Nonadherence to medications
- Alcohol
- Tobacco
- NSAIDs

Gastric Ulcers

Ultimately, the most important reason to scope a patient is to exclude GU as a cause of the pain because of the possibility of cancer. The only way to exclude cancer is with biopsy. You can test for *H. pylori* with noninvasive methods and treat it, but you cannot exclude gastric cancer noninvasively.

What Is Different about GU versus DU?

- GU pain is more often **worsened by food**.
- GU is routinely **biopsied**.
- GU is associated with **cancer in 4%**.
- Routinely **repeating the endoscopy** to confirm healing is standard with GU.

NON-ULCER DYSPEPSIA

Non-ulcer (functional) dyspepsia is **epigastric pain that has no identified etiology**. This disorder can only be diagnosed after endoscopy. The pain of non-ulcer dyspepsia (NUD) can be identical to gastritis, PUD, gastric cancer, or reflux disease. If the patient is **under 45 years old, treat empirically** with antisecretory therapy such as PPIs and scope only if symptoms do not resolve. Endoscopy is definitely not indicated initially for those under 45. For those over 55, endoscopy is definitely indicated to exclude cancer. Between 45 and 55, the answer is unclear, so this type of case is unlikely to appear in Step 2.

Scope patients with dyspepsia if:

- Patient is over 45 to 55 years old
- "Alarm" symptoms are present (dysphagia, weight loss, anemia)

The cause of NUD is unknown. NUD is the most common cause of epigastric pain. The best initial therapy is with PPIs.

NUD is **not** definitely associated with *Helicobacter pylori*; however, if symptoms do not resolve with initial therapy and *H. pylori* is present, you should try to treat it.

There is no definite benefit to treating NUD with antibiotics to eradicate *Helicobacter*. Only about 10% of patients will experience an improvement in symptoms after *Helicobacter* is treated.

Non-ulcer dyspepsia is epigastric pain with a normal endoscopy.

GASTRINOMA (ZOLLINGER-ELLISON SYNDROME)

Less than 1% of those with ulcer disease have a gastrinoma.

"WHAT IS THE MOST LIKELY DIAGNOSIS?"

Look for a patient with ulcers that are:

- **Large** (>1–2 cm)
- **Recurrent** after *Helicobacter* eradication
- **Distal** in the duodenum
- **Multiple**

> Gastrinoma is often associated with **diarrhea** because **acid inactivates lipase**.

DIAGNOSTIC TESTS

Laboratory Tests

Once endoscopy confirms the presence of an ulcer, the most accurate diagnostic test is:

- **High gastrin levels** off antisecretory therapy (PPIs or H2 blockers) **with gastric acidity**
- High gastrin levels despite a high gastric acid output
- Persistent high gastrin levels despite injecting secretin

Any one of these 3 can be used to confirm the diagnosis of gastrinoma. The single most accurate test is always a functional test such as looking at the response to secretin.

> Hypercalcemia is the clue for multiple endocrine neoplasia from hyperparathyroidism.

Imaging

Once a diagnosis of gastrinoma is confirmed, the most important issue is to exclude metastatic disease. Ultrasound, CT, and MRI of the abdomen have poor sensitivity.

Somatostatin receptor scintigraphy (nuclear octreotide scan) is combined with **endoscopic ultrasound** to exclude metastatic disease.

> Gastrinoma is associated with a massive increase in the number of somatostatin receptors in the abdomen.

TREATMENT

Local disease is removed surgically. Metastatic disease is unresectable and is treated with lifelong PPIs to block acid production.

DIABETIC GASTROPARESIS

Long-standing diabetes leads to gastric dysmotility. Distention of the stomach and intestines is normally the most important stimulant to motility. Gastroparesis is an autonomic neuropathy leading to dysmotility. Dysmotility is from the inability to **sense** stretch in the GI tract.

"WHAT IS THE MOST LIKELY DIAGNOSIS?"

Look for a diabetic patient with chronic abdominal discomfort, "bloating," and constipation. There is also anorexia, nausea, vomiting, and early satiety.

A 64-year-old patient with diabetes for 20 years comes to the office with several months of abdominal fullness, intermittent nausea, constipation, and a sense of "bloating." On physical examination, a "splash" is heard over the stomach on auscultation of the stomach when moving the patient.

What is the most appropriate next step in the management of this patient?

a. Abdominal CT scan
b. Colonoscopy
c. Erythromycin
d. Upper endoscopy
e. Nuclear gastric emptying study

Answer: The correct answer is (C). When the diagnosis of diabetic gastroparesis seems clear, there is no need to do diagnostic testing unless there is a failure of therapy. Erythromycin and metoclopromide increase gastrointestinal motility. The most accurate test for diabetic gastroparesis is the nuclear gastric emptying study, although it is rarely needed.

GASTROINTESTINAL BLEEDING

A 69-year-old woman comes to the emergency department with multiple red/black stools over the last day. Her past medical history is significant for aortic stenosis. Her pulse is 115 per minute and her blood pressure is 94/62 mm Hg. The physical examination is otherwise normal.

What is the most appropriate next step in the management of this patient?

a. Colonoscopy
b. Nasogastric tube placement
c. Upper endoscopy
d. Bolus of normal saline
e. CBC
f. Bolus of 5% dextrose in water
g. Consult gastroenterology
h. Check for orthostasis

STOP

Answer: The correct answer is (D). The precise etiology of severe GI bleeding is not as important as a fluid resuscitation. There is no point in checking for orthostasis with the person's systolic blood pressure under 100 mm Hg or when there is a tachycardia at rest. Endoscopy should be performed, but it is not as important to do first as fluid resuscitation. When blood pressure is low, normal saline (NS) or Ringer lactate are better fluids to give than 5% dextrose in water (D5W). D5W does not stay in the vascular space to raise blood pressure as well as NS.

> USMLE Step 2 CK really wants you to know the order in which to do things. Sequence is indispensible.

ETIOLOGY

The most common cause of upper GI bleeding is **ulcer disease**, but it can also be caused by: gastritis, esophagitis, duodenitis, cancer, and varices.

The most common cause of lower GI bleeding is **diverticulosis**, but it can also be caused by:

- Angiodysplasia (arteriovenous malformation, or AVM)
- Polyps or cancer
- Inflammatory bowel disease
- Hemorrhoids
- Upper GI bleeding with rapid transit from high volume

> Assessing blood pressure is the most important initial management for GI bleeding.

Physical Findings

Orthostasis is defined as:

- More than a 10-point rise in pulse when going from lying down to sitting or standing up

or

- Blood pressure drop of 20 points or more when sitting up

Severity of Blood Loss Based on Hemodynamics	
Physical finding	**Percentage of blood loss**
Orthostasis	15%–20%
Pulse >100 per minute	30%
Systolic BP <100 mm Hg	30%

Variceal Bleeding

The only form of GI bleeding in which physical examination helps determine etiology is variceal bleeding. The presence of the signs of liver disease helps establish the diagnosis. Variceal bleeding is suspected when the case describes:

- Vomiting blood +/– black stool
- Spider angiomata and caput medusa

> Initial management of GI bleeding is **not based on the etiology**; it is **based on the severity.**

- Splenomegaly
- Palmar erythema
- Asterixis

DIAGNOSTIC TESTS

For acute bleeding, especially when the bleeding is severe, **it is far more important to replace fluids** and check the hematocrit, platelet count, and coagulation tests such as the prothrombin time (PT) or INR than it is to do an endoscopy.

Nasogastric Tube

The nasogastric (NG) tube can decompress the stomach by clearing out blood, which helps visualization during endoscopy. **Variceal bleeding may be the best time to use an NG tube**.

- If the stool is black but there is no hematemesis, an NG tube showing red blood tells you to use octreotide and arrange urgent endoscopy for possible "banding" of varices.

> If upper endoscopy will be done anyway, there is a limited role for an NG tube.

- Ten percent of those with red blood from the rectum have high-volume upper GI bleeding with "rapid transit time." NG tube can rapidly identify upper GI bleeding and hence, who needs upper endoscopy for banding before colonoscopy.

▶**TIP**

NG tube placement has very limited benefit. There is **no therapy to be delivered through the NG tube**, but it can guide where to start with endoscopy.

> Eighty percent of GI bleeding will stop spontaneously if the fluid resuscitation is adequate. Most patients die of inadequate fluid replacement.

Additional Diagnostic Tests for GI Bleeding	
Test	**Indication**
Nuclear bleeding scan	Endoscopy unrevealing in a massive acute hemorrhage
Angiography	Specific vessel or site of bleeding needs to be identified prior to surgery or embolization of the vessel; used only in massive, nonresponsive bleeding
Capsule endoscopy	Small bowel bleeding; upper and lower endoscopy do not show the etiology
CT or MRI of abdomen	Not useful in GI bleeding
EKG	Shows ischemia in severe bleeding

TREATMENT

1. **Fluid replacement** with high volumes (1 to 2 liters an hour) of saline or Ringer lactate in those with acute, severe bleeding
2. **Packed red blood cells** if the **hematocrit is below 30** in those who are older or suffer from coronary artery disease; if the patient is young, transfusion may not be needed until the hematocrit is very low (under 20–25)
3. **Fresh frozen plasma** if the PT or INR is elevated and active bleeding is occurring
4. **Platelets** if the count is **below 50,000 and** there is **bleeding**
5. **Octreotide for variceal bleeding**
6. Endoscopy to determine the diagnosis and administer some treatment (band varices, cauterize ulcers, inject epinephrine into bleeding gastric vessels)
7. IV PPI for upper GI bleeding
8. Surgery to remove the site of bleeding if fluids, blood, platelets, and plasma will not control the bleeding

▶ **TIP**

Platelets are transfused when the count is under 50,000/μl when there is active bleeding. You would not transfuse platelets to prevent a spontaneous bleed unless the count were much lower (below 10,000–20,000).

Esophageal and Gastric Varices

What do you do in addition to **fluids, blood, platelets, plasma**?

1. **Octreotide** (somatostatin) decreases portal pressure.
2. **Banding** performed by endoscopy obliterates esophageal varices.
3. Transjugular intrahepatic portosystemic shunting (**TIPS**) is used to decrease portal pressure in those who are not controlled by octreotide and banding.
4. **Propranolol** is used to **prevent** subsequent episodes of bleeding. Propranolol will not do anything for the current episode of bleeding.

> Sclerotherapy is **never** the right answer if **banding is technically possible.**

DIARRHEA

Antibiotic Associated Diarrhea

Although clindamycin may be associated with the highest incidence of antibiotic associated diarrhea and *Clostridium difficile* (C. diff), any antibiotic can potentially cause diarrhea. Blood and white cells may be present in the stool. It usually presents several days or weeks after the start of antibiotics. The best initial test is a stool C. diff toxin test. Metronidazole is the best initial therapy. If there is no response to metronidazole, the next step in management is to switch to oral vancomycin.

A 75-year-old man is admitted to the hospital with pneumonia. Several days after the start of antibiotics, he begins to have diarrhea. The stool C. diff toxin is positive and he is started on metronidazole, which leads to resolution of diarrhea over a few days. Two weeks later the diarrhea recurs and the C. diff toxin is again positive.

What is the most appropriate next step in the management of this patient?

a. Retreat with metronidazole orally
b. Use vancomycin orally
c. Sigmoidoscopy and treat only if pseudomembranes are found
d. Intravenous metronidazole
e. Wait for stool culture
f. Intravenous vancomycin

Answer: The correct answer is (A). Recurrent episodes of C. diff-associated diarrhea are best treated with another course of metronidazole. Intravenous metronidazole is used only if oral therapy cannot be used, such as in a patient with an adynamic ileus. Stool is never cultured for C. diff because it simply will not grow in culture. The difficulty in culturing C. diff is the source of the name of the organism. Endoscopy looking for pseudomembranes will diagnose antibiotic associated diarrhea, but is not a necessary step given the availability of stool toxin assay.

> Intravenous vancomycin is always wrong for antibiotic associated diarrhea since it will not pass the bowel wall.

▶ **TIP**

Switching to oral vancomycin is the answer when the case does not respond to metronidazole.

Malabsorption

Celiac disease is one of the most common types of malabsorption and can present as an adult. Chronic pancreatitis has a very similar presentation with fat malabsorption. Rare causes of fat malabsorption are tropic sprue and Whipple disease. All of these present with steatorrhea, defined as stool that is oily, greasy, floating, and foul smelling.

All forms of fat malabsorption present with deficiency of fat-soluble vitamins such as vitamins A, D, E, and K. Hence, they can all present with the following:

[handwritten: EtOH ABSORBED IN STOMACH]
[handwritten: B12 Terminal ileum]

Deficiencies and Manifestations	
Deficiency	**Manifestation**
Vitamin D	Hypocalcemia, osteoporosis
Vitamin K	Bleeding, easy bruising
Vitamin B_{12}	Anemia, hypersegmented neutrophils, neuropathy

[handwritten: ↳ SCHILLING TEST   STAGE 1=GIVE B12   STAGE 2 GIVE B12 + IF]

[handwritten: CELIAC SPRUE
Anti ENDOMYSIAL
Bx DUODENUM = BLUNTING OF VILLI]

▶ **TIP**

Fat malabsorption frequently presents with **weight loss**.

PRESENTATION

There is nothing **clinically** to distinguish tropic sprue from celiac disease (gluten-sensitive enteropathy).

Whipple Disease

→ BACTRIM FOR 1 YEAR

Whipple disease also presents with:

- Arthralgias
- Ocular findings
- Neurologic abnormalities (dementia, seizures)
- Fever
- Lymphadenopathy

DIAGNOSTIC TESTS

One of the main distinctions between chronic pancreatitis and gluten sensitive enteropathy is the presence of **iron deficiency**. This is because iron needs an intact bowel wall to be absorbed, but does not need pancreatic enzymes to be absorbed.

Unique Tests

Celiac disease:

- Anti-tissue transglutaminase (first test)
- IgA antigliadin antibody
- Antiendomysial antibody

The **most accurate diagnostic test** for celiac disease is a **small bowel biopsy** that shows flattening of the villi. Whipple disease and tropic sprue are also most accurately diagnosed with a bowel wall biopsy showing the specific organism.

Chronic Pancreatitis

Specific diagnostic tests are:

- **Abdominal x-ray:** 50% to 60% sensitive for calcification of the pancreas
- **Abdominal CT scan:** 80% to 90% sensitive for pancreatic calcification
- **Secretin stimulation testing:** This is the most accurate diagnostic test. Place a nasogastric tube; an unaffected pancreas will **release a large volume of bicarbonate-rich fluids** after the intravenous injection of secretin.

FECAL ELASTASE → LOW = CHRONIC PANC

PSEUDOCYSTS
CANCER

> Vitamin B$_{12}$ needs an intact bowel wall **and** pancreatic enzymes to be absorbed.

> Celiac disease gives dermatitis herpetiformis in 10% of cases.

> Bowel biopsy is essential in celiac disease to exclude lymphoma.

> The abdominal x-ray is very specific for chronic pancreatitis when the test is abnormal.

PANC. CA (EXOCRINE)

- PAINLESS JAUNDICE
- PALPABLE NON-TENDER GALLBLADDER
- PANCREATITIS
  TOBACCO
  FAM Hx
  HIGH FAT DIET
  DIABETES
  ♂
  OBESITY
  SEDENTARY LIFESTYLE

MARKERS
  CA 19-9
  CEA

IMAGING
  - ERCP
  - CT
  - ENDOSCOPIC U/S

TREATMENT
  RESECT w/ WHIPPLE
  ADJUVANT CHEMO

INSULINOMA
  HYPOGLYCEMIA
  ↑ C-PEPTIDE
  HARD TO SCAN
  RESECT

GLUCAGONOMA
  HYPERGLYCEMIA
  "REFRACTORY DM"
  HARD TO FIND
  RESECT

VIPoma
  LIKE CHOLERA

Figure 8.4: Chronic pancreatitis leads to calcification of the pancreas, visible in 50% to 60% of patients. *Source: Conrad Fischer, MD.*

Figure 8.5: Abdominal CT scan has greater sensitivity and specificity in the detection of calcifications of the pancreas. *Source: Conrad Fischer, MD.*

D-xylose testing: old test to distinguish pancreatitis from bowel wall abnormalities. D-xylose test results are normal in pancreatic disorders.

Treatment	
Disease	**Specific treatment**
Chronic pancreatitis	Enzyme replacement STOP EtOH/TOB OPIOIDS
Celiac disease	Avoid gluten-containing foods such as wheat, oats, rye, or barley
Whipple disease	Ceftriaxone, trimethoprim/sulfamethoxazole
Tropic sprue	Trimethoprim/sulfamethoxazole

Carcinoid Syndrome

Carcinoid syndrome presents with intermittent diarrhea in association with:

- **Flushing**
- **Wheezing**
- **Cardiac abnormalities** of the **right side** of the heart

The best initial diagnostic test is the urinary 5-hydroxyindoleacetic acid (5 HIAA) test. **Therapy is with octreotide**, which is a synthetic version of somatostatin used to control the diarrhea.

Lactose Intolerance

No weight loss is associated with lactose intolerance because lactose is only one of several sugars to absorb. Lactose intolerance does not alter the absorption of any other nutrient such as fat so there is **no deficiency in calories**. Vitamins are absorbed normally. The stool osmolality is increased, but the usual way to make the diagnosis is simply to remove all milk-containing products from the diet and wait a single day for resolution of symptoms. Avoiding milk products except yogurt is the therapy. Using **oral lactase replacement** is also good therapy and is available over the counter.

[handwritten: MCC. CHRONIC DIARRHEA]

IRRITABLE BOWEL SYNDROME

Irritable bowel syndrome (IBS) is a **pain syndrome** that can have **diarrhea, constipation,** or **both.** There is no specific diagnostic test and it is a diagnosis of exclusion in association with a complex of symptoms. **IBS is not associated with weight loss.** Pain does not automatically mean malabsorption.

The **pain** of IBS is:

- **Relieved by a bowel movement**
- **Less at night**
- **Relieved by a change in bowel habit** such as diarrhea

[handwritten: → RULE OUT EVERYTHING ELSE]

TREATMENT

1. Fiber in the diet
2. Antispasmodic agents such as:
   - **Hyoscyamine**
   - **Dicyclomine**
3. Tricyclic antidepressants (eg, amitriptyline)
4. Antimotility agents such as loperamide for diarrhea
5. Lubiprostone (chloride channel activator that increases bowel movement frequency)

> IBS is **not** associated with blood or white cells in the stool.

INFLAMMATORY BOWEL DISEASE

Inflammatory bowel disease (IBD) is an idiopathic disorder that presents with diarrhea, blood in the stool, weight loss, and fever. Both Crohn disease (CD) and ulcerative colitis (UC) have extraintestinal manifestations that can be identical in both diseases. These are:

- Arthralgias
- Uveitis, iritis

> Erythema nodosum is an indicator of disease activity.

- Skin manifestation (erythema nodosum, pyoderma gangrenosum)
- Sclerosing cholangitis (more frequent in UC)

Both forms of IBD can lead to colon cancer. The risk of colon cancer is related to the duration of involvement of the colon. CD that involves the colon has the same risk of colon cancer as UC.

Differences between CD and UC	
Crohn disease	**Ulcerative colitis**
Skip lesions	Curable by surgery
Transmural granulomas	Entirely mucosal
Fistulas and abscesses	No fistulas, no abscesses
Masses and obstruction	No obstruction
Perianal disease	No perianal disease

▶ **TIP**

Frequent question: **When** should screening occur?

Answer: After 8 to 10 years of colonic involvement, with colonoscopy every 1 to 2 years.

DIAGNOSTIC TESTS

Endoscopy is the most accurate test when the disease can be reached by a scope. For CD that is mainly in the small bowel, radiologic tests such as barium studies will detect the lesions. When the diagnosis is still unclear, serologic testing may be helpful. All IBD is associated with anemia.

ANCA and ASCA Results in IBD		
Test	**Crohn disease**	**Ulcerative colitis**
Antineutrophil cytoplasmic antitibody (ANCA)	Negative	Positive
Antisaccharomyces cerevesiae antibody (ASCA)	Positive	Negative

TREATMENT

Acute exacerbations of disease are treated with steroids in both CD and UC. Chronic maintenance of remission is with 5-ASA derivatives such as mesalamine. Asacol (mesalamine; Procter & Gamble, Cincinnati, Ohio) is used for UC and Pentasa (mesalamine; Shire, Wayne, Pennsylvania) for CD. Rowasa (mesalamine; Alaven, Marietta, Georgia) is for UC largely limited to the rectum.

→ **Azathioprine and 6-mercaptopurine are used to wean patients off of steroids** when the disease is so severe that severe recurrences develop as the steroids are stopped.

Perianal CD is treated with ciprofloxacin and metronidazole.

Fistulae and severe disease unresponsive to other agents is treated with anti-tumor necrosis factor (TNF) agents such as **infliximab**. Surgery is done for fistulae only if there is no response to anti-TNF agents.

Neither form of IBD is routinely treated with surgery. UC can be cured, however, with colectomy. In CD, surgery is used exclusively for bowel obstruction. CD will tend to recur at the site of the surgery.

DIVERTICULAR DISORDERS

Diverticulosis   Mcc. Acute GI Blee in >40 y.o.

Outpocketings of the colon are so common on a standard meat-filled diet as to be routinely expected in those above 65 to 70 years of age. Vegetarians rarely develop diverticulosis. Diverticulosis is asymptomatic most of the time. Patients may present with left lower quadrant abdominal pain, constipation, bleeding, and sometimes infection (diverticulitis).

The most accurate test is colonoscopy. Barium studies are acceptable, but not as accurate.

Bran, psyllium, methylcellulose, and increased **dietary fiber** are used to decrease the rate of progression and complications.

Diverticulitis

The "most likely diagnosis" question is easily answered when presented with an older patient with:

- Left lower quadrant pain and **tenderness**
- **Fever**
- **Leukocytosis**
- Palpable mass sometimes occurs

Symptoms such as nausea, constipation, and bleeding can be present, but are too nonspecific to be useful in establishing a diagnosis. The best initial test is a CT scan.

> Colonoscopy and barium enema are **dangerous** in acute diverticulitis because of increased risk of perforation. Infection weakens the colonic wall.

TREATMENT

Treatment for diverticulitis is with antibiotics that will cover the *E. coli* and anaerobes that are present in the bowel such as:

- **Ciprofloxacin combined with metronidazole**

Or the beta-lactam/beta-lactamase combinations such as:

- Amoxicillin/clavulanate

- Ticarcillin/clavulanate
- Piperacillin/tazobactam

Surgery is the answer when there is:

- No response to medical therapy
- Frequent recurrences of infection
- Perforation, fistula formation, abscess, strictures, or obstruction

Who is more likely to get a recommendation of surgery: young or old patients? Younger patients should have the colon resected more often because of the greater total number of recurrent episodes that will occur. Diverticular disease does **not** disappear despite treating episodes of diverticulitis or the use of fiber in the diet.

> Patients with acute diverticulitis should not be fed.

COLON CANCER SCREENING

Ninety-five percent of colon cancer deaths are preventable with screening.

Which of the following is the most effective method of screening for colon cancer?

a. Colonoscopy
b. Sigmoidoscopy
c. Fecal occult blood testing (FOBT)
d. Barium enema
e. Virtual colonoscopy with CT scanning
f. Capsule endoscopy

Answer: The correct answer is (A). Since 40% of colon cancer occurs proximal to the rectum and sigmoid colon, sigmoidoscopy is not nearly as sensitive in detecting lesions as colonoscopy. Barium studies, CT colonoscopy, and capsule endoscopy do not allow for biopsy. FOBT has more false positives and false negatives than colonoscopy. In addition, a positive FOBT must be followed up with colonoscopy.

Capsule endoscopy is used to detect sources of bleeding in the small bowel not reachable by endoscopy.

> Virtual colonoscopy is **never** the correct answer for anything.

Frequency of Screening

Routine testing: Patients should have a colonoscopy every 10 years beginning at age 50.

Screening with a Family History of Colon Cancer

Single family member: Begin 10 years earlier than the age at which the family member developed their cancer or age **40**, whichever is **younger**.

Three family members, 2 generations, 1 premature (before 50): Hereditary nonpolyposis colon cancer syndrome (HNPCC) comprises these factors. Start screening at age 25 with colonoscopy every 1 to 2 years.

[handwritten margin note: CEA TUMOR MARKER (ALSO IN GASTRIC CA & PANCREATIC CA)]

Familial adenomatous polyposis (FAP): FAP is defined as the presence of thousands of polyps with an abnormal genetic test known as the adenomatous polyposis coli (APC) test. **Start screening with sigmoidoscopy at age 12** every year.

Previous single adenomatous polyp: Patient should have a colonoscopy every 3 to 5 years.

Previous history of colon cancer: Patient should have colonoscopy at 1 year after resection, then at 3 years, then every 5 years.

Other Polyposis Syndromes

Peutz-Jeghers Syndrome

Peutz-Jeghers syndrome is characterized by multiple hamartomatous polyps in association with:

- **Melanotic spots** on the lips and skin
- Increased frequency of breast cancer
- Increased gonadal and pancreatic cancer

Gardner Syndrome

APC ABNORMAL

Gardner syndrome is colon cancer in association with:

- **Osteomas**
- Desmoid tumors
- Other soft tissue tumors

Turcot Syndrome   *"TURBAN ON HEAD"*

APC ABNORMAL

Turcot syndrome is colon cancer in association with:

- CNS malignancy

Juvenile Polyposis

Juvenile polyposis is colon cancer in association with:

- Multiple hamartomatous polyps

> None of these polyposis syndromes (Peutz-Jeghers syndrome, Gardner syndrome, Turcot syndrome, juvenile polyposis) requires increased frequency of screening.

ACUTE PANCREATITIS

DEFINITION/ETIOLOGY

Acute pancreatitis is an acute inflammation of the pancreas, with over 90% caused by alcoholism and cholelithiasis.

Less common causes of acute pancreatitis include:

- **Trauma**
- Hypertriglyceridemia
- Hypercalcemia

- Infection
- Drug toxicity (pentamidine, didanosine, azathioprine, estrogens)
- Drug allergy (sulfa drugs such as furosemide and **hydrochlorothiazide**)
- Ductal obstruction, endoscopic retrograde cholangiopancreatography (ERCP), cystic fibrosis
- Scorpion sting

> Pancreatitis: a stone, a stricture, tumor, and obstruction.

PRESENTATION/"WHAT IS THE MOST LIKELY DIAGNOSIS?"

Acute epigastric **pain** + **tenderness** + nausea/**vomiting** = **pancreatitis**

In severe cases there is hypotension and fever.

▶ **TIP**

The pain of pancreatitis goes **straight through** to the back "like a spear" stabbed into the abdomen. Cholecystitis pain goes **around the side** to the back.

Which of the following is associated with the worst prognosis in pancreatitis?

a. Elevated amylase
b. Elevated lipase
c. Intensity of the pain
d. Low calcium
e. C-reactive protein (CRP) rising

Answer: The correct answer is (D). Severe pancreatic damage decreases lipase production and release leading to fat malabsorption in the gut. Calcium binds with fat (saponifies) in the bowel, leading to calcium malabsorption. Although amylase and lipase are elevated in pancreatitis, there is no correlation between the height of these enzyme levels and disease severity.

> CRP has never shown definite correlation with severity in any disease.

Pain intensity is subjective and does **not** correlate with the degree of organ damage.

DIAGNOSTIC TESTS

The **best initial tests** are amylase and lipase.

The **most specific test** is CT scan.

Disease severity strongly correlates with the degree of necrosis seen on CT scanning. Needle biopsy is indispensible in determining the presence of infection in those who have extensive necrosis.

> Greater than 30% necrosis = "extensive" necrosis

Laboratory Tests

- **CBC:** Leukocytosis, drop in hematocrit over time with rehydration
- Elevated LDH and AST

- Hypoxia, hypocalcemia
- Elevated urinary trypsinogen activation peptide

Imaging

- CT or MRI scan are best. These also detect pseudocysts.
- ERCP is useful in determining the etiology of the disease (stones, stricture, tumor).
- Plain x-ray shows a sentinel loop of bowel (air-filled piece of small bowel in left upper quadrant).
- Ultrasound has very poor accuracy; overlying bowel blocks precise imaging. → GOOD TO FIND STONES THOUGH

> Abdominal CT scan is always performed with IV and oral contrast to better define and outline abdominal structures.

TREATMENT

- NPO (no food)
- IV hydration
- Analgesia
- PPIs decrease pancreatic stimulation from acid entering the duodenum

If there is more than **30% necrosis on CT** or MRI, **adding antibiotics such as imipenem** may decrease mortality by decreasing the development of infected, necrotic pancreatitis. Severe necrosis is an indication for needle biopsy to determine the presence of infection.

Pseudocysts are drained with a needle if they are enlarging or painful.

ERCP is used to:

- Remove obstructing stones and dilate strictures
- Place stents

> Infected, necrotic pancreatitis should be resected with surgical debridement to prevent ARDS and death.

LIVER DISEASE

All forms of chronic liver disease can produce:

- Ascites
- Coagulopathy (all clotting factors except VIII are made in liver)
- **Asterixis** and encephalopathy
- Hypoalbuminemia and edema
- Spider angiomata and palmar erythema
- Portal hypertension leading to varices
- **Thrombocytopenia** from splenic sequestration
- Renal insufficiency (hepatorenal syndrome)
- **Hepatopulmonary syndrome**

Ascites

Paracentesis should be performed if there is:

- New-onset ascites
- Abdominal pain and tenderness
- Fever

Portal hypertension from cirrhosis is the etiology of the ascitic fluid if there is a low albumin level in the fluid. The difference or "gradient" between the serum and ascites is also called the serum ascites albumin gradient (SAAG). If the SAAG is above 1.1, it is highly suggestive of portal hypertension.

SAAG: Correlating Level with Specific Diseases	
<1.1 g/dL	**>1.1 g/dL**
• Infections (except SBP) • Cancer • Nephrotic syndrome	• Portal hypertension • CHF • Hepatic vein thrombosis • Constrictive pericarditis

Spontaneous Bacterial Peritonitis

Spontaneous bacterial peritonitis (SBP) is **infection without a perforation** of the bowel. We don't actually know how the bacteria gets there. *E coli* is the most common organism. Anaerobes are rarely the cause of SBP. Pneumococcus, a respiratory pathogen, causes SBP for unknown reasons.

Best initial test: **Cell count with more than 250 neutrophils** is the basis upon which we start therapy.

Gram stain is almost always negative. Fluid culture is the most accurate test, but the results are never available at the time we have to make a treatment decision.

LDH level is too nonspecific.

Treatment of SBP is with **cefotaxime**.

SBP frequently recurs. When the ascites fluid albumin level is quite low, prophylactic norfloxacin or trimethoprim/sulfamethoxazole is used to prevent SBP.

Treatment of Specific Features of Cirrhosis

Feature	Treatment
Ascites and edema	Spironolactone and other diuretics. Serial paracenteses for large-volume ascites.
Coagulopathy and thrombocytopenia	FFP and/platelets only if bleeding occurs
Encephalopathy	Lactulose and neomycin
Hypoalbuminemia	No specific therapy
Spider angiomata and palmar erythema	No specific therapy
Varices	Propranolol and banding via endoscopy
Hepatorenal syndrome	Somatostatin (octreotide), midodrine
Hepatopulmonary syndrome	No specific therapy

Hepatopulmonary Syndrome

This is lung disease and hypoxia entirely on the basis of liver failure. Look for **orthodeoxia**, which is hypoxia upon sitting upright. There is no specific therapy.

SPECIFIC CAUSES OF CIRRHOSIS

Alcoholic Liver Disease

This is a diagnosis of exclusion. There is no specific therapy. The most accurate test, as with most of the causes of cirrhosis except for sclerosing cholangitis, is a liver biopsy.

Alcohol, like all drugs causing liver disease, gives a greater elevation in AST compared to ALT. Viral hepatitis gives a higher ALT than AST. Binge drinking gives a sudden rise in GGTP.

Primary Biliary Cirrhosis

Answer primary biliary cirrhosis (PBC) as the "most likely diagnosis" when the question describes:

- Woman in 40s or 50s   *ASSOCIATED WITH AUTO IMMUNE DISEASE*
- Fatigue and itching
- Normal bilirubin with an elevated alkaline phosphatase

Most unique features of PBC are:

- Xanthelasma/xanthoma
- Osteoporosis

AMA Ab's

DIAGNOSTIC TESTS/TREATMENT

A liver biopsy is the most accurate test. The most accurate **blood** test is the **antimitochondrial antibody**. Bilirubin and IgM levels do not elevate until the disease is very far advanced. Treat PBC with **ursodeoxycholic acid**.

Primary Sclerosing Cholangitis

Over 80% of primary sclerosing cholangitis (PSC) occurs in association with inflammatory bowel disease. Look for:

- Pruritus
- Elevated alkaline phosphatase and GGTP as well as elevated bilirubin level

Early PSC can look just like PBC. The bilirubin level can be normal in early disease.

The most accurate test is an ERCP that shows beading, narrowing, or strictures in the biliary system. You can diagnose PSC from a biopsy if it was done for other reasons, but biopsy is not essential for establishing the diagnosis. Treat with cholestyramine or ursodeoxycholic acid, the same as PBC.

> PSC is the **only** cause of cirrhosis for which a biopsy is **not** the most accurate test.

▶ TIP
PSC does **not** improve or resolve with resolution of the IBD. Even after a colectomy in ulcerative colitis, the patient may still progress to needing a liver transplantation.

Alpha 1-Antitrypsin Deficiency

Look for the combination of **liver disease** and **emphysema (COPD)** in a **young patient** (under 40) who is a **nonsmoker**. They may throw in a family history of COPD at an early age. Treat by replacing the enzyme. The most frequently asked question is "What is the most likely diagnosis?"

Hemochromatosis

This is a genetic disorder leading to **overabsorption of iron in the duodenum**. The mutation is the C282y gene.

Men present earlier than women because **menstruation delays the onset** of liver fibrosis and cirrhosis.

> Hemochromatosis **may be found on routine testing** with mildly abnormal liver function tests (LFTs) or iron levels.

PRESENTATION

Look for a patient in his 50s with mild increases in AST and alkaline phosphatase and:

- Fatigue and joint pain (pseudogout)
- Erectile dysfunction in men, and amenorrhea in women (from pituitary involvement)
- Skin darkening

> *Vibrio vulnificus, Yersina,* and *Listeria* infections occur because these organisms feed on iron.

- Diabetes
- Cardiomyopathy

DIAGNOSTIC TESTS

The best initial test is iron studies that show:

- Increased serum iron and ferritin
- Decreased iron binding capacity

The most accurate test is a liver biopsy for increased iron. The EKG may show conduction defects and the echocardiogram can show dilated or restrictive cardiomyopathy.

A 54-year-old man has been evaluated in the office for fatigue, erectile dysfunction, and skin darkening. He is found to have transferrin saturation (iron divided by TIBC) above 50%. His AST is 2 times the upper limit of normal.

What would you do next to confirm the diagnosis?

a. Echocardiography
b. Glucose level
c. Abdominal MRI and HFE (C282y) gene testing
d. Liver biopsy
e. Prussian blue stain of the bone marrow
f. Deferoxamine
g. Deferasirox

Answer: The correct answer is (C). MRI will show increased iron deposition in the liver. An abnormal MRI combined with an abnormal genetic test for hemochromatosis can spare the patient the need for a liver biopsy. There is an association with diabetes; however, glucose levels will not confirm a diagnosis of hemochromatosis. Prussian blue is the stain of blood cells for iron. Prussian blue is also used to diagnose sideroblastic anemia.

Iron chelation therapy is used in hemochromatosis for those who:

1. Cannot be managed with phlebotomy
2. Are anemic and have hemochromatosis from overtransfusion such as thalassemia

Deferoxamine and deferasirox should not be started until the diagnosis is confirmed. Deferasirox is a huge breakthrough medication because it is effective orally. Deferoxamine has to be given lifelong by injection.

TREATMENT

Phlebotomy is clearly the best therapy for those with overabsorption of iron.

> Liver fibrosis can resolve if phlebotomy is begun before cirrhosis develops.

Chronic Hepatitis B and C

There are no specific physical findings to allow you to answer "What is the most likely diagnosis?" without blood testing. Both chronic hepatitis B and C are associated with developing cirrhosis and liver cancer. Both can be associated with polyarteritis nodosa.

DIAGNOSTIC TESTS

Chronic hepatitis B has surface antigen positive for longer than 6 months as a matter of definition. Most cases are e-antigen positive as well. Hepatitis B DNA level by PCR is the best way to determine viral replication activity. Biopsy to detect "bridging necrosis" no longer has any significant meaning.

In over 80% of patients with hepatitis C, the infection persists as chronic infection. Since the acute viral illness is not felt with hepatitis C, there is no precise way to determine the time course of the infection. Most patients with chronic hepatitis C were never symptomatic. Hence, you cannot ask how long someone has had it and get a precise answer. Hepatitis C PCR RNA viral load is the most accurate way of determining disease activity.

> ▶ **TIP**
>
> The questions on chronic hepatitis are most likely to be treatment questions.

TREATMENT

Treat chronic hepatitis B with any **one** of the following agents:

- Adefovir
- Lamivudine
- Telbivudine
- Entecavir
- Tenofovir
- Interferon

To treat chronic hepatitis C, use a **combination** of interferon and ribavirin.

Adverse Effects of Hepatitis Medications	
Drug	**Adverse effects**
Interferon	Arthralgias, thrombocytopenia, depression, leukopenia
Ribavirin	Anemia
Adefovir	Renal dysfunction
Lamivudine	None

Wilson Disease

This is a disorder of abnormally decreased copper excretion from the body. Because of a decrease in ceruloplasmin, copper is not excreted and it builds up in the body in the liver, kidney, red blood cells, and the nervous system.

"WHAT IS THE MOST LIKELY DIAGNOSIS?"

In addition to all the previously described features of cirrhosis and hepatic insufficiency, you will answer Wilson disease as the diagnosis if you see:

Terms such as chronic "active" or chronic "persistent" hepatitis are no longer relevant.

Liver biopsy determines the degree of inflammation and fibrosis. Biopsy can help you understand the urgency for treatment if fibrosis is present or worsening.

*Combination therapy has **not** been proven to be more effective than monotherapy in hepatitis B.*

- Neurological symptoms: psychosis, tremor, dysarthria, ataxia, or seizures
- **Coombs negative hemolytic anemia**
- Renal tubular acidosis or nephrolithiasis

▶ **TIP**

Wilson disease gives psychosis and delusions—**not** the encephalopathic features or delirium that you would get with any form of liver failure.

Diagnostic Tests

The best initial test is a **slit-lamp** examination for **Kayser-Fleischer rings**, a brownish ring around the eye from copper deposition. Liver biopsy is more sensitive and specific and will detect abnormally increased hepatic copper.

Copper deposits in Descemet's membrane

Figure 8.6: Copper deposits in the Descemet membrane give a brownish ring around the outer edge of the cornea. *Source: Nishith Patel.*

The most accurate diagnostic test is looking at an abnormally increased amount of copper excretion into the urine after giving penicillamine.

Treatment

Penicillamine will chelate copper and remove it from the body. Additional therapies are:

- **Zinc: interferes with intestinal copper absorption**
- Trientine: an alternate copper-chelating compound

> Decreased ceruloplasmin level is not the most accurate test. This is the most common wrong answer. All plasma proteins can be decreased in those with liver dysfunction and cirrhosis.

Autoimmune Hepatitis

Look for young women with signs of liver inflammation with a positive ANA. More specific tests are liver-kidney microsomal antibodies and **anti-smooth muscle antibodies**. The most accurate test is the liver biopsy. Treat with prednisone and or azathioprine.

Nonalcoholic Steatohepatitis or Nonalcoholic Fatty Liver Disease

Nonalcoholic steatohepatitis is an extremely common cause of mildly abnormal liver function tests. The biopsy is the most accurate test and shows the microvesicular fatty deposits you would find in alcoholic liver disease, but without the history of alcohol use.

This disorder is associated with:

- Obesity
- Diabetes
- Hyperlipidemia
- Corticosteroid use

The most important issue is to exclude more serious liver disease. Management is with correcting the underlying causes previously described. There is no specific drug therapy to reverse it.

NEUROLOGY

9

STROKE

DEFINITION

Stroke is the sudden onset of a neurological deficit from the death of brain tissue. Stroke is the third most common cause of death in the United States. The **risk factors** for stroke are the same as those for myocardial infarction: **hypertension**, **diabetes**, **hyperlipidemia**, and **tobacco** smoking. *& HYPER COAGUABLE*

TIA = STROKE < 24 HOURS

ETIOLOGY

Stroke is caused by a **sudden blockage in the flow of blood to the brain** in 85% of cases and by bleeding in 15% of cases. A cerebral vessel is blocked either by a thrombosis occurring in the vessel or by an embolus to the vessel. **Emboli** originate from:

- **Heart:** atrial fibrillation, valvular heart disease, or a DVT paradoxically getting into the brain through a patent foramen ovale (PFO).
- **Carotid stenosis**

PRESENTATION

Middle cerebral artery (MCA) stroke (more than 90% of cases):

- **Weakness or sensory loss** on the **opposite (contralateral) side** of the stroke.
- **Homonymous hemianopsia:** loss of visual field on the opposite side of the stroke. A left-sided MCA stroke results in loss of the right visual fields. The eyes can't see the right side, so the eyes deviate to the left. Hence the **eyes "look towards the side of the lesion."**
- **Aphasia** if the stroke occurs on the same side as the speech center. This is the left side in 90% of patients.

Speech is controlled by the same side as "handedness." Right-handed people (left brain dominant) have a speech center on the left-hand side of the brain.

AICA
- FACIAL PARALYSIS
- DEAFNESS / TINNITUS
- NYSTAGMUS / VERTIGO

PICA (WALLENBERG)
- CONTRALATERAL PAIN/TEMP LOSS IN BODY
- IPSILATERAL FACE LOSS OF PAIN/TEMP
- IPSILAT ATAXIA & PAST POINTING

Anterior cerebral artery (ACA) stroke:

- **Personality/cognitive defects such as confusion**
- **Urinary incontinence**
- **Leg more than arm weakness** CONTRALATERAL

Posterior cerebral artery (PCA) stroke:

- **Ipsilateral sensory** loss of the face, ninth and 10th cranial nerves
- **Contralateral sensory** loss of the limbs
- Limb **ataxia**
  VISUAL DEFECTS

DIAGNOSTIC TESTS

RULE OUT HEMORRHAGIC STROKE

The **best initial test in any kind of stroke is a CT scan** of the head without contrast. The most accurate test is an MRI. CT scan is done first, not because it is the most sensitive test for stroke, but in order to exclude hemorrhage as a cause of the stroke prior to initiating treatment. CT scan needs 4 to 5 days to reach greater than 95% sensitivity. MRI needs only 24 to 48 hours to reach greater than 95% sensitivity.

FIND CAUSE
- CAROTID DOPPLER
- ECHO
- MRI ???
- ANGIOGRAM

Figure 9.1: Nonhemorrhagic stroke is characterized by edema without blood. *Source: Mohammad Maruf, MD.*

TREATMENT

The best initial therapy for a nonhemorrhagic stroke is:

- **Less than 3 hours since onset of stroke: thrombolytics** ➜
- **More than 3 hours since onset of stroke: aspirin**
- **Hemorrhagic stroke: nothing**
  ↳ MANNITOL / HYPERVENTILATE / HOB TO 30°
  ↳ REVERSE ANTICOAGULATION
  ↳ NEUROSURG ?

FIRST TIA - ASPIRIN

If the patient is already on aspirin at the time of the stroke, the answer is:

- **Add** dipyridamole

or

- **Switch** to clopidogrel   *ESPECIALLY W/ CAD*
  (PLAVIX)

> Hemorrhagic stroke has no treatment to reverse it. Surgical drainage will not help.

Figure 9.2: Acute blood appears white on a CT scan. Contrast is not needed to detect blood. *Source: Saba Ansari, MD.*

Evaluation of Causes of Stroke and Their Treatment

Echocardiogram:

- Surgical replacement or repair of certain damaged valves
- Thrombi: heparin followed by warfarin to an INR of 2 to 3

EKG: Atrial fibrillation or flutter is treated with warfarin to an INR of 2 to 3 as long as the arrhythmia persists.

Holter monitor (24 to 48 hour ambulatory EKG): If the initial EKG is normal, a Holter monitor should be performed to detect atrial arrhythmias with greater sensitivity.

Carotid duplex ultrasound: Carotid stenosis is a frequent cause of emboli to the brain. If a patient has **symptomatic cerebrovascular disease and more than 70% stenosis** is detected, surgical correction of the narrowing should be performed. Endarterectomy is superior to carotid angioplasty. **Endarterectomy has no value for milder stenosis (under 50%).** It is unclear if endarterectomy will benefit moderate stenosis (50%–70%).

> Carotid **angioplasty and stenting** is of no proven value for stroke patients. It is always a wrong answer.

▶ TIP

USMLE Step 2 CK will stay away from controversial or unclear areas such as the management of moderate carotid stenosis (50%–70%). Your question will be clear: Definitely operate with more than 70% stenosis and do **not** operate with less than 50% stenosis.

Control of Risk Factors for Stroke

- Diabetes to a hemoglobin A1C below 7%
- Hypertension   < 140/90
- Reduce LDL to below 100 if carotid stenosis is the cause of the stroke   HDL >35
- Tobacco smoking should be stopped
- EXERCISE
- ASPIRIN

> Carotid stenosis is considered an equivalent of coronary artery disease, so control the LDL to less than 100 mg/dL.

HEADACHE

"WHAT IS THE MOST LIKELY DIAGNOSIS?"

Tension headache is, by far, the most common cause of headache. It is a diagnosis of exclusion. You must exclude:

MIGRAINES ♀
CLUSTER ♂

No B.C. TO ♀ w/ MIGRAINE Ē AURA

SCAN IF:
- *WORSENING OVER DAYS*
- *ONSET AFTER 50 Yo*
- *PAPILLADEMA*
- *SEIZURES AMS.*
- *FOCAL NEURO*
- *VOMITING BEFORE HA*

- **Migraine:** visual disturbance (flashes, sparks, stars, luminous hallucinations), photophobia, aura, relationship to menses, association with food *TYRAMINE* (chocolate, red wine, cheese). May be precipitated by emotions. Associated with nausea and vomiting. *USUALLY PRESENT FROM YOUNG AGE | UNILATERAL*
- **Cluster headache:** frequent, short duration, high intensity headaches, with men affected 10 times more than women.
- **Giant cell (temporal) arteritis:** visual disturbance, systemic symptoms such as muscle pain, fatigue, and weakness. Jaw claudication.
- **Pseudotumor cerebri:** associated with obesity, venous sinus thrombosis, oral contraceptives, and vitamin A toxicity. Mimics a brain tumor with nausea and vomiting.

Physical Examination

- **Tension headache:** no physical findings   *BILATERAL*
- **Migraine:** no physical findings usually, but rare cases have aphasia, numbness, dysarthria, or weakness   *UNILATERAL*
- **Cluster headache:** red, tearing eye with rhinorrhea; Horner syndrome occasionally
- **Giant cell (temporal) arteritis:** visual loss, tenderness of the temporal area
- **Pseudotumor cerebri:** papilledema with diplopia from sixth cranial nerve (abducens) palsy

> Evaluate for glaucoma with headache and a red eye.

HA + EOM PALSY = CAVERNOUS SINUS THROMBOSIS

DIAGNOSTIC TESTS

Tension headache, migraine, and cluster headache have **no specific diagnostic tests**. Head CT or MRI is done to exclude intracranial mass lesions if the diagnosis is unclear or the syndrome has recently started. There is no need to perform imaging if there is a clear history of headache of a particular type.

Pseudotumor cerebri: The diagnosis cannot be made without a CT or MRI to exclude an intracranial mass lesion and a lumbar puncture **(LP) showing increased pressure**. Only the pressure is abnormal. The CSF itself is normal.
> 200 mm

Giant cell arteritis is associated with a markedly **elevated ESR** and the most accurate test is a **biopsy**.

It is critical to start steroids without waiting for biopsy in giant cell arteritis.

TREATMENT

- **Tension headache:** NSAIDs and other analgesics
- **Migraine:** triptans or ergotamine as abortive therapy
- **Cluster headache:** triptans, ergotamine, or 100% oxygen as abortive therapy
- **Giant cell (temporal) arteritis:** prednisone
- **Pseudotumor cerebri: weight loss; acetazolamide** to decrease production of cerebrospinal fluid. Steroids help. Repeated lumbar puncture rapidly lowers intracranial pressure. Place a ventriculoperitoneal shunt if medical therapy does not control it.

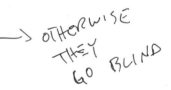
→ OTHERWISE THEY GO BLIND

Abortive Therapy for Migraine and Cluster Headache

Both of these can be rapidly interrupted by either **ergotamine or one of the triptans** (eg, sumaptriptan, eletriptan, almotriptan, zolmitriptan). The main difference is that 100% oxygen, prednisone, and lithium are effective at interrupting cluster headaches, but not migraines. The reason for this is not clear.

Prophylactic (Preventive) Therapy for Migraine

Patients experiencing 3 or more migraine headaches per month should be started on treatment to prevent them. The **best preventive therapy is propranolol**.

Other preventive medications are:

- Calcium channel blockers
- Tricyclic antidepressants (amitriptyline)
- SSRIs
- Botulinum toxin injections

Since cluster headaches happen in short bursts (hence the name "cluster") and then resolve for months to years, preventive therapy is not as clear. All forms of preventive therapy take several weeks to begin to work, and the cluster has usually resolved by the time they would be effective.

TRIGEMINAL NEURALGIA

Trigeminal neuralgia is an idiopathic disorder of the fifth cranial nerve resulting in severe, overwhelming pain in the face. Attacks of pain can be precipitated by chewing, touching the face, or pronouncing certain words in which the tongue strikes the back of the front teeth. Patients describe the pain as feeling as if a knife is being stuck into the face. There is no specific diagnostic test. **Treat with oxcarbazepine or carbamazepine.** Baclofen and lamotrigine have also been effective. If medications do not control the pain, surgical decompression can be curative.

POSTHERPETIC NEURALGIA

Herpes zoster reactivation, or shingles, is associated with a pain syndrome after resolution of the vesicular lesions in about 15% of cases. **Treatment with antiherpetic medications** such as acyclovir, famciclovir, or valganciclovir seems to **reduce the incidence of postherpetic neuralgia**, but steroids do not.

> There is no clear routinely effective treatment for peripheral neuropathy.

The pain is treated with tricyclic antidepressants, gabapentin, pregabalin, carbamazepine, or phenytoin until an effective therapy is found. Topical capsaicin is helpful. Most antiepileptic medications have some beneficial effect in neuropathic pain such as postherpetic neuralgia or peripheral neuropathy. However, none seem to work in more than 50% to 70% of patients at best.

Prevention of Herpes Zoster (Shingles)

Zoster vaccine is indicated in all persons above the age of 60 to prevent herpes zoster (shingles). This vaccine is similar to the varicella vaccine routinely administered to children to prevent chicken pox or varicella, except that the dose is much higher.

SEIZURES

Generalized tonic-clonic seizures are caused by:

- Hyponatremia or hypernatremia
- Hypoxia — BABIES
- Hypoglycemia
- Any CNS infection (encephalitis, meningitis, abscess)
- Any CNS anatomic abnormality (trauma, stroke, tumor)
- Hypocalcemia
- Uremia (elevated creatinine)
- Hepatic failure
- Alcohol, barbiturate, and benzodiazepine withdrawal
- FEVER IN KIDS < 5
- MEDS
  ↳ BUPROPION | BUSPIRONE | ENFLURANE | THEOPHYLLINE (OD)
- WITHDRAW OF MEDS
  ↳ BENZOS | BARBITURATE | ALCOHOL | ANTI-CONVULSANT

- Toxoplasmosis / Cystosarcosis
- Vitamin B6 deficiency especially with isoniazid
- Cocaine toxicity
- Hypomagnesemia (rare)

DIAGNOSTIC TESTS

An **electroencephalogram would not be the right answer unless all of these tests were done and were normal** including a CT or MRI of the head. There is no point in doing an EEG to identify the cause of a seizure if there is a clear metabolic, toxic, or anatomic defect causing the seizure. In other words, what would be the point of doing an EEG if the patient had hyponatremia or a brain lesion? You have already found the cause of the seizure.

Finger stick BG

Delirium, Stupor, and Coma

These terms represent variations on a spectrum of abnormalities of altered consciousness or unresponsiveness to stimuli. All of the metabolic, toxic, and CNS anatomic problems previously listed can cause confusion or difficulty with arousal described as delirium, stupor, obtundation, or coma. When the condition is severe enough, a seizure occurs. Confusion is to coma and seizure, as angina is to myocardial infarction.

> Seizures of unclear etiology are called epilepsy. If there is a clear cause, it is not epilepsy.

Treatment of Status Epilepticus

This is the only seizure treatment that is truly clear. The best initial therapy for a persistent seizure is a **benzodiazepine** such as lorazepam or diazepam intravenously. If the seizure persists, **then give phenytoin or fosphenytoin**. Fosphenytoin and phenytoin have the same efficacy, but **fosphenytoin has fewer adverse effects** compared to phenytoin. Like lidocaine, phenytoin is a class 1b antiarrhythmic medication. When given intravenously, it is associated with hypotension and AV block. Fosphenytoin does not have these adverse effects and can therefore be given more rapidly.

If benzodiazepines and fosphenytoin do not stop the seizure, then administer phenobarbital. Finally, the ultimate therapy for unresolving seizure is to use a neuromuscular blocking agent such as succinylcholine, vecuronium, or pancuronium to allow you to intubate the patient and then give general anesthesia such as midazolam or propofol. The patient must be placed on a ventilator before the administration of propofol, which can stop breathing.

> Neuromuscular blocking agents (eg, succinylcholine) do not stop the seizure; they just stop muscular contraction or the external manifestations of the seizure.

Classification of Seizure Disorders

Partial seizure: Like the name implies, this is a seizure that is focal to one part of the body. For instance, a patient may have a seizure that is limited just to an arm or leg. Partial seizures can either be simple (intact consciousness) or complex (loss of consciousness).

Tonic-clonic seizure: This is a generalized seizure with varying phases of muscular rigidity (tonic) followed by jerking of the muscles of the body for several minutes (clonic).

Absence (petit-mal) seizure: Consciousness is impaired only briefly. The patient often remains upright and gives a normal appearance or seems to be staring into space. Absence seizures occur more often in children.   *3 Hz*

Treatment of Status Epilepticus

1. Benzodiazepine
2. Fosphenytoin
3. Phenobarbital
4. General anesthesia

Treatment/Antiepileptic Drugs

Indications for Treatment

It is not necessary to begin antiepileptic drugs for a single seizure. The exceptions in which you should start after a single seizure are:

- Presentation in status epilepticus
- Abnormal EEG
- Family history of seizures

Choice of Antiepileptic Drugs

The treatment of status epilepticus is clear. The **best treatment of epilepsy is not clear**. A number of medications are effective, but none is clearly superior to the others. In other words, phenytoin, valproic acid, and carbamazepine all have nearly equal efficacy. You cannot be asked to choose between them based on efficacy.

Alternate treatment is with gabapentin, topiramate, lamotrigine, oxcarbazepine, or levetiracetam.

Ethosuximide is the best therapy for absence seizures.   *VALPROATE 2ND LINE*

If seizures are not controlled with a single agent, an alternate medication should be tried. If seizures are still not controlled, adding a second drug may help. If multiple medications do not control the seizure, surgical correction of a seizure focus may lead to resolution of recurrences.

PHENYTOIN — GINGIVAL HYPERPLASIA

ALMOST ALL - SJS (LAMOTRIGINE IS M.C.)

P450 INDUCERS

B ARBS
C ARBAMAZEPINE
G RISEOFULVIN
P HENYTOIN
Q UINIDINE
R IFAMPIN
S + JOHN'S WORT

> Alcohol withdrawal seizures are not treated with long-term antiepileptic drugs.

Discontinuance of Medication

The standard of care is to wait until the patient has been **seizure-free for 2 years**. A sleep deprivation EEG is the best way to tell if there is the possibility of recurrence. Sleep deprivation can elicit abnormal activity on an EEG, but the test lacks high sensitivity.

A 38-year-old man is evaluated for seizures. He achieves partial control with the addition of a second antiepileptic medication. He drives to work each day.

What do you do about his ability to drive?

a. Confiscate his license
b. Allow him to drive if he is seizure-free for 1 year
c. Allow him to drive as long as his seizure history is noted on his license
d. Recommend that he find an alternate means of transportation
e. Do not let him leave the office unless he is picked up by someone; no further driving
f. Allow him to drive as long as he is accompanied

*Answer: The correct answer is (D). You do **not** have the right, as a physician, to confiscate a patient's driver's license. The rules on seizure disorder and motor vehicles vary from state to state. Reporting his condition to the department of motor vehicles does not have the same clarity as, for instance, reporting child abuse, in which the doctor is legally protected for all reports made in good faith. You cannot hold a patient (incarcerate) for seizures in the way that you can for tuberculosis. Being accompanied in a car does not prevent seizures.*

SUBARACHNOID HEMORRHAGE

DEFINITION/ETIOLOGY

Subarachnoid hemorrhage (SAH) is caused by rupture of an aneurysm that is usually located in the anterior portion of the circle of Willis. Aneurysms are present in 2% of routine autopsies. The vast majority never rupture. They are more frequent in those with:

- Polycystic kidney disease   *VIA HTN?*
- Tobacco smoking
- Hypertension
- Hyperlipidemia
- High alcohol consumption

RUPTURED ANEURYSM
AVM's
TRAUMA

What provokes a rupture is not clear in the majority of cases.

"WHAT IS THE MOST LIKELY DIAGNOSIS?"

Look for the sudden onset of an extremely **severe headache** with meningeal irritation (**stiff neck, photophobia**) and **fever**. Fever is secondary to blood irritating the meninges. **Loss of consciousness occurs in 50%** from the sudden increase in intracranial pressure. Focal neurological complications occur in as many as 30%.

> **How SAH differs from meningitis:**
> - Very sudden in onset
> - Loss of consciousness

DIAGNOSTIC TESTS

Best initial test: CT without contrast (95% sensitive).

Most accurate test: lumbar puncture showing blood.

Xanthochromia is a yellow discoloration of CSF from the breakdown of red blood cells (RBCs) in the CSF. LP is necessary only for the 5% that have a falsely negative CT scan. The CSF in SAH will have an increased number of WBCs, which can mimic meningitis. However, the ratio of WBCs to RBCs will be normal in SAH. When the WBC count exceeds the normal ratio, you should suspect meningitis.

> Normal ratio: **One WBC** for every **500 to 1000 RBCs**.

Figure 9.3: Head CT without contrast is 95% sensitive in the detection of SAH. Lumbar puncture is 100% sensitive. *Source: Saba Ansari, MD.*

Electrocardiographic Findings with Intracranial Bleeding

The EKG may show large or inverted T waves suggestive of myocardial ischemia (cerebral T waves). This is thought to be from excessive sympathetic activity.

Angiography is used to determine the site of the aneurysm in order to guide repair of the lesion. The diagnosis of SAH is based on CT and sometimes LP.

> Contrast on CT or MRI improves detection of mass lesions such as cancer or abscess. **Don't use contrast when looking for blood.**

The only way to tell precisely which vessel ruptured is with CT angiography, standard angiography with a catheter, or MRA.

> 50% of those who rebleed will die.

TREATMENT

No treatment is able to reverse the hemorrhage.

1. **Nimodipine** (calcium channel blocker) prevents subsequent ischemic stroke.
2. **Embolization** (coiling) uses a catheter to "clog up" the site of bleeding to prevent a repeated hemorrhage. An interventional neuroradiologist places platinum wire into the site of hemorrhage. **Embolization is superior to surgical clipping** in terms of survival and complications.
3. **Ventriculoperitoneal shunt:** SAH is associated with hydrocephalus. Place a shunt only if hydrocephalus develops.
4. **Seizure prophylaxis:** Phenytoin is generally given to prevent seizures. If the question asks "Which of the following is most likely to decrease mortality?" phenytoin is not the answer. If the question asks "Which of the following is indicated?" antiepileptic therapy is the answer.

▶ **TIP**

Why tell you about surgical clipping if embolization is a better choice? When the truly right treatment (embolization) is not one of the choices, you choose the one **closest** to being right.

A woman comes to the emergency department with a severe headache starting one day prior to admission. On physical examination she has a temperature of 103°F, nuchal rigidity, and photophobia. Her head CT is normal. LP shows CSF with 1250 white blood cells and 50,000 red blood cells.

What is the most appropriate next step in the management of this patient?

a. Angiography
b. Ceftriaxone and vancomycin
c. Nimodipine
d. Embolization
e. Surgical clipping
f. Repeat the CT scan with contrast
g. Neurosurgical consultation

*Answer: The correct answer is **(B)**. The number of WBCs in the CSF in this patient far exceeds the normal ratio of 1 WBC to each 500 to 1000 RBCs. With 50,000 RBCs, there should be no more than 50 to 100 WBCs. The presence of 1250 WBCs indicates an infection, and ceftriaxone and vancomycin are the best initial therapy for bacterial meningitis. **Contrast is not useful when looking for blood**. Try never to answer "consultation" for anything.*

NORMAL PRESSURE HYDROCEPHALUS
   WET   WOBBLY   WEIRD
   FIBROSIS OF ARACHNOID GRANULATIONS   AFTER   SAH & CHRONIC MENINGITIS
      CT SCAN   &   LP
      VP SHUNT

► **TIP**

"Consultation" is the right answer only when you want to do a particular procedure and the procedure is not given as a choice. If the right answer is "embolization" and is not listed, but "interventional neuroradiology consultation" is one of the choices, then the right answer in that case is "consultation."

SPINE DISORDERS

Anterior Spinal Artery Infarction

Anterior spinal artery infarction presents with:

- **Loss of all function except for the posterior column** (position and vibratory sensation intact)
- **Flaccid paralysis** below the level of the infarction
- **Loss of deep tendon reflexes** (DTRs) at the level of the infarction
- Evolves into spastic paraplegia several weeks later
- Loss of pain and temperature
- Extensor plantar response

There is no specific therapy.

Subacute Combined Degeneration of the Cord

- From B12 deficiency or neurosyphilis.
- Position and vibratory sensation are lost.

Spinal Trauma

Acute onset of limb weakness and/or sensory disturbance below the level of the injury with the severity in proportion to the degree of injury. **Sphincter function impaired**. Loss of DTRs at the level of the injury followed by hyperreflexia below the level of the trauma. **Treat with glucocorticoids**.

Brown-Séquard Syndrome

After unilateral hemisection of spinal cord from an injury (such as a knife wound cutting half the cord), patients lose **pain and temperature on the contralateral** side from the injury, and lose motor function as well as **position and vibratory sense on the ipsilateral side** of the injury. There is no treatment.

TREATMENT

Empiric therapy with penicillin plus metronidazole plus ceftriaxone (or cefepime) is acceptable while waiting for the results of culture. Vancomycin can be used instead of penicillin, particularly if there has been recent neurosurgery and the risk of staphylococci, especially resistant staphylococci, is greater.

> **Biopsy** for culture is **indispensible** in precise treatment of brain abscess. Avoid prolonged empiric therapy.

NEUROCUTANEOUS DISEASES

Tuberous Sclerosis

- **Neurological abnormalities:** seizures, progressive psychomotor retardation, slowly progressive mental deterioration
- **Skin:**
  - **Adenoma sebaceum** (reddened facial nodules)
  - **Shagreen patches** (leathery plaques on the trunk)
  - Ash leaf (hypopigmented) patches

- **Retinal lesions**
- Cardiac rhabdomyomas

There is no specific treatment. Control seizures.

Neurofibromatosis (von Recklinghausen Disease)

- **Neurofibromas:** soft, flesh-colored lesions attached to peripheral nerves
- **Eighth cranial nerve tumors**
- Cutaneous hyperpigmented lesions (**café au lait spots**)
- **Meningioma and gliomas**

There is **no specific treatment**. Eighth cranial nerve lesions may need surgical decompression to help preserve hearing.

Figure 9.6: The lesions of neurofibromatosis are flesh-colored, soft, and nontender. *Source: Mohammad Maruf, MD.*

Sturge-Weber Syndrome

Presents with:

- **Port-wine stain of the face**
- **Seizures**
- CNS: homonymous hemianopsia, hemiparesis, mental subnormality

Skull x-ray shows calcification of angiomas. There is no treatment beyond controlling seizures.

ESSENTIAL TREMOR

Essential tremor occurs at **both rest and with intention** (reaching for things). The tremor is greatest in the hands, but can affect the head as well. The examination is otherwise normal. The tremor may affect some manual skills such as handwriting or the use of a computer keyboard. Caffeine makes it worse. The **best therapy** for essential tremor is **propranolol.**

▶ **TIP**

Tremor at rest and exertion improved with a drink of alcohol is the key to the diagnosis.

PARKINSONISM

DEFINITION

Parkinsonism is the loss of cells in the substantia nigra resulting in a **decrease in dopamine**, which leads to a significant movement disorder presenting with tremor and gait disturbance.

ETIOLOGY

Although there are many causes of parkinsonism, it is important for you to remember only the ones that will help you answer the "What is the most likely diagnosis?" question. For instance, gait disturbance with a history of repeated head trauma from boxing or the use of antipsychotic medications such as thorazine will help you establish the diagnosis. Other causes are encephalitis, reserpine, or metoclopromide.

The most common cause of parkinsonism is idiopathic.

▶ **TIP**

There is no test for parkinsonism. The diagnosis is based entirely on the clinical presentation.

PRESENTATION

Look for a patient age 50 to 60 or older who presents with a **tremor, muscular rigidity, bradykinesia** (slow movements), and a shuffling gait with unsteadiness on turning and a tendency to fall. **Cogwheel rigidity** is the slowing of movement on passive flexion or extension of an extremity. Facial expression is limited (**hypomimia**) and writing is small (**micrographia**). **Postural instability** is orthostatic hypotension. This happens because the same slowness that results in bradykinesia results in the inability of the pulse and blood pressure to reset appropriately. When an unaffected person stands up, the pulse speeds up within seconds. This is impaired in parkinsonism, leading to lightheadedness when getting up from a seated position.

▶ **TIP**

The most frequent parkinsonism question is treatment. Know the drugs.

TREATMENT

Mild disease:

- **Anticholinergic medications** (benztropine and trihexyphenidyl) relieve tremor and rigidity. It is unclear why blocking acetylcholine improves symptoms of insufficient dopamine. **Adverse effects of dry mouth, worsening prostate hypertrophy, and constipation** occur more frequently in older patients.

- **Amantadine** may work by increasing the release of dopamine from the substantia nigra. Definitely the answer in older patients (above 60) intolerant of anticholinergic medications.

Severe disease (inability to care for themselves, orthostatic):

- **Dopamine agonists:** pramipexole and ropinirole are the best initial therapy in severe parkinsonism. Bromocriptine and cabergoline are older agents that are not used as frequently because of adverse effects.

- **Levodopa/carbidopa:** the most effective medication. **Associated with "on/off" phenomena** which results in episodes of insufficient dopamine ("off") characterized by bradykinesia. The "on" effect is too much dopamine, resulting in dyskinesia.

- **COMT inhibitors** (tolcapone, entacapone) **extend the duration of levodopa/carbidopa by blocking the metabolism of dopamine**. Used only in those treated with levodopa/carbidopa. Use when there are "on/off" phenomena to even out the dopamine level, or when the response to therapy is inadequate.

- **MAO inhibitors** (rasagiline, selegiline) as a single agent or an adjunct to levodopa/carbidopa. They **block metabolism of dopamine**.

> Avoid tyramine-containing foods (eg, cheese) with MAO inhibitors; they precipitate hypertension.

- **Deep brain stimulation:** electrical stimulation is highly effective in some patients.

Which of the following is most likely to slow the progression of parkinsonism?

a. Pramipexole
b. Levodopa/carbidopa
c. Rasagiline
d. Tolcapone
e. Amantandine

Answer: The correct answer is (C). Only the MAO inhibitors are associated with the possibility of retarding the progression of parkinsonism.

A 70-year-old man with extremely severe parkinsonism comes by ambulance to the emergency department secondary to psychosis and confusion developing at home. He is maintained on levodopa/carbidopa, ropinirole, and tolcapone.

What is the most appropriate next step in management?

a. Stop levodopa/carbidopa
b. Start clozapine
c. Stop ropinirole
d. Stop tolcapone
e. Start haloperidol

Answer: The correct answer is (B). When a patient has very severe parkinsonism, you cannot stop medications because the patient will become "locked in" with severe bradykinesia. Psychosis and confusion are a known adverse effect of antiparkinsonian treatment. Use antipsychotic medications with the fewest extrapyramidal (antidopaminergic) effects. Clozapine has fewer adverse effects than haloperidol.

> Lewy body dementia = parkinsonism with dementia

> Shy-Drager syndrome = parkinsonism predominantly with orthostasis

Spasticity

Painful, contracted muscles from damage to the central nervous system is called spasticity. Spasticity is often associated with MS. No single treatment is universally effective. **Baclofen**, **dantrolene**, and the central acting alpha agonist **tizanadine** may all work.

RESTLESS LEG SYNDROME

Patients report an uncomfortable sensation in the legs that is "creepy and crawly" at night. The **discomfort** is worsened by caffeine and **relieved by moving the legs**. This can happen during sleep; a patient is sometimes brought in by a bed partner who is being kicked at night. **Treat with dopamine agonists such as pramipexole.**

USUALLY IDIOPATHIC
2° TO : IRON DEFICIENCY

HUNTINGTON DISEASE   ↓ Ach

Huntington disease (HD) is a hereditary disease characterized by CAG trinucleotide repeat sequences on chromosome 4.   A.D.

"WHAT IS THE MOST LIKELY DIAGNOSIS?"

HD is the answer when you see:

- Choreaform **movement disorder** (dyskinesia)
- **Dementia**
- **Behavior changes** (irritability, moodiness, antisocial behavior)
- Onset between the ages of 30 and 50 with a family history of HD

The movement disorder of HD starts with "fidgetiness" or restlessness progressing to dystonic posturing, rigidity, and akinesia.

> Movement disorder may be troubling in HD, but it is far worse to progress to no movement at all (rigidity).

DIAGNOSTIC TESTS/TREATMENT

There is **no specific diagnostic test in HD**; the symptom triad (movement/memory/mood) establishes the diagnosis. No treatment reverses HD. Dyskinesia is treated with **tetrabenazine**. Psychosis is treated with **haloperidol or quetiapine**.

DOPAMINE ANTAGONISTS

> Head CT or MRI shows caudate nucleus involvement.

TOURETTE DISORDER

Tourette is an idiopathic disorder of:

- **Vocal tics, grunts, and coprolalia**
- Motor tics (sniffing, blinking, frowning)
- Obsessive-compulsive behavior

There are no specific diagnostic tests. Treat with haloperidol, clonazepam, pimozide, or other neuroleptic medications.

MULTIPLE SCLEROSIS

DEFINITION/ETIOLOGY

Multiple sclerosis (MS) is an idiopathic disorder exclusively of CNS (brain and cord) white matter. MS is more common in white women who live in colder climates.

"WHAT IS THE MOST LIKELY DIAGNOSIS?"

Look for multiple neurological deficits of the CNS affecting any aspect of CNS functioning. The most common presentation is blurry vision or visual disturbance from optic neuritis.

After optic neuritis, the most common abnormalities are motor and sensory. The least common abnormalities are cognitive defects and dementia. Sexual function remains relatively intact.

Other findings:

- Fatigue
- Spasticity and hyperreflexia
- Cerebellar deficits

> Internuclear ophthalmoplegia (INO) is the inability to adduct one eye with nystagmus in the other eye. INO is characteristic of MS.

DIAGNOSTIC TESTS

1. **MRI** is both the best **initial** test and the **most accurate** test.
2. Lumbar puncture shows CSF with a mild elevation in protein and fewer than 50 to 100 WBCs. **Oligoclonal bands** are found in about **85%** of patients. Oligoclonal bands are not specific to MS.

Figures 9.7, 9.8: MS plaques appear white and are exclusively in the white matter of the CNS.
Source: Saba Ansari, MD.

> Visual and auditory evoked potentials are always the wrong answer.

▶ TIP

Oligoclonal bands are the answer in the 3% to 5% of patients with an equivocal or nondiagnostic MRI.

TREATMENT

> Steroids shorten the duration of exacerbation.

High-dose **steroids** are the best initial therapy for acute exacerbations of disease.

Drugs that Prevent Relapse and Progression

- Glatiramer (copolymer 1)
- Beta-interferon

- Natalizumab
- Mitoxantrone
- Azathioprine
- Cyclophosphamide

A patient develops worsening neurological deficits with the use of a chronic suppressive medication. The MRI shows new, multiple white matter hypodense lesions.

Which of these medications is most likely to have caused this? **Natalizumab**, an inhibitor of alpha-4 intergrin. It has occasionally been associated with the development of **progressive multifocal leukoencephalopathy (PML)**.

> Glatiramer and beta-interferon are the best first choice for prevention of relapse.

MOTOR NEURON DISEASE AND AMYOTROPHIC LATERAL SCLEROSIS

DEFINITION/ETIOLOGY

The cause of amyotrophic lateral sclerosis (ALS) is unknown. It is a loss exclusively of upper and lower motor neurons.

"WHAT IS THE MOST LIKELY DIAGNOSIS?"

Look for **weakness** of unclear etiology starting in the 20s to 40s with a unique combination of upper and lower motor neuron loss. The most common initial presentation is with **difficulty in chewing and swallowing** and a **decrease in gag reflex**. This leads to pooling of saliva in the pharynx and frequent episodes of aspiration. A **weak cough** leads to death in many patients within 3 to 5 years after diagnosis.

> In ALS, there is no sensory loss and the sphincters are spared.

Presentation of Amyotrophic Lateral Sclerosis	
Upper motor neurons	**Lower motor neurons**
Weakness	Weakness
Spasticity	Wasting
Hyperreflexia	Fasciculations
Extensor plantar responses	

DIAGNOSTIC TESTS/TREATMENT

Electromyography reveals loss of neural innervation in multiple muscle groups. CPK levels are elevated. **Riluzole** reduces glutamate buildup in neurons and may prevent progression of disease. **Baclofen treats spasticity**. **CPAP** and **BiPAP** help with respiratory difficulties secondary to muscle weakness. **Tracheostomy and maintenance on a ventilator** is often necessary when the disease advances.

> In ALS, the most common cause of death is respiratory failure.

CHARCOT-MARIE-TOOTH DISEASE

Charcot-Marie-Tooth (CMT) is a genetic disorder with loss of both motor and sensory innervation leading to:

- Distal weakness and sensory loss
- Wasting in the legs
- Decreased deep tendon reflexes
- Tremor

Foot deformity with a **high arch** is common (pes cavus). The legs look like inverted champagne bottles. The most accurate test is **electromyography** and there is **no treatment**.

PERIPHERAL NEUROPATHY

The **most common cause** of peripheral neuropathy is **diabetes mellitus**. Other causes include uremia, alcoholism, and paraproteinemias like monoclonal gammopathy of unknown significance.

The best initial therapy is **pregabalin** or **gabapentin**. **Tricyclic antidepressants** and most seizure medications (phenytoin, carbamazepine, lamotrigine) are effective in some people.

Specific Peripheral Nerve Neuropathies		
Nerve	**Precipitating event described in the stem**	**Manifestations/Presentation**
Ulnar	Biker, pressure on palms of hands, trauma to the medial side of elbow	Wasting of hypothenar eminence, pain in fourth and fifth fingers
Radial	Pressure of inner, upper arm; falling asleep with arm over back of chair ("Saturday night palsy"); using crutches and pressure in the axilla	Wrist drop
Lateral cutaneous nerve of thigh	Obesity, pregnancy, sitting with crossed legs	Pain/numbness of outer aspect of one thigh
Tarsal tunnel (Tibial nerve)	Worsens with walking	Pain/numbness in ankle and sole of foot
Peroneal	High boots, pressure on back of knee	Weak foot with decreased dorsiflexion and eversion
Median	Typists, carpenters, working with hands	Thenar wasting, pain/numbness in first 3 fingers

Facial (Seventh Cranial) Nerve Palsy or Bell Palsy

Most cases of facial palsy are idiopathic. Some identified causes are Lyme disease, sarcoidosis, herpes zoster, and tumors.

MY LOVELY BELL HAD AN STD

PRESENTATION

Paralysis of the entire side of the face is classic. Stroke will paralyze only the lower half of the face because the upper half of the face receives innervation from both cerebral hemispheres. There is difficulty with closing the eye. If the patient **can** wrinkle her forehead on the affected side, worry about stroke. If the patient **cannot** wrinkle his forehead on the affected side, it is Bell.

Two additional features are:

- **Hyperacusis:** Sounds are extra loud because the seventh cranial nerve normally supplies the stapedius muscle, which acts as a "shock absorber" on the ossicles of the middle ear.
- **Taste disturbances:** The seventh cranial nerve supplies the sensation of taste to the anterior two-thirds of the tongue.

> Eating is "sloppy" because of difficulty closing the lips.

▶ TIP

Look for statements that "the face feels stiff" or "pulled to one side" to answer "What is the most likely diagnosis?"

DIAGNOSTIC TESTS

No test is usually done because of the characteristic presentation of paralysis of half of the face. The most accurate test (if asked) is electromyography and nerve conduction studies.

TREATMENT

60% of patients have full recovery even without treatment. The best initial therapy is prednisone. Acyclovir does not help. *& EYE CARE*
VALACYCLOVIR ??

A 38-year-old carpenter comes with pain near his ear that is quickly followed by weakness of one side of his face. Both the upper and lower parts of his face are weak, but sensation is intact.

What is the most common complication of his disorder?

a. Corneal ulceration
b. Aspiration pneumonia
c. Sinusitis
d. Otitis media
e. Deafness
f. Dental caries

Answer: The correct answer is (A). Corneal ulceration occurs with seventh cranial nerve palsy because of difficulty in closing the eye, especially at night. This leads to dryness of the eye and ulceration. This is prevented by taping the eye shut and using lubricants in the eye. Dental caries don't happen because although there is drooling from difficulty closing the mouth, saliva production is normal. Rather than deafness, sounds are extra loud. Aspiration does not occur because gag reflex and cough are normal.

ACUTE INFLAMMATORY POLYNEUROPATHY (GUILLAIN-BARRÉ SYNDROME)

DEFINITION

Guillain-Barré Syndrome (GBS) is an **autoimmune** damage of **multiple peripheral nerves**. By definition, there is no CNS involvement. A circulating antibody attacks the myelin sheaths of the peripheral nerves, removing their insulation. GBS is associated with *Campylobacter jejuni* infection.

"WHAT IS THE MOST LIKELY DIAGNOSIS?"

Look for **weakness in the legs that ascends** from the feet and moves toward the chest, associated with a loss of DTRs. A few patients have a mild sensory disturbance. The main problem is that when GBS hits the diaphragm, it is associated with **respiratory muscle weakness**. Autonomic dysfunction with hypotension, hypertension, or tachycardia can occur.

> Ascending weakness + loss of reflexes = GBS

DIAGNOSTIC TESTS

The most specific diagnostic test is **nerve conduction studies/electromyography**. These will show a decrease in the propagation of electrical impulses along the nerves.

CSF shows **increased protein** with a **normal cell count**.

Tests of Respiratory Muscle Involvement

When the diaphragm is involved, there is a decrease in forced vital capacity and peak inspiratory pressure. Inspiration is the "active" part of breathing and the patient loses the strength to inhale. PFTs tell who might die from GBS.

> Death from GBS, although rare, is from dysautonomia and respiratory failure.

TREATMENT

Intravenous immunoglobulin (IVIG) or plasmapheresis are equal in efficacy.

▶ **TIP**

Prednisone is a wrong answer for GBS; it does not help.

Combining IVIG and plasmapheresis is a wrong answer.

A woman comes to the emergency department with bilateral leg weakness developing over the last few days. She has lost her knee jerk and ankle jerk reflexes. The weakness started in her feet and progressed up to her calves and then her thighs. She is otherwise asymptomatic.

Which of the following is the most urgent step?

a. Pulmonary function testing
b. Arterial blood gas
c. Nerve conduction study
d. Lumbar puncture
e. Peak flow meter

*Answer: The correct answer is (A). The most dangerous thing that can happen with GBS is dysautonomia or involvement of the respiratory muscles. Peak **inspiratory** pressure or a decrease in forced vital capacity (FVC) is the earliest way to detect impending respiratory failure. If you wait until there is CO_2 accumulation on an ABG, it is too late. Nerve conduction studies are the most accurate test, but their results are not as important as answering the question "Do you know who is going to die from respiratory failure?" Peak flow assesses **expiratory** function, which is not greatly impaired in GBS; peak flow is best used to assess obstructive disease such as COPD or asthma.*

MYASTHENIA GRAVIS

LAMBERT EATON — PARANEOPLASTIC BETTER WITH USE

DEFINITION

Myasthenia gravis (MG) is a disorder of muscular weakness from the production of antibodies against acetylcholine receptors at the neuromuscular junction.

PRESENTATION/"WHAT IS THE MOST LIKELY DIAGNOSIS?"

Look for a question describing "**double vision** and **difficulty chewing**" or "weakness of limb muscles **worse at the end of the day**."

This is because the extraocular muscles and mastication (maseter) are often the only 2 muscular activities universally done by people (ie, watching TV and eating).

Physical examination reveals ptosis, weakness with sustained activity, and **normal pupillary responses**.

> Severe myasthenia affects respiratory muscles.

DIAGNOSTIC TESTS

Best initial test: acetylcholine receptor antibodies (80%–90% sensitive). This is a better first answer than edrophonium testing.

Do CHEST X-RAY TO CHECK FOR THYMOMA

Edrophonium: short-acting inhibitor of acetylcholinesterase. The temporary bump up in acetylcholine levels is associated with a clear improvement in motor function that lasts for a few minutes.

Most accurate test: Electromyography shows decreased strength with repetitive stimulation.

▶ **TIP**

Questions often ask, "What imaging test should be done?" Answer: **chest something**. Chest x-ray, CT, or MRI are done to look for thymoma or thymic hyperplasia.

TREATMENT

Best initial treatment: **Neostigmine** or **pyridostigmine**. These are longer acting versions of edrophonium.

Thymectomy in myasthenia is like splenectomy in idiopathic thrombocytopenic purpura. It markedly improves recurrent, hard-to-control disease.

If these medications do not control the disease, the "most appropriate next step in management" is a thymectomy if the patient is under age 60. If the patient is over age 60, prednisone is used. Azathioprine, cyclophosphamide, or mycophenolate are used in order to get the patient off of steroids before serious adverse effects occur.

Management of Acute Myasthenic Crisis

Acute myasthenic crisis presents with severe, overwhelming disease with profound weakness or respiratory involvement. It is **treated with IVIG or plasmapheresis**.

BENIGN ESSENTIAL TREMOR → FINE TREMOR → FAMILIAL → ALCOHOL/β-BLOCKERS

DUCHENE'S MD → XR → No inflammation → GOWER'S → ↑ CPK/DNA TESTING → STEROIDS

MGM STUDIOS — METS, GLIOBLASTOMA, MENINGIOMA, SCHWANNOMA

NEPHROLOGY

10

DIAGNOSTIC TESTS IN NEPHROLOGY

▶ **TIP**

The "**best initial test**" in nephrology is a **urinalysis** and the **blood urea nitrogen (BUN) and creatinine**.

Urinalysis

The urinalysis (urine analysis or UA) measures chemical reactions associated with:

- Protein
- White cells (direct microscopic examination) or leukocyte esterase (dipstick)
- Red cells
- Specific gravity and pH
- Nitrites (indicates presence of Gram-negative bacteria on dipstick)

The dipstick gives some quantitative values as well. This means it is not just positive or negative, but can give an approximation of the quantity of the protein, white cells, and red cells. This can be described either as a direct number (eg, 300 mg protein) or a scale: 0, 1+, 2+, 3+, or 4+.

▶ **TIP**

Do not worry about knowing the precise scale. Every USMLE Step 2 CK test comes with the range of normal values attached so you will be able to assess severity.

Protein

It is normal to excrete a very tiny amount of protein. The tubules secrete slight amounts of protein normally known as **Tamm-Horsfall** protein. This should be less than 30 to 50 mg per 24 hours. Greater amounts of protein can be associated with either tubular disease or glomerular disease. Very **large amounts of protein** can only be excreted with **glomerular disease**.

> Severe proteinuria means glomerular damage.

In terms of proteinuria, the problem with using the scale of "trace" through 4+ is that UA measures only the amount of protein excreted at a particular moment in the day. It does not give an average or total amount of protein excreted over 24 hours because renal function itself varies during the day based on bodily position and physical activity. It is like the difference between an EKG and a Holter monitor. **Transient proteinuria** is present in 2% to 10% of the population, with most of this being **benign** without representing pathology. If **proteinuria persists** and is not related to prolonged standing (**orthostatic proteinuria**), a **kidney biopsy** should be performed.

> Standing and physical activity increase urinary protein excretion.

Assuming constant protein excretion throughout the day, 1+ protein is about one gram excreted per 24 hours, 2+ protein is about 2 grams per 24 hours, and so on. The 2 methods to assess the total amount of protein in a day are:

> Urine dipstick for protein detects only **albumin**.

- Single protein to creatinine ratio
- 24-hour urine collection

These tests are considered **equal** in accuracy. However, since the 24-hour urine is much harder to collect, it is rarely performed.

> ▶ **TIP**
>
> To assess proteinuria:
>
> - UA is the initial test.
> - Protein-to-creatinine ratio is more accurate at determining the amount.

Protein-to-Creatinine Ratio

A protein-to-creatinine (P/Cr) ratio of one is equivalent to one gram of protein on a 24-hour urine. A P/Cr ratio of 2.5 is equivalent to 2.5 grams of protein found on a 24-hour urine. The **P/Cr ratio can be superior in accuracy to a 24-hour urine** because of technical difficulties in collecting a full day's worth of urine. If you collect a little less, it will underestimate the true excretion. If you add a single extra urination, you might overestimate the protein excretion.

> Biopsy determines the cause of proteinuria.

> ▶ **TIP**
>
> If both P/Cr ratio and 24-hour urine are in the choices, choose the **P/Cr ratio. It is faster** and technically easier to perform.

Microalbuminuria

The presence of **tiny amounts** of protein that are too small to detect on the UA is called **microalbuminuria**. This is very important to detect in diabetic patients. Long-term **microalbuminuria leads to worsening renal function** in a diabetic patient and should be treated.

A diabetic patient is evaluated with a UA that shows no protein. Microalbuminuria is detected (level between 50 and 300 mg per 24 hours).

What is the next best step in the management of this patient?

a. Enalapril
b. Kidney biopsy
c. Hydralazine
d. Renal consultation
e. Low-protein diet
f. Repeat UA annually and treat when trace protein is detected

Answer: The correct answer is (A). ACE inhibitors or angiotensin receptor blocker (eg, losartan, valsartan) are the best initial therapy for any degree of proteinuria in a diabetic patient. They decrease the progression of proteinuria and delay the development of renal insufficiency in diabetic patients. Hydralazine is not as effective and has more adverse effects. Low-protein diets are less effective than ACE inhibitors. Do not consult for initiating medications like ACE inhibitors.

> *TREAT MICROALBUMINEMIA WITH ACE INHIBITORS OR ARBs IN DIABETICS*

> Kidney biopsy is especially important in kidney disease in a diabetic patient with no ophthalmic findings.

> Bence–Jones protein in myeloma is not detectable on a dipstick. Use immunoelectrophoresis.

White Blood Cells

White blood cells detect inflammation, **infection**, or allergic **interstitial nephritis**. You cannot distinguish neutrophils from eosinophils on a UA. Neutrophils indicate infection. **Eosinophils** indicate allergic or acute **interstitial nephritis**. It is very useful if eosinophils are found because of their specificity. It is less important if they are absent, because the sensitivity of the test is limited. Microscopic examination gives a precise numerical count of the number of white cells present.

> *PMN = INFECTION*
> *EOS = ALLERGY OR INT NEPHRITIS*

> NSAID-induced renal disease does not show eosinophils.

▶ **TIP**

Wright and Hansel stains detect eosinophils in the urine. They are the answer for allergic interstitial nephritis.

> *WRIGHT & HANSEL FOR EOSINOS IN URINE*

Hematuria

Hematuria is indicative of:

- **Stones** in bladder, ureter, or kidney
- Hematologic disorders that cause bleeding (**coagulopathy**)
- **Infection** (cystitis, pyelonephritis)
- **Cancer** of bladder, ureters, or kidney
- Treatments (cyclophosphamide gives hemorrhagic cystitis)

- **Trauma**; simply "banging" the kidney or bladder makes them shed red cells
- **Glomerulonephritis**

False positive tests for hematuria on UA are caused by **hemoglobin or myoglobin** in the urine.

> *A woman is admitted to the hospital with trauma and dark urine. The dipstick is markedly positive for blood.*
>
> *What is the best initial test to confirm the etiology?*
>
> *a. Microscopic examination of the urine*
> *b. Cystoscopy*
> *c. Renal ultrasound*
> *d. Renal/bladder CT scan*
> *e. Abdominal x-ray*
> *f. Intravenous pyelogram*
>
> *Answer: The correct answer is **(A)**. Hemoglobin and myoglobin make the dipstick positive for blood, but no red cells are seen on microscopic examination of the urine. Abdominal x-ray detects small bowel obstruction (ileus) but is very poor at detecting stones or cancer. **Renal CT** is the most accurate test for **stones**, but would not be done until the etiology of the positive dipstick had been confirmed as blood.*

▶ **TIP**

Intravenous pyelogram (IVP) is always wrong. It is slower and the contrast is renal toxic.

▶ **TIP**

[handwritten: DYSMORPHIC RBC's = GLOMERULONEPHRITIS]

When "dysmorphic" red cells are described, the correct answer is glomerulonephritis.

When Is Cystoscopy the Answer?

The answer is **cystoscopy** when there is **hematuria** without infection or prior trauma and:

Cystoscopy is the most accurate test of the bladder.

- The renal ultrasound or CT does not show an etiology.
- **Bladder** sonography shows a **mass** for possible biopsy.

[handwritten: CYTOSCOPY IF: → No INFECTION or TRAUMA → RENAL U.S. IS (NEG) → BLADDER SONOGRAPHY IS (POS)]

Casts

These are microscopic collections of material clogging up the tubules and being excreted in the urine.

Types of Urinary Casts and Their Significance

Type of cast	Association
Red cell	Glomerulonephritis
White cell	Pyelonephritis
Eosinophil	Acute (allergic) interstitial nephritis
Hyaline	Dehydration concentrates the urine and the normal Tamm-Horsfall protein precipitates or concentrates into a cast.
Broad, waxy	Chronic renal disease
Granular "muddy-brown"	Acute tubular necrosis; they are collections of dead tubular cells

> Casts are very useful if found, but they are often not present.

HYALINE = DEHYDRATION

WAXY = CHRONIC

▶ **TIP**

The presence of a cast helps answer the "most likely diagnosis" question because they are specific.

ACUTE KIDNEY INJURY

DEFINITION

Acute kidney injury (AKI), formerly called acute renal failure (ARF), which you may encounter as a synonym, is defined as a decrease in creatinine clearance resulting in a sudden rise in BUN and creatinine. The definition is not based on a specific number of BUN and creatinine.

ETIOLOGY

AKI is categorized into 3 types:

- Prerenal azotemia (decreased perfusion)
- Postrenal azotemia (obstruction)
- Intrinsic renal disease (ischemia and toxins)

Prerenal azotemia: These are problems of **inadequate perfusion** of the kidney in which the kidney itself is normal. Any cause of hypoperfusion or hypovolemia will raise the BUN and creatinine, with the BUN rising more than the creatinine.

- **Hypotension** (systolic below 90 mm Hg) from sepsis, anaphylaxis, bleeding, dehydration
- **Hypovolemia:** diuretics, burns, pancreatitis
- Renal artery stenosis: Even though the blood pressure may be high, the kidney is underperfused.

→ NORMAL VOLUME, BUT BAD HEART → CARDIOGENIC SHOCK

- "Relative hypovolemia" from decreased pump function: CHF, constrictive pericarditis, tamponade
- Hypoalbuminemia *↓ ALBUMIN = LOSS OF FLUID INTO TISSUE*
- Cirrhosis
- **NSAIDs** constrict the afferent arteriole.
- **ACE inhibitors** cause efferent arteriole vasodilation.

> **Management** of prerenal and postrenal azotemia is based on correcting the underlying cause.

Postrenal azotemia: Obstruction of any cause damages the kidney by blocking filtration at the glomerulus. Causes of postrenal azotemia include:

- **Prostate hypertrophy** or cancer
- **Stone** in the ureter
- Cervical **cancer**
- Urethral **stricture**
- Neurogenic (atonic) bladder
- Retroperitoneal **fibrosis** (look for bleomycin, methylsergide, or radiation in the history)

> You must obstruct **both** kidneys for the creatinine to rise.

Prerenal and postrenal azotemia combined account for 80% of acute kidney. **The majority are reversible.**

The major force favoring filtration is the hydrostatic pressure in the glomerular capillary. If hydrostatic pressure in Bowman space rises, you cannot filter fluid. Unilateral obstruction causes renal failure if the person has only one kidney.

> The kidney in prerenal and postrenal disease would function normally if transplanted into another person.

Intrinsic renal disease: The most common cause is **acute tubular necrosis** (ATN) from toxins or prolonged ischemia of the kidney. Glomerulonephritis is rarely acute, but when the kidney is injured from any cause, there is always a greater risk of AKI. For example, a few hours of hypotension might not damage a normal kidney at all, but with underlying renal damage, it may cause AKI. Other causes are:

- Acute (allergic) interstitial nephritis (commonly from medications such as penicillin)
- Rhabdomyolysis and hemoglobinuria
- Contrast agents, aminoglycosides, cisplatin, amphotericin, cyclosporine, and **NSAIDs:** most common toxins causing AKI from ATN

> *NSAIDs = M.C. TOXIN LEADING TO AKI VIA ATN*

- Crystals such as hyperuricemia, hypercalcemia, or hyperoxaluria
- Proteins such as Bence-Jones protein from myeloma
- Poststreptococcal infection

PRESENTATION

AKI may present with only an asymptomatic rise in BUN and creatinine. When symptomatic, the patient feels:

- **Nauseated** and **vomiting**
- Tired/**malaise**

- Weak
- Short of breath and edema from fluid overload

Very **severe disease** presents with:

- **Confusion**
- Arrhythmia from hyperkalemia and acidosis $\uparrow K^+$ $\uparrow H^+$
- Sharp, pleuritic chest pain from **pericarditis**

> There is no pathognomonic physical finding of AKI.

▶ **TIP**

No symptoms are specific enough to answer the "most likely diagnosis" question without lab testing.

Presentation of Postrenal Azotemia

Enlargement (distention) of the **bladder** and massive diuresis after Foley (urinary) catheter placement are specific to urinary obstruction. This is the closest you will get to a specific presentation for any form of AKI.

DIAGNOSTIC TESTS

The best initial test is the BUN and creatinine. With completely dead kidneys, the creatinine will rise about one point (1 mg/dL) a day. If the BUN:creatinine ratio is above 20:1, the etiology is either prerenal or postrenal damage of the kidney. Intrinsic renal disease has a ratio closer to 10:1. Renal sonogram is the best initial imaging test. Sonography does not need contrast. Contrast should be avoided in renal insufficiency.

BUN : Cr
20:1 — PRERENAL (or POST)
10:1 — INTRINSIC

Prerenal azotemia is usually a clear diagnosis with the question describing:

- **BUN: creatinine** ratio above **20:1**

and

- Clear history of **hypoperfusion or hypotension**

Postrenal azotemia is usually a clear diagnosis with the question describing:

- **BUN: creatinine** ratio above **20:1**

and

- **Distended bladder** or massive **release of urine** with catheter placement

and

- Bilateral or unilateral **hydronephrosis** on sonogram (ultrasound)

▶ **TIP**

Kidney biopsy is rarely the right answer for AKI. Although the biopsy is the most accurate test of allergic interstitial nephritis or poststreptococcal glomerulonephritis, it is rare for either of these to actually need biopsy.

Tests for AKI of Unclear Etiology

When the cause of AKI is not clear, the "next best diagnostic step" is:

- Urinalysis
- Urine sodium (UNa)
- Fractional excretion of sodium ($F_E Na$)
- Urine osmolality

> ▶ **TIP**
>
> If all of these are choices, always go with urinalysis first.

Urine Sodium and Fractional Excretion of Sodium

Decreased blood pressure (or decreased intravascular volume) normally will increase aldosterone. Increased aldosterone increases sodium reabsorption. It is normal for urine sodium to decrease when there is decreased renal perfusion because aldosterone levels rise.

> ▶ **TIP**
>
> You can answer all the questions on USMLE Step 2 CK without knowing the mathematical formula for $F_E Na$.

Urine Osmolality

When **intravascular volume** is **low**, normally ADH levels should rise. A **healthy** kidney will **reabsorb more** water to fill the vasculature and increase renal perfusion.

When more water is reabsorbed from the urine, will the urine be more concentrated, or dilute? **Increased** water **reabsorption** leads to an **increase in urine osmolality**: more **concentrated** urine.

Normal tubule cells reabsorb water. In **ATN, the urine cannot be concentrated** because the tubule **cells are damaged**. The urine produced in ATN is similar in osmolality to the blood (about 300 mOsm/L). This is called **isosthenuria**. Urine osmolality in ATN is **inappropriately low**. Isosthenuria is especially problematic when the patient is dehydrated.

Isosthenuria means the urine is the same (*iso*) strength (*sthenos*) as the blood. The term *isosthenuria* is used interchangeably with the phrase *renal tubular concentrating defect*.

Dehydration should **normally increase urine concentration** (osmolality). If there is damage to the tubular cells from ischemia or toxins, the kidney loses the ability to absorb sodium and water because a live, functioning cell is necessary to absorb sodium and water. In **ATN**, the body **inappropriately loses sodium** (UNa above 20) and water (UOsm below 300) into the urine.

Healthy person with **fluid overload** → **low urine osmolality** or dilute urine

Healthy person with **dehydration** → **high urine osmolality** or concentrated urine

---

Prerenal azotemia: low UNa (below 20) = low $F_E Na$ (less than 1%)

Urine sodium and $F_E Na$ give you the same information.

A 20-year-old African American man comes for a screening test for sickle cell. He is found to be heterozygous (trait or AS) for sickle cell.

What is the best advice for him?

a. Nothing needed until he has a painful crisis
b. Avoid dehydration
c. Hydroxyurea
d. Folic acid supplementation
e. Pneumococcal vaccination

Answer: The correct answer is (B). The only significant manifestation of sickle cell trait is a defect in renal concentrating ability or isosthenuria. These patients will continue to produce inappropriately dilute, high-volume urine despite dehydration. Hydroxyurea is used to prevent painful crises when they occur more than 4 times a year. Painful crises rarely occur in sickle cell trait. They do not have hemolysis, so there is no need for additional folic acid supplementation. Splenic function is abnormal only in those who are homozygous, so pneumococcal vaccination is not routinely indicated.

Classification of Acute Renal Failure by Laboratory Testing		
Test	**Prerenal azotemia**	**Acute tubular necrosis**
BUN:creatinine	>20:1	<20:1
Urine sodium (UNa)	<20 mEq/L	>20 mEq/L
Fractional excretion of sodium (F_ENa)	<1%	>1%
Urine osmolality (UOsm)	>500 mOsm/kg	<300 mOsm/kg

Urine specific gravity correlates to urine osmolality.
High UOsm = high specific gravity

Acute Tubular Necrosis (ATN)

DEFINITION

ATN is an injury to the kidneys from ischemia and/or toxins resulting in sloughing off of tubular cells into the urine. Sodium and water reabsorptive mechanisms are lost with the tubular cells. Proteinuria is not significant since protein, not tubules, spills into the urine when glomeruli are damaged.

ETIOLOGY

Knowing the causes of ATN is critical, since there is no specific diagnostic test to prove the etiology. You cannot do a blood level of a drug or a biopsy to prove that a particular toxin caused the renal failure.

▶ **TIP**

Acute renal failure and a toxin in the history are your clues to the "What is the most likely diagnosis?" question for ATN.

Specific Causes of ATN

A patient comes with fever and acute, left lower quadrant abdominal pain. Blood cultures on admission grow E. coli *and* Candida albicans. *She is started on vancomycin, metronidazole and gentamicin, and amphotericin. She has a CT scan that identifies diverticulitis. After 36 hours, her creatinine rises dramatically.*

Which of the following is most likely the cause of her renal insufficiency?

a. Vancomycin
b. Gentamicin
c. Contrast media
d. Metronidazole
e. Amphotericin

Answer: The correct answer is **(C)**. *Radiographic* **contrast** *media has a very* **rapid onset of injury**. *Creatinine rises the* **next day. Vancomycin, gentamicin,** *and* **amphotericin** *are all potentially nephrotoxic, but they would not cause renal failure with just 2 or 3 doses. They need 5 to 10 days to result in nephrotoxicity. Metronidazole is hepatically excreted and does not cause renal failure.*

A 74-year-old blind man is admitted with obstructive uropathy and chest pain. He has a history of hypertension and diabetes. His creatinine drops from 10 mg/dL to 1.2 mg/dL 3 days after catheter placement. The stress test shows reversible ischemia.

What is the most appropriate management?

a. Coronary artery calcium score on CT scan
b. One to two liters of normal saline hydration prior and during angiography
c. N-acetylcysteine prior to angiography
d. Mannitol during angiography
e. Furosemide during angiography
f. Intravenous sodium bicarbonate before and during angiography

Answer: The correct answer is **(B)**. **Saline hydration** *has the* **most proven benefit** *at preventing contrast-induced nephrotoxicity. Mannitol and furosemide may or may not prevent nephrotoxicity. There is minimal data to support their use. N-acetylcysteine and sodium bicarbonate have some benefit, but the evidence is not as clear as that with saline.* **Calcium scoring on** *CT scan is still* **considered experimental**. *It does not provide sufficient information to eliminate angiography.*

How to Answer Questions Correctly When Your Real-life Experience Disagrees with What You Read Here

The last question may distress those of you who regularly see your attendings use N-acetylcysteine and bicarbonate to prevent renal failure from contrast. This is a case in which a person with no clinical experience in the area will do better than a person regularly in the hospital. They are using these substances because:

- The risk of precipitating worse renal failure is very real when using contrast.

- Contrast-enhanced procedures are often unavoidable.
- These are generally benign substances.
- We have nothing else to offer beyond hydration.

Extra-Difficult Question—How to Get a 280 on Step 2 CK

A patient with mild renal insufficiency undergoes angiography and develops a 2 mg/dL rise in creatinine from ATN despite the use of saline hydration before and after the procedure.

What do you expect to find on laboratory testing?

a. Urine sodium 8 (low), $F_E Na$ >1%, urine specific gravity 1.035 (high)
b. Urine sodium 58 (high), $F_E Na$ >1%, urine specific gravity 1.005 (low)
c. Urine sodium 5 (very low), $F_E Na$ <1%, urine specific gravity 1.040 (very high)
d. Urine sodium 45 (high), $F_E Na$ >1% urine specific gravity 1.005 (low)

Answer: The correct answer is (C). Although **contrast-induced** *renal failure is a form of* **ATN**, *the urinary* **lab values are an exception** *from the other forms of ATN.* **Contrast causes spasm of the afferent arteriole** *that leads to renal tubular dysfunction. There is tremendous reabsorption of sodium and water, leading the specific gravity of the urine to become very high. This results in profoundly low urine sodium. The usual finding in ATN from nephrotoxins would be UNa above 20, $F_E Na$ greater than 1%, but a low specific gravity. Specific gravity correlates with urine osmolality.*

A patient with extremely severe myeloma with a plasmacytoma is admitted for combination chemotherapy. Two days later, the creatinine rises.

What is the most likely cause?

a. Cisplatin
b. Hyperuricemia
c. Bence-Jones proteinuria
d. Hypercalcemia
e. Hyperoxaluria

Answer: The correct answer is (B). Two days after chemotherapy, the creatinine rises in a person with a hematologic malignancy. This is most likely from **tumor lysis syndrome** *leading to* **hyperuricemia**. *Cisplatin, as with most* **drug toxicities**, *would not produce a* **rise in creatinine for 5 to 10 days**. *Bence-Jones protein and hypercalcemia both cause renal insufficiency, but it would not be rapid and it would not happen as a result of treatment. Treatment for myeloma would end up decreasing both the calcium and Bence-Jones protein levels because they are produced from the leukemic cells. Cancer cells do not release oxalate.*

What would have prevented this event? **Allopurinol, hydration, and rasburicase** should be given **prior to chemotherapy** to **prevent renal failure** from tumor lysis syndrome.

A patient who is suicidal ingests an unknown substance and develops renal failure 3 days later. Her calcium level is also low and the urinalysis shows an abnormality.

What did she take?

a. Aspirin
b. Acetaminophen
c. Ethylene glycol
d. Ibuprofen
e. Opiates
f. Methanol

*Answer: The correct answer is (C). **Ethylene glycol** is associated with acute kidney injury based on **oxalic acid** and **oxalate** precipitating within the **kidney tubules** causing ATN. Oxalate crystal appears as **envelope-shaped crystals**. The calcium level is low because it precipitates as calcium oxalate. Aspirin is renal toxic but does not lower calcium levels and has no abnormality on urinalysis. **Acetaminophen is hepatotoxic**. Ibuprofen and all **NSAIDS are renal toxic** by constricting the afferent arteriole, causing allergic interstitial nephritis and papillary necrosis. They have no impact on calcium levels and the only time something would be found in the urine is in the case of papillary necrosis. Papillary necrosis causes sudden flank pain and fever. **Methanol causes inflammation of the retina** and has no renal toxicity. **Opiates are associated with focal-segmental glomerulonephritis**, not AKI. In addition, that is only with the impurities found with injection drug use, certainly not opiate medications.*

Toxins Producing ATN

Toxins have an **increased likelihood** of developing ATN **if there is hypoperfusion** of the kidney and if there is **underlying renal insufficiency** such as from hypertension or diabetes. The risk of ATN is directly proportional to **increasing age** of the patient.

Summary of Causes of ATN

- Nonoliguric renal injury is caused by aminoglycoside antibiotics, amphotericin, cisplatin, vancomycin, acyclovir, and cyclosporine. **Slower onset:** usually **5 to 10 days**. Dose dependent: the more administered, the sicker the patient gets. **Low magnesium level** may increase **risk of aminoglycoside** or cisplatin **toxicity.**
- **Contrast** media cause **immediate renal toxicity**. This can best be **prevented with saline hydration**. N-acetylcysteine and sodium bicarbonate are not consistently proven as beneficial.
- Hemoglobin and **myoglobin** (rhabdomyolysis)
- **Hyperuricemia** from tumor lysis syndrome acutely. Long-standing hyperuricemia from gout can cause chronic renal failure.
- **Precipitation of calcium oxalate in the renal cortex** from **ethylene glycol** overdose
- **Bence-Jones** protein is directly **toxic to renal tubules**.
- **NSAIDs**

> The body loses 1% of renal function for every year past the age of 40.

Rhabdomyolysis

Rhabdomyolysis is caused by **trauma**, prolonged **immobility**, snake bites, seizures, and **crush injuries**. The best initial test to confirm the diagnosis is a urinalysis. The **UA** will be **positive only on dipstick** for large amounts of **blood**, but **no cells will be seen** on microscopic examination.

Urine dipstick cannot tell the difference between:

- **Hemoglobin**
- **Myoglobin**
- **Red blood cells**

Creatine phosphokinase (CPK) levels are **markedly elevated**, but it is the findings on UA that tell you myoglobin is spilling into the urine. The most **specific test** is a **urine test for myoglobin**. **Hyperkalemia** occurs from the release of potassium from damaged cells because 95% of potassium in the body is intracellular. **Hyperuricemia** occurs for the same reason it does in tumor lysis syndrome. When **cells break down**, **nucleic acids** are **released** from the cell's nuclei and are rapidly **metabolized to uric acid**. Damaged muscle releases phosphate. **Hypocalcemia** occurs from increased calcium binding to damaged muscle.

> Why doesn't hemolysis cause hyperuricemia? RBCs have no nuclei.

Treat with:

- **Saline** hydration
- **Mannitol** as an osmotic diuretic
- **Bicarbonate**, which drives potassium back into cells and may prevent precipitation of myoglobin in the kidney tubule

The concept is that myoglobin is a severe oxidant stress on the tubular cells. Saline and mannitol increase urine flow rates to decrease the amount of contact time between the myoglobin and the tubular cells.

> Don't treat hypocalcemia in rhabdomyolysis if asymptomatic. In recovery, the calcium will come back out of the muscles.

A man comes to the emergency department after a triathlon, followed by status epilepticus. He takes simvastatin at triple the recommended dose. His muscles are tender and the urine is dark. Intravenous fluids are started.

What is the next best step in the management of this patient?

a. CPK level
b. EKG
c. Potassium replacement
d. Urine dipstick
e. Urine myoglobin

*Answer: The correct answer is (B). EKG is done to **detect life-threatening hyperkalemia**. Your question may have "potassium level" as the answer. CPK level, urine dipstick for blood and myoglobin should all be done, but the EKG will see if he is about to die of a fatal arrhythmia from hyperkalemia. Potassium replacement in a person with rhabdomyolysis would be fatal.*

TREATMENT

> More urine output with diuretics does not mean renal failure is reversing.

There is **no therapy proven to benefit ATN**. Patients should be managed with hydration, if they are volume depleted, and correction of electrolyte abnormalities. **Diuretics increase urine output**, **but do not change overall outcome**.

▶ TIP

Answering **treatment questions for ATN** is based on recognizing the most **common wrong answers**:

> Correct the underlying cause in ATN.

- Low-dose dopamine
- Diuretics
- Mannitol
- Steroids

All of these are ineffective in reversing ATN.

When Is Dialysis the Answer?

Dialysis is initiated if there is:
- COAGULOPATHY
- Fluid overload
- Encephalopathy
- Pericarditis
- Metabolic acidosis < 7.2
- Hyperkalemia

Initiating **dialysis** is **not based** on a specific level of **BUN or creatinine**. It is based on the development of **life-threatening conditions** like these that cannot be corrected another way.

Hypocalcemia, for example, is life-threatening (**seizures**, prolonged QT interval leading to **arrhythmia**) but you do not dialyze; you **give vitamin D and calcium**.

A patient develops ATN from gentamicin. She is vigorously hydrated and treated with high doses of diuretic, low-dose dopamine, and calcium acetate as a phosphate binder. Urine output increases but she still progresses to end-stage renal failure. She also becomes deaf.

What caused her hearing loss?

a. Hydrochlorothiazide
b. Dopamine
c. Furosemide
d. Chlorthalidone
e. Calcium acetate

Answer: The correct answer is (C). Furosemide causes ototoxicity by damaging the hair cells of the cochlea, resulting in sensorineural hearing loss. This is related not only to the total dose, but how fast it is injected. It essentially "burns" the inner ear. Aminoglycoside antibiotics also cause hearing loss. Furosemide in ATN adds no proven overall benefit. It does add ototoxicity to the gentamicin.

Hepatorenal Syndrome

Hepatorenal syndrome is renal failure developing secondary to liver disease. The kidneys are intrinsically normal. Look for:

- Severe liver disease (**cirrhosis**)
- New-onset renal failure with no other explanation
- Very **low urine sodium** (less than 10–15 mEq/dL)
- F_ENa below 1%
- **Elevated BUN: creatinine ratio (greater than 20:1)**

Treatment is with:

- Albumin
- Midodrine
- Octreotide

> Lab values in hepatorenal syndrome fit in with prerenal azotemia.

Atheroemboli

ETIOLOGY

Cholesterol plaques in the aorta or near the coronary arteries are sometimes large and fragile enough that they can be "**broken off**" when these vessels are manipulated during **catheter procedures**. **Cholesterol emboli** lodge in the kidney, leading to AKI. Look for **blue/purplish skin lesions** in fingers and toes, **livedo reticularis**, and ocular lesions.

Figure 10.1: Livedo reticularis.
Source: Farshad Bagheri, MD.

> Peripheral **pulses are normal** in atheroemboli. They are too small to occlude vessels such as the radial or brachial artery.

DIAGNOSTIC TESTS

Look for:

- Eosinophilia
- Low complement levels
- **Eosinophiluria**
- Elevated ESR

Biopsy of one of the **purplish skin lesions** is the **most accurate diagnostic test**. It shows cholesterol crystals, but this result **does not change management** because there is **no specific therapy** to reverse atheroembolic disease.

Acute (Allergic) Interstitial Nephritis

DEFINITION

Acute (allergic) interstitial nephritis (AIN) is a form of acute renal failure that damages the tubules occurring on an idiosyncratic (idiopathic) basis. Antibodies and **eosinophils attack the cells lining the tubules** as a reaction to **drugs (70%)**, infection, and autoimmune disorders.

ETIOLOGY

Although any medication can cause AIN, certain medications are more allergenic (allergy-inducing) than others. The most common medications are:

- **Penicillins** and cephalosporins
- **Sulfa drugs** (including diuretics like furosemide and thiazides, which are sulfa derivatives)
- Phenytoin

NSAIDS ?

- Rifampin
- Quinolones
- Allopurinol
- Proton pump inhibitors

Some medications are just not allergenic. For example, it is extremely rare to have a rash from calcium channel blockers, SSRIs, or beta blockers. These drugs are also almost never associated with AIN, toxic epidermal necrolysis, or hemolysis.

The medications that cause AIN are the same as those that cause:

- Drug allergy and rash
- Stevens-Johnson syndrome
- Toxic epidermal necrolysis
- Hemolysis

▶ **TIP**

Why learn these allergies as separate diseases? They are the same process, with different target organs affected.

Allergenic substances affect:

- Skin
- Kidney
- Red cells

In addition to drugs, AIN is also caused by infections and autoimmune disease like systemic lupus erythematosus (SLE), Sjögren, and sarcoidosis.

PRESENTATION/"WHAT IS THE MOST LIKELY DIAGNOSIS?"

Look for acute renal failure (rising BUN and creatinine) with:

- **Fever** (80%)
- **Rash** (50%)
- Arthralgias
- Eosinophilia and **eosinophiluria** (80%)

DIAGNOSTIC TESTS

- Elevated BUN and creatinine with ratio below 20:1
- White and red cells in the urine

Eosinophils are not found in the urine with AKI from NSAIDs

STOP

> Urine sodium and osmolality are not uniformly up or down in AIN. They cannot help establish the diagnosis.

1. STOP DRUG
2. GLUCOCORTICOIDS IF NOT RESOLVING

The **most accurate test is the Hansel** or **Wright stain**, which is how you determine whether **eosinophils** are present. The UA is able to detect only WBCs, RBCs, and protein; **it is not sufficiently accurate to determine that they are eosinophils**.

Treatment

AIN usually resolves spontaneously with stopping the drug or controlling the infection. Severe disease is managed with dialysis, which may be temporary. When the creatinine continues to rise after stopping the drug, giving glucocorticoids (prednisone, hydrocortisone, methylprednisolone) is the answer.

ANALGESIC NEPHROPATHY

Analgesic nephropathy presents with:

- **ATN** from direct toxicity to the tubules
- **AIN**
- **Membranous glomerulonephritis**
- **Vascular insufficiency** of the kidney from **inhibiting prostaglandins**. Prostaglandins dilate the afferent arteriole. **NSAIDs constrict the afferent arteriole** and decrease renal perfusion. This is asymptomatic in healthy patients. When patients are older and have underlying renal insufficiency from diabetes and/or hypertension, then NSAIDs can tip them over into clinically apparent renal insufficiency.
- **Papillary necrosis**

There is no specific diagnostic test to determine NSAIDs caused the disease previously described. **Exclude other causes and look for NSAIDs in the history.**

Papillary Necrosis

DEFINITION/ETIOLOGY

Papillary necrosis is a **sloughing off of the renal papillae**. It is caused by toxins such as **NSAIDs**, or sudden vascular insufficiency leading to death of the cells in the papillae and their dropping off the internal structure of the kidney.

Patients who are otherwise healthy don't get papillary necrosis. The case must describe a reason for underlying renal damage, even if the baseline BUN and creatinine levels are normal. Remember that a patient must lose at least 60% to 70% of renal function before the creatinine even begins to rise. Look for **extra NSAID use** with a history of:

- **Sickle cell disease**
- Diabetes
- Urinary obstruction
- Chronic pyelonephritis

PRESENTATION

Papillary necrosis can be very hard to distinguish from pyelonephritis. Look for **the sudden onset of flank pain**, fever, and hematuria in a patient with one of the diseases previously listed.

DIAGNOSTIC TESTS

The best initial test is a UA that shows red and white cells and may show necrotic kidney tissue. The urine culture will be normal (no growth). The **most accurate test is a CT scan** that shows the abnormal internal structures of the kidney from the loss of the papillae.

TREATMENT

There is **no specific therapy**. You cannot reattach the sloughed-off part of the kidney.

> Papillary necrosis can give grossly visible **necrotic material** passed **in the urine**. These are the renal papillae.

Differences between Pyelonephritis and Papillary Necrosis		
	Pyelonephritis	**Papillary necrosis**
Onset	Few days	Few hours
Symptoms	Dysuria	Necrotic material in urine
Urine culture	Positive	Negative
CT scan	Diffusely swollen kidney	"Bumpy" contour of interior where papillae were lost
Treatment	Antibiotics such as ampicillin/gentamicin or fluoroquinolones	No treatment

SUMMARY OF TUBULAR DISEASE

- Generally, tubular diseases are **acute**.
- Tubular diseases are caused by **toxins** (drugs, myoglobin, hemoglobin, oxalate, urate, NSAIDS, contrast).
- **None of them ever cause nephrotic syndrome** or give massive proteinuria.
- **Biopsy is not needed** to establish a diagnosis.
- They are **not treated with steroids** (like all drug allergies, AIN usually resolves spontaneously).
- Additional **immunosuppressive medications** (cyclophosphamide, mycophenolate) are **not used**.
- Treat tubular diseases by **correcting hypoperfusion** and **removing the toxin**.

Acute = Tubular = Toxin

Tubular Diseases

- Acute
- Toxins
- None nephrotic
- No biopsy usually
- No steroids
- Never additional immunosuppressive agents

GLOMERULAR DISEASES

General Answers to Glomerular Disease Questions

- Glomerular diseases are generally **chronic**.
- Glomerular diseases are generally **not caused by toxins or hypoperfusion**.
- **All of them** can cause **nephrotic syndrome**.
- **Biopsy is the most accurate test** to establish a diagnosis (though not always needed).
- They are **often treated with steroids** (several resolve spontaneously).
- **Additional immunosuppressive** medications (cyclophosphamide, mycophenolate) are **frequently used**.

Glomerular = Slow = Sample = Steroids = Immunosuppressives

Glomerular Diseases

- Chronic
- **Not from toxins/drugs**
- All potentially **nephrotic**
- **Biopsy sample**
- **Steroids often**

DIAGNOSTIC TESTS

All forms of glomerulonephritis have:

- UA with **hematuria**
- **"Dysmorphic"** red cells (deformed as they "squeeze" through an abnormal glomerulus)
- **Red cell casts**
- Urine sodium and F_ENa are low
- **Proteinuria**

The degree or **amount** of proteinuria is the main difference between **glomerulonephritis** and **nephrotic** syndrome.

Individual Glomerular Diseases

Every type of glomerulonephritis causes proteinuria, red cells, red cell casts in urine, hypertension, and edema, so you will need to know what is different or unique about each disease. It is like an IQ test: Which of these is different from the others?

→ ## Goodpasture Syndrome

Goodpasture also presents with **lung** and **kidney** involvement, but unlike Wegener granulomatosis (WG), there is **no upper respiratory tract involvement**. Goodpasture is also limited to just the lung and kidney, so signs of systemic vasculitis are absent. There is **no skin, joint, GI, eye, or neurological involvement**.

CRESCENTIC

DIAGNOSTIC TESTS/TREATMENT

The best initial test is antiglomerular basement membrane antibodies. The most accurate test is a lung or kidney biopsy. **Anemia is often present** from chronic blood loss from hemoptysis. The chest x-ray will be abnormal but is insufficient to confirm the diagnosis.

Treat with **plasmapheresis and steroids**. Cyclophosphamide can be helpful.

Kidney biopsy in Goodpasture syndrome shows "linear deposits."

→ ## IgA Nephropathy (Berger Disease)

IgA nephropathy is the **most common cause of acute glomerulonephritis** in the United States. Look for an Asian patient with recurrent episodes of **gross hematuria** 1 to 2 **days** after an upper respiratory tract infection (**synpharyngitic**). This actually helps, because IgA disease is the most common cause of glomerulonephritis and all the other causes have some specific physical findings.

Poststreptococcal glomerulonephritis follows pharyngitis by 1 to 2 **weeks**.

IgA = DAYS
PSGN = WEEKS

▶ **TIP**

There are **no unique physical findings** in IgA nephropathy to allow you to answer the "most likely diagnosis" question.

DIAGNOSTIC TESTS

IgA levels are increased in only 50%. The **most accurate test is a kidney biopsy**.

Proteinuria levels correspond to severity of disease and likelihood of progression.

More proteinuria = worse progression

TREATMENT

There is **no treatment proven to reverse the disease**. Thirty percent will completely resolve. Between 40% and 50% will slowly progress to end-stage renal disease.

Severe **proteinuria** is treated with **ACE inhibitors and steroids**. Fish oil is of uncertain benefit.

Postinfectious Glomerulonephritis

The most common organism leading to postinfectious glomerulonephritis (PIGN) is *Streptococcus*, but almost any infection can lead to abnormal activation of the immune system and PIGN. Poststreptococcal glomerulonephritis (PSGN) **follows throat infection or skin infection (impetigo) by 1 to 3 weeks.**

PRESENTATION

Patients present with:

- **Dark (cola-colored) urine**
- Edema that is often **periorbital**
- **Hypertension**
- Oliguria

DIAGNOSTIC TESTS

A UA with **proteinuria**, red cells, and **red cell casts** tells you that glomerulonephritis is present. PSGN from group A beta hemolytic streptococci (pyogenes) is confirmed first by antistreptolysin O (ASO) titers and anti-DNAse antibody titers. Biopsy is the most accurate test, but you should **not routinely do a kidney biopsy** because the blood test is sufficiently accurate and the disorder usually resolves spontaneously.

> Complement levels are low in PSGN.

TREATMENT

Management of PSGN does not reverse the glomerulonephritis. Use supportive therapies such as:

- **Antibiotics**
- **Diuretics** to control fluid overload

> Less than 5% of those with PSGN will progress.

Alport Syndrome

Alport syndrome is a congenital **defect of collagen** that results in glomerular disease combined with:

- Sensorineural **hearing loss**
- **Visual disturbance** from loss of the collagen fibers that hold the **lens of the eye** in place

There is **no specific therapy** to reverse this defect of type IV collagen.

Polyarteritis Nodosa

DEFINITION

Polyarteritis nodosa (PAN) is a **systemic vasculitis** of small and medium-sized arteries that most commonly affects the kidney. Virtually every organ in the body can be affected, but it tends to **spare the lung**. Although it is of unknown etiology, it can be **associated with hepatitis** B and all patients with PAN should be tested.

PRESENTATION

Besides the presentation of **glomerulonephritis**, PAN presents with nonspecific symptoms of **fever, malaise, weight loss, myalgias, and arthralgia** developing over weeks to months—as does almost every type of vasculitis. The most common organ systems involved are:

> PAN spares the lungs.

Gastrointestinal: Abdominal pain, bleeding, nausea, and vomiting occur. **Pain can be worsened by eating** because of mesenteric vasculitis.

> Damage to small blood vessels around nerves starves them into neuropathy.

Neurologic: Vasculitis damages the blood vessels surrounding larger peripheral nerves such as the peroneal, ulnar, radial, and brachial nerves. When more than one large peripheral nerve is involved, it is called "**mononeuritis multiplex.**" When presented with **stroke in a young person**, you should look for vasculitis.

> PAN is nonspecific. There is no single finding that allows you to answer the "most likely diagnosis" question.

Skin: Vasculitis of any cause leads to purpura (large) and petechiae (small). PAN also gives ulcers, **digital gangrene, and livedo reticularis.**

Cardiac disease is present in about one-third of patients.

> Stroke or MI in a young person suggests PAN.

DIAGNOSTIC TESTS

Blood tests will show:

- Anemia and leukocytosis
- Elevated ESR and C-reactive protein
- **ANCA: not present in most cases**
- ANA and rheumatoid factor: sometimes present in low titer

Angiography of the renal, mesenteric, or hepatic artery showing aneurysmal dilation in association with new-onset hypertension and characteristic symptoms is the best initial test that has specificity for PAN. Angiography is a clear answer as a diagnostic test when the most involved organ is not easily accessible for a biopsy (such as the kidney).

The **most accurate diagnostic test is a biopsy** of a symptomatic site such as skin, nerves, or muscles.

> There is no blood test to confirm PAN.

TREATMENT

Prednisone and cyclophosphamide are the standard of care and they lower mortality.

Treat hepatitis B when it is found.

Lupus Nephritis

SLE can give **any degree of renal involvement**. The kidneys in SLE can be normal or present with **mild, asymptomatic proteinuria**. Severe disease presents with **membranous glomerulonephritis**. Long-standing SLE may simply "scar" the kidneys and biopsy will **show glomerulosclerosis**, which has no active inflammatory component but may lead to such damage as to require dialysis.

Biopsy is the most accurate test of lupus nephritis. **Biopsy is indispensible in determining therapy.** Mild inflammatory changes may respond to glucocorticoids. Severe, proliferative disease such as membranous nephropathy is treated with **glucocorticoids combined with either cyclophosphamide or mycophenolate**.

Amyloidosis

Amyloid is an **abnormal protein** produced in association with:

- **Myeloma**
- Chronic inflammatory diseases
- Rheumatoid arthritis
- Inflammatory bowel disease
- Chronic infections

There is also a primary form of amyloidosis in which the protein is produced for unknown reasons. The kidney is the primary target of the protein.

Biopsy is the most accurate test. You will see **green birefringence with Congo red staining**.

Treat amyloidosis by trying to control the underlying disease. When this is unsuccessful or there is no primary disease to control, the treatment of amyloidosis is with **melphalan and prednisone**.

Nephrotic Syndrome

DEFINITION

Nephrotic syndrome is a measure of the **severity** of proteinuria in association with any form of glomerular disease. Nephrotic syndrome occurs when proteinuria is so massive that the liver can no longer increase the production of albumin to compensate for urinary losses. Massive proteinuria leads to:

- Edema
- Hyperlipidemia
- Thrombosis: from urinary loss of the natural anticoagulants protein C, protein S, and antithrombin

---

> Any form of glomerular disease can produce nephrotic syndrome.

> Biopsy is not performed to diagnose lupus, but rather to guide intensity of therapy.

> Amyloid, HIV nephropathy, polycystic kidneys, and diabetes give **large kidneys** on sonogram and CT scan.

> Nephrotic syndrome is not based on the etiology; it is based on the severity.

ETIOLOGY

Overall, diabetes and hypertension are the most common causes of nephrotic syndrome. Any of the glomerular diseases just described may lead to such massive protein loss that nephrotic syndrome develops.

In addition to systemic disease, there are a number of diseases limited to the kidney that produce nephrotic syndrome. It is better to describe "associations" rather than "causes," since we do not know what causes nephrotic syndrome. The associations are:

Cancer (solid organ): membranous

Children: minimal change disease

Injection drug use and AIDS: focal-segmental

NSAIDs: minimal change disease and membranous

SLE: Any of them

> The major difference between "nephritic" and "nephrotic" is the amount of proteinuria.

PRESENTATION

Nephrotic syndrome presents with generalized **edema**. **Infections are more frequent** because of increased urinary loss of immunoglobulins and complement. **Clots are more common** from loss of antithrombin, protein C, and protein S.

> CHF leads to edema of dependent areas like the legs. Nephrotic patients are edematous everywhere.

DIAGNOSTIC TESTS

The **best initial test is a urinalysis**.

Protein levels on a UA roughly correspond to the amount of protein excreted over 24 hours; however, since renal function varies with the time of day, as well as posture (flat or upright), the **UA is not sufficiently accurate**. You can have trace proteinuria on one UA and 2+ protein on another.

The urine **albumin/creatinine ratio** gives a measure of the average protein produced over 24 hours. A ratio of 2:1 means 2 grams of protein excreted over 24 hours. A ratio of 5.4 to 1 means 5.4 grams excreted over 24 hours.

The **urine albumin/creatinine spot urine ratio is equal to a 24-hour urine** in terms of accuracy and is much easier to obtain.

Renal biopsy is the most accurate test of the cause of nephrotic syndrome. Although there are certain associations with each form of nephrotic syndrome, only the biopsy can distinguish between the forms:

- Focal-segmental
- Membranous
- Membranoproliferative
- Minimal change
- Mesangial

> UA only detects albumin as a protein.

> Periorbital edema is characteristic of nephrotic syndrome

> UA shows Maltese crosses, which are lipid deposits in sloughed-off tubular cells.

By definition, nephrotic syndrome is:

- **Hyperproteinuria (more than 3.5 grams per 24 hours)**
- **Hypoproteinemia**
- **Hyperlipidemia** → *LEADS TO ACCELERATED ATHEROSCLEROSIS*
- **Edema**

Lipid levels rise because the lipoprotein signals that turn off the production of circulating lipid are now lost in the urine. With loss of these lipoproteins that surround chylomicrons and VLDLs, all lipid levels in the blood will rise.

TREATMENT

The best **initial therapy** for nephrotic syndrome is **glucocorticoids**. If there is no response after several weeks of therapy, other immunosuppressive medications such as **cyclophosphamide** are used.

ACE inhibitors or ARBs (angiotensin receptor blockers) are used to try to control proteinuria.

Edema is managed with **salt restriction and diuretics**. **Hyperlipidemia is managed with statins** as you would any form of hyperlipidemia.

END-STAGE RENAL DISEASE

DEFINITION

End-stage renal disease (ESRD), or chronic renal failure, is defined as that form of kidney failure **so severe as to need dialysis** or renal transplantation. **ESRD is not defined as a particular BUN or creatinine.** ESRD is defined as the loss of renal function leading to a collection of symptoms and laboratory abnormalities also known as **uremia**. Uremia is a term interchangeable with the conditions for which dialysis is the answer as therapy.

ETIOLOGY

Any form of tubular or glomerular damage can cause ESRD. Overall, diabetes and hypertension are, by far, more common than all the other causes of renal failure combined. ESRD usually implies disease that has been present for years; however, rapidly progressive glomerulonephritis is so named because it can lead to ESRD over weeks.

> Diabetes and hypertension are the most common causes of ESRD.

PRESENTATION

Uremia is defined as the presence of:

- Metabolic **acidosis**
- **Fluid** overload
- **Encephalopathy**
- **Hyperkalemia**
- **Pericarditis**

Each of these is an indication for dialysis. Although pericarditis is the least common, these events usually occur at the same time when creatinine clearance drops below the level at which acids, fluid, and potassium can be excreted.

> Peritoneal dialysis and hemodialysis are equally effective at removing wastes from the body.

Manifestations of Renal Failure

Anemia: Loss of erythropoietin leads to normochromic, normocytic anemia.

Hypocalcemia: The kidney transforms the less active 25-hydroxy-vitamin D into the much more active 1,25-dihydroxy-vitamin D. Without 1,25 dihydroxy form of vitamin D, the body will not absorb enough calcium from the gut.

Osteodystrophy: Low calcium leads to **secondary hyperparathyroidism**. High parathyroid hormone levels remove calcium from bones, making them soft and weak.

Bleeding: Platelets do not work normally in a uremic environment. They do not degranulate. If a platelet does not release the contents of its granules, it will not work.

Infection: The same defect occurs with neutrophils. Without degranulation, neutrophils will not effectively combat infection.

Pruritus: unclear reasoning; urea accumulating in skin causes itching

Hyperphosphatemia: Phosphate is normally excreted through kidneys. **High parathyroid hormone levels release phosphate from bones**, but the body is unable to excrete it.

Hypermagnesemia: from loss of excretory ability

> Cardiac disease kills triple the number that infection does in ESRD.

Accelerated atherosclerosis and hypertension: The immune system (lymphocytes) helps keep arteries clear of lipid accumulation. White cells don't work normally in a uremic environment. This is the most common cause of death in those on dialysis.

Endocrinopathy: Women are **anovulatory**. Men have **low testosterone**. **Erectile dysfunction** is common. Insulin levels tend to go up because insulin is excreted renally. However, insulin resistance also increases. Glucose levels therefore can be up or down.

> Anemia from ESRD is the only time erythropoietin is always used.

Treatment of the Manifestations of ESRD	
Manifestation	**Treatment**
Anemia	Erythropoietin replacement and iron supplementation
Hypocalcemia and osteomalacia	Replace vitamin D and calcium
Bleeding	DDAVP increases platelet function; use only when bleeding
Pruritus	Dialysis and ultraviolet light
Hyperphosphatemia	Oral binders: see "Treatment of Hyperphosphatemia"
Hypermagnesemia	Restriction of high-magnesium foods, laxatives, and antacids
Atherosclerosis	Dialysis
Endocrinopathy	Dialysis, estrogen and testosterone replacement

TREATMENT OF HYPERPHOSPHATEMIA

Oral phosphate binders will prevent phosphate absorption from the bowel. Treatment of hypocalcemia will also help because it is the hyperparathyroidism that causes increased phosphate release from bone. When vitamin D is replaced to control hypocalcemia, it is critical to also give phosphate binders; otherwise vitamin D will increase GI absorption of phosphate.

Use:

- Calcium acetate
- Calcium carbonate
- Sevelamer
- Lanthanum

> Use sevelamer and lanthanum when the calcium level is high.

> **Never** use aluminum-containing phosphate binders. **Aluminum causes dementia.**

Kidney Transplantation

Only 50% of ESRD patients will be suitable for transplantation. The donor does not have to be alive or related, although these are both better.

> HLA-identical, related donor kidneys last 24 years on average.

Survival by Method			
	1 year	**3 years**	**5 years**
Living, related donor	95%	88%	72%
Deceased donor	90%	78%	58%
Dialysis alone	Variable	Variable	30%–40%
Diabetics on dialysis	Variable	Variable	20%

THROMBOTIC THROMBOCYTOPENIC PURPURA AND HEMOLYTIC UREMIC SYNDROME

Thrombotic thrombocytopenic purpura (TTP) and hemolytic uremic syndrome (HUS) are different variants of what is probably the same disease. TTP is associated with HIV, cancer, and drugs such as cyclosporine, ticlopidine, and clopidogrel. HUS is more common in children and the most frequently tested association is *E. coli* 0157:H7 and *Shigella*. Both TTP and HUS are associated with:

- Intravascular hemolysis
- Renal insufficiency
- Thrombocytopenia

The hemolysis is visible on smear with **schistocytes,** helmet cells, and **fragmented red cells**.

TTP is associated with:

- Neurological symptoms
- Fever

TTP does not have to have all 5 manifestations to establish a diagnosis. In fact, **the only indispensible finding to establish the diagnosis is the intravascular hemolysis**.

Figure 10.2: Fragmented red cells, or schistocytes, are characteristic of intravascular hemolysis. *Source: Abhay Vakil, MD.*

Most cases of **HUS from *E. coli* will resolve spontaneously**. Plasmapheresis is generally urgent in TTP. Severe HUS also needs urgent plasmapheresis. If plasmapheresis is not one of the choices, use **infusions of fresh frozen plasma (FFP)**. Steroids do **not** help.

▶ **TIP**

Platelet transfusion is never the correct choice for TTP or HUS.

CYSTIC DISEASE

The single most important point in cystic disease is how to recognize a cyst that is potentially malignant and needs to be aspirated. If any of the qualities of a complex cyst are found, it should be aspirated to exclude malignancy.

Comparing Benign (Simple) Cysts and Potentially Malignant Cysts		
	Simple cyst	**Complex cysts (potential malignancy)**
Echogenicity	Echo free	Mixed echogenicity
Walls	Smooth, thin	Irregular, thick
Demarcation	Sharp	Lower density on back wall
Transmission	Good through to back	Debris in cyst

Polycystic Kidney Disease

Polycystic kidney disease (PCKD) presents with:

- Pain
- Hematuria
- Stones
- Infection
- Hypertension

What is the most common cause of death from PCKD?

a. Intracerebral hemorrhage
b. Stones
c. Infection
d. Malignancy
e. Renal failure

Answer: The correct answer is (E). Renal failure occurs in PCKD from recurrent episodes of pyelonephritis and nephrolithiasis causing progressive scarring and loss of renal function. PCKD does not have malignant potential. Only 10% to 15% of affected people have cerebral aneurysms, most of which do not rupture. Connective tissue is weak throughout the body. These patients may have:

- *Liver cysts (most common site outside the kidney)*
- *Ovarian cysts*
- *Mitral valve prolapse*
- *Diverticulosis*

> No therapy exists to prevent or reverse cysts of any type.

SODIUM DISORDERS

Hypernatremia

ETIOLOGY

Hypernatremia occurs when there is **loss of free water**. Examples are:

- **Sweating**
- Burns
- Fever
- **Pneumonia:** from insensible losses from hyperventilation
- Diarrhea
- Diuretics

Diabetes insipidus (DI) leads to **high-volume water loss** from **insufficient or ineffective antidiuretic hormone (ADH)**. Any CNS disorder (stroke, tumor, trauma, hypoxia, infection) can damage the production of ADH in the hypothalamus or storage in the posterior pituitary, leading to central diabetes insipidus (CDI).

Nephrogenic DI is a **loss of ADH effect** on the collecting duct of the kidney. This is much less common. Nephrogenic DI is caused by **lithium** or demeclocycline, **chronic kidney disease, hypokalemia, or hypercalcemia.** They make **ADH ineffective** at the tubule.

High-volume **nocturia** is the first clue to the **presence of DI.**

PRESENTATION

DI and hypernatremia of any cause presents with **neurological** symptoms such as **confusion, disorientation, lethargy,** and **seizures.** If uncorrected, severe hypernatremia causes **coma** and irreversible **brain damage.**

Sodium disorders cause **CNS** problems.

▶ **TIP**

Polyuria is high urine volume. Frequency just means increased attempts at voiding. The volume in urinary frequency might be very small (such as in urethritis or cystitis).

DIAGNOSTIC TESTS

High serum sodium is nearly equivalent to hyperosmolality since the majority of osmolality is sodium. Fluid losses from the skin, kidneys, or stool generally lead to:

Increased urine volume despite dehydration and hyperosmolality of the blood suggests DI.

- Decreased urine volume (high urine volume in DI)
- Increased urine osmolality (decreased urine osmolality in DI)
- Decreased urine sodium

Water Deprivation Test

The best initial test for DI is preventing the patient from drinking, then observing urine output and urine osmolality. With **DI,** urine **volume stays high** and urine **osmolality** stays **low** despite vigorous urine production and despite developing dehydration.

Response to ADH administration:

- **CDI: sharp decrease in urine volume,** increase in osmolality
- NDI: No change in urine volume or osmolality with ADH administration

The single most accurate test of CDI vs. NDI is an **ADH level.** The **ADH level is low in CDI,** and markedly **elevated in NDI.**

A "positive" water deprivation test means urine volume stays high despite withholding water.

Comparison of Central versus Nephrogenic Diabetes Insipidus		
	CDI	**NDI**
Polyuria and nocturia	Yes	Yes
Urine osmolality and sodium	Low	Low
Positive water deprivation test	Yes	Yes
Response to ADH	Yes	No
ADH level	Low	High

TREATMENT

1. Fluid loss: **Correct the underlying cause** of fluid loss.
2. **CDI: Replace ADH** (vasopressin also known as DDAVP).
3. **NDI:**

   - Correct **potassium and calcium**.
   - Stop lithium or demeclocycline.
   - Give hydrochlorothiazide or NSAIDs for those still having NDI despite these interventions.

Complications of Therapy

If sodium levels are brought down too rapidly, cerebral edema will occur. This is from the shift of fluids from the vascular space into the cells of the brain. Cerebral edema presents with worsening confusion and seizures.

Hyponatremia

ETIOLOGY

Hyponatremia is characterized according to overall **volume status** of the body.

Hypervolemia   *↑ VOLUME*

The most common causes of hyponatremia with a hypervolemic state are:

- **CHF**
- **Nephrotic syndrome**
- **Cirrhosis**

These are cases in which **intravascular volume depletion** leads to **increased ADH levels**. Pressure receptors in the **atria and carotids sense the decrease in volume and stimulate ADH production** and release. Although the sodium level drops, it is more important to maintain vascular volume and organ perfusion.

Look For:
Edema
JVD
Ascites
CHF

> Perfusion is more important than normal sodium.

Hypovolemia   *↓ VOLUME*

Fluid Loss

- **Sweating**
- Burns
- Fever
- **Pneumonia:** from insensible losses from hyperventilation
- Diarrhea
- Diuretics

All of these are also causes of hypernatremia; however, they cause hyponatremia if there is **chronic replacement with free water**. A little sodium and a lot of water are lost in urine, which is then replaced with free water that has no sodium. Over time, this process **depletes the body of sodium** and the serum sodium level drops.

Addison disease or loss of adrenal function also causes hyponatremia because of loss of aldosterone. Aldosterone causes sodium reabsorption. If the body **loses aldosterone, it loses sodium.**

Euvolemia

The most common causes of hyponatremia with euvolemia (normal volume status) are:

- Pseudohyponatremia (hyperglycemia)
- Psychogenic polydipsia
- Hypothyroidism
- Syndrome of inappropriate ADH release (SIADH)

R TA
A LDOSTERONE (ADDISON'S)
T HYROID
S IADH

Hyperglycemia: Very **high glucose** levels lead to a **decrease in sodium levels**. Hyperglycemia acts as an osmotic draw on fluid inside the cells. Free water leaves the cells to correct the hyperosmolar serum. This drops the sodium level. The management is to correct the glucose level.

↑GLU = ↑H$_2$O OUTSIDE CELL = Na DILUTION

For every 100 mg/dL of glucose above normal, there is a 1.6 mEq/L decrease in sodium.

$$\frac{GLU - 100}{100} \times 1.6 = \text{AMOUNT TO ADD TO Na FOR ACTUAL READING}$$

Psychogenic polydipsia: Massive ingestion of free water above 12 to 24 liters a day will overwhelm the kidney's ability to excrete water. The minimum urine osmolality is 50 mOsm/kg. The body can produce 12 to 24 liters of urine a day, depending on whether you can get the urine osmolality down to 50 or 100 mOsm/kg.

> 12-24 LITERS/DAY

▶ **TIP**

Look for a history **of bipolar disorder to suggest psychogenic polydipsia.**

BIPOLAR → PSYCHOGENIC POLYDIPSIA

Hypothyroidism: Thyroid hormone is needed to excrete water. If the thyroid hormone level is low, free water excretion is decreased.

SIADH: Any **lung** or **brain disease** can cause **SIADH** for unclear reasons. Certain drugs such as SSRIs, sulfonylureas, vincristine, cyclophosphamide, or tricyclic antidepressants can cause SIADH. Certain cancers, especially small-cell cancer of the lung, produce ADH. Pain causes SIADH.

PRESENTATION

Hyponatremia presents entirely with **CNS symptoms**:

- Confusion
- Lethargy
- Disorientation
- Seizures
- Coma

If the sodium levels drop very fast, the patient can immediately seize. **Slow drops** may be entirely **asymptomatic** even if the level is very low.

> Symptoms of hyponatremia are dependent on how fast it occurs.

> Sodium means CNS symptoms.

DIAGNOSTIC TESTS

In SIADH, the urine is inappropriately concentrated (**high urine osmolality**). The urine sodium is inappropriately high in SIADH. The uric acid level and BUN are low in SIADH.

The most accurate test is a high ADH level.

Response to Hyponatremia		
	Normal levels	**SIADH**
Urine osmolality	Low (<100 mOsm/kg)	High
Urine sodium	Low (<20 mEq/L)	High (>40 mEq/L)

TREATMENT

Clinical Manifestations of Hyponatremia by Severity		
Degree of hyponatremia	**Specific manifestation**	**Management**
Mild hyponatremia	No symptoms	Restrict fluids
Moderate	Minimal confusion	Saline and loop diuretic
Severe	Lethargy, seizures, coma	Hypertonic saline, conivaptan, tolvaptan

▶ **TIP**

The treatment answer is not based on the sodium level; it is based on the symptoms.

ADH antagonists: Tolvapatan and conivaptan are antagonists of ADH. They are the answer as part of urgent therapy for severe, symptomatic SIADH. They are only for urgent treatment in hospital. No oral version is available.

Chronic SIADH: SIADH can be from an underlying disorder that cannot be corrected such as metastatic cancer. **Demeclocycline treats chronic SIADH.** **Demeclocycline blocks** the action of **ADH** at the collecting duct of the kidney tubule.

Complications of Treatment

Correction of sodium must occur slowly. "Slowly" is defined as under 0.5 to 1 mEq per hour or 12 to 24 mEq per day. If the sodium level is brought up to normal too rapidly, the neurological disorder known as **central pontine myelinolysis** or **osmotic demyelinization** occurs.

POTASSIUM DISORDERS

Hyperkalemia

High potassium levels (hyperkalemia) are an absolutely indispensible portion of your knowledge because of the **life-threatening nature of potassium disorders.**

Margin notes:

SIADH = Too much ADH = retain H₂O

Losing same amount of Na, so urine Na is ↑ but serum Na is ↓ from dilution

In SIADH, saline without a diuretic makes it worse.

CPM = dehydration of the brain

Severe hyperkalemia can stop the heart in seconds if the level is high enough.

ETIOLOGY

Pseudohyperkalemia (falsely elevated levels):

- **Hemolysis**
- Repeated fist clenching with tourniquet in place
- **Thrombocytosis** or **leukocytosis** will leak out of cells in the lab specimen

None of these causes of hyperkalemia needs further treatment or investigation beyond repeating the sample.

Decreased excretion:

- **Renal failure**
- **Aldosterone decrease:**
  - **ACE inhibitors**/ARBs
  - Type IV renal tubular acidosis (hyporeninemic, hypoaldosteronism)
  - Spironolactone and eplerenone (aldosterone inhibitors)
  - Triamterene and amiloride (potassium-sparing diuretics)
  - Addison disease

Release of potassium from tissues:

- Any **tissue destruction**, such as hemolysis, **rhabdomyolysis**, or **tumor lysis** syndrome, can release potassium.
- **Decreased insulin:** Insulin normally drives potassium into cells.
- **Acidosis:** Cells will pick up hydrogen ions (acid) and release potassium in exchange.
- Beta blockers and digoxin: These drugs inhibit the sodium/potassium ATPase that normally brings potassium into the cells.
- Heparin increases potassium levels, presumably through increased tissue release.

> Since 95% of potassium in the body is intracellular, shifting potassium out of cells can easily be fatal.

PRESENTATION

Potassium disorders interfere with muscle contraction and cardiac conductance. Look for:

- Weakness
- **Paralysis** when severe
- **Ileus** (paralyzes gut muscles)
- Cardiac rhythm disorders

> Hyperkalemia does not cause seizures.

DIAGNOSTIC TESTS

Besides a potassium level, testing is aimed at looking for the causes previously described. **The most urgent test in severe hyperkalemia is an EKG.**

HYPERKALEMIA = ECG

The EKG in severe hyperkalemia shows:

- **Peaked T waves**
- Wide QRS
- PR interval prolongation

TREATMENT

Handwritten left margin:
HYPERKALEMIA (↑ SERUM K⁺)
→ CaCl | Ca GLUCONATE
→ INSULIN + GLUCOSE
→ BICARB IF CAUSED BY ACIDOSIS

Life-Threatening Hyperkalemia (Abnormal EKG)
1. Calcium chloride or calcium gluconate — *PROTECTS HEART BUT DOESN'T HELP* ↑
2. Insulin and glucose to drive potassium back into cells
3. Bicarbonate: drives potassium into cells but should be used most when acidosis causes hyperkalemia

Removing Potassium from the Body

Sodium polystyrene sulfonate (**Kayexalate**; Sanofi-Aventis, Bridgewater, New Jersey) **removes potassium from the body** through the bowel. The patient ingests Kayexalate orally and over several hours it will bind potassium in the gut and remove it from the body.

Insulin and bicarbonate lower the potassium level through redistribution into the cells.

Other methods to lower potassium are:

- Inhaled beta agonists (albuterol)
- Loop diuretics
- Dialysis

> Calcium is only used if the EKG is abnormal to protect the heart. It does not lower the potassium level.

> Insulin does not remove potassium from the body.

> Sodium = CNS symptoms
> Hyperkalemia = muscular and cardiac symptoms

▶ TIP

When there is hyperkalemia and an abnormal EKG, the "most appropriate next step" is clearly calcium chloride or gluconate.

Hypokalemia

ETIOLOGY

Decreased intake: This is unusual because the kidney can decrease potassium excretion to extremely small amounts.

Shift into cells:

Handwritten: CELL ⟶ K⁺ SERUM, H⁺ →

- Alkalosis (hydrogen ions come out of the cell in exchange for potassium entering)
- Increased insulin
- Beta adrenergic stimulation (accelerates sodium/potassium ATPase)

Renal loss:

- Loop diuretics
- Increased aldosterone

- Primary hyperaldosteronism (Conn syndrome)
- Volume depletion raises aldosterone
- Cushing syndrome
- Bartter syndrome (genetic disease causing salt loss in loop of Henle)
- Licorice

- Hypomagnesemia: There are magnesium-dependent potassium channels. When magnesium is low, they open and spill potassium into the urine.

$\downarrow Mg^{2+} = $ URINARY LOSS OF K^+

- Renal tubular acidosis (RTA) types I and II

Gastrointestinal loss:

- Vomiting
- Diarrhea
- Laxative abuse

PRESENTATION

Hypokalemia leads to problems with muscular contraction and cardiac conduction. Potassium is essential for proper neuromuscular contraction. Hypokalemia presents with:

- Weakness
- Paralysis
- Loss of reflexes

> Muscular abnormalities may be so severe as to cause rhabdomyolysis.

EKG findings

U waves are the most characteristic finding of hypokalemia.

Other findings are ventricular ectopy (PVCs), flattened T waves, and ST depression.

> Hypokalemia does **not** cause seizures.

TREATMENT

There is no **maximum rate of oral potassium replacement**. The gastrointestinal system cannot absorb potassium faster than the kidneys can excrete it, so you cannot go too far too fast. **Intravenous potassium replacement, however, can cause a fatal arrhythmia** if it is done too fast. You must allow time for potassium to equilibrate into the cells.

> Intravenous potassium replacement must be very slow.

A patient is admitted with vomiting and diarrhea from gastroenteritis. His volume status is corrected with intravenous fluids and the diarrhea resolves. His pH is 7.40 and his serum bicarbonate has normalized. Despite vigorous oral and intravenous replacement, his potassium level fails to rise.

What should you do?

a. Consult nephrology
b. Magnesium level
c. Parathyroid hormone level
d. Intracellular pH level
e. 24-hour urine potassium level

K⁺

K⁺

Mg²⁺

URINE

Answer: The correct answer is (B). Hypomagnesemia can lead to increased urinary loss of potassium. If magnesium is replaced, it will close up the magnesium-dependent potassium channels and stop urinary loss. Although magnesium is necessary for parathyroid hormone release, this would have nothing to do with potassium levels. Try not to consult on Step 2. You are supposed to handle anything that is based on knowledge. Consultations are generally indicated only for procedures such as catheterization or endoscopy. Although there will be increased potassium on a 24-hour urine with hypomagnesemia, there is no point in performing this test because you still have to detect and treat hypomagnesemia.

A woman with ESRD and glucose 6-phosphate dehydrogenase deficiency skips dialysis for a few weeks and then is crushed in a motor vehicle accident. She is taking dapsone and has recently eaten fava beans. What is the most urgent step?

a. Initiate dialysis
b. EKG
c. Bicarbonate administration
d. Insulin administration
e. Kayexalate
f. Urine dipstick
g. CPK levels
h. Urine myoglobin

Answer: The correct answer is (B). All of these interventions may be helpful in a person with life-threatening hyperkalemia. The most important step is to determine if there are EKG changes from hyperkalemia. If the EKG is abnormal, she needs calcium chloride or gluconate in order to protect her heart while the other interventions are performed. Kayexalate and dialysis take hours to remove potassium from the body. Bicarbonate and insulin work in 15 to 20 minutes, but they are not as instantaneous in effect as giving calcium.

▶ **TIP**

Protect the heart first in potassium disorders.

ACID-BASE DISTURBANCES

Renal Tubular Acidosis

DEFINITION

Renal tubular acidosis (RTA) is a metabolic acidosis with a normal anion gap. The anion gap is defined as sodium minus chloride plus bicarbonate.

$$(Na^+) \text{ minus } (Cl^- \text{ and } HCO_3^-)$$

A normal anion gap is between 6 and 12. The difference between the cations and the anions is predominantly from negative charges that are on albumin. The 2 most important causes of a metabolic acidosis with a normal anion gap are:

- RTA
- Diarrhea

The anion gap is normal in both of these because the chloride level rises. Hence, they are also referred to as hyperchloremic metabolic acidosis. The anion gap increases from ingested substances such as ethylene glycol or methanol, or organic acids such as lactate that are anionic and drive down the chloride level.

Distal RTA (Type I)

The **distal tubule** is responsible for **generating new bicarbonate** under the influence of aldosterone. Drugs such as **amphotericin** and **autoimmune diseases** such as SLE or Sjögren syndrome can damage the distal tubule. If new bicarbonate cannot be generated at the distal tubule, then acid cannot be excreted into the tubule, raising the pH of the urine.

In an alkaline urine, there is **increased formation of kidney stones** from calcium oxalate.

No acid into the tubule makes the urine basic.

Distal RTA calcifies the kidney parenchyma (nephrocalcinosis).

DIAGNOSTIC TESTS

The best initial test is a UA looking for an abnormally **high pH above 5.5.** The most accurate test is to infuse acid into the blood with ammonium chloride. A healthy person will be able to excrete the acid and will decrease the urine pH. Those with distal RTA cannot excrete the acid and the urine pH will remain basic (over 5.5) despite an increasingly acidic serum.

Treatment of Distal RTA

Replace bicarbonate that will be absorbed at the proximal tubule. Since the majority of bicarbonate is absorbed at the proximal tubule, distal RTA is relatively easy to correct. Just give more bicarbonate and the proximal tubule will absorb it and correct the acidosis.

RTA does not mean the tubule is always acidic.

Proximal RTA (Type II)

Normally 85% to 90% of filtered bicarbonate is reabsorbed at the proximal tubule. Damage to the proximal tubule from amyloidosis, myeloma, Fanconi syndrome, acetazolamide, or heavy metals **decreases the ability of the kidney to reabsorb most of filtered bicarbonate**. Bicarbonate is lost in the urine until the body is so depleted of bicarbonate that the distal tubule can absorb the rest. When this happens, the urine pH will become low (at or below 5.5). Chronic metabolic acidosis leaches calcium out of the bones and they become soft (osteomalacia).

DIAGNOSTIC TESTS

The **urine pH is variable in proximal RTA**. First it is basic (above 5.5) until most bicarbonate is lost from the body, then it is low (below 5.5). The most accurate test is to evaluate bicarbonate malabsorption in the kidney by giving bicarbonate and testing the urine pH. Because the kidney cannot absorb bicarbonate, the urine pH will rise.

Both proximal and distal RTA are hypokalemic. Potassium is lost in the urine.

TREATMENT

Because bicarbonate is not absorbed well in proximal RTA, it is difficult to treat it with bicarbonate replacement and massive doses are necessary. **Thiazide diuretics cause volume depletion. Volume depletion will enhance bicarbonate reabsorption.**

Hyporeninemia, Hypoaldosteronism (Type IV RTA)

Type IV RTA occurs most often in diabetes. There is a decreased amount or effect of aldosterone at the kidney tubule. This leads to loss of sodium and retention of potassium and hydrogen ions. Test for type IV RTA by finding a persistently high urine sodium despite a sodium-depleted diet. In addition, hyperkalemia is a main clue to answering "What is the most likely diagnosis?"

> Fludrocortisone is the steroid with the highest mineralocorticoid or "aldosteronelike" effect.

▶ **TIP**

Just because RTA is difficult does not mean it isn't tested. RTA is tested. Learn it.

Types of Renal Tubular Acidosis (RTA)			
	Proximal (type II)	**Distal (type I)**	**Type IV**
Urine pH	Variable	High >5.5	<5.5
Blood potassium level	Low	Low	High
Nephrolithiasis	No	Yes	No
Diagnostic test	Administer bicarbonate	Administer acid	Urine salt loss
Treatment	Thiazides	Bicarbonate	Fludrocortisone

Urine Anion Gap

DEFINITION

The **urine anion gap (UAG) is a way to distinguish between diarrhea and RTA** as causes of normal anion gap metabolic acidosis.

$$UAG = sodium\ minus\ chloride$$

or

$$Na^+\ minus\ Cl^-$$

Acid excreted by the kidney is buffered off as NH_4Cl or ammonium chloride. The more acid excreted, the greater the amount of chloride found in the urine. In RTA there is a defect in acid excretion into the urine, so the amount of chloride in the urine is diminished. This gives a positive number when calculating Na^+ minus Cl^-.

> RTA has a positive UAG.

In diarrhea, the ability to excrete acid through the kidney remains intact. Because diarrhea is associated with metabolic acidosis, the kidney tries to compensate by increasing acid excretion. Hence, in diarrhea there is more acid in the urine. Acid (H^+) is excreted with chloride. So, in diarrhea, more acid in the urine means more chloride in the urine. Na^+ minus Cl^- will become a negative number in diarrhea.

> Diarrhea has a negative UAG.

Metabolic Acidosis

Normal anion gap (6–12): RTA and diarrhea

Elevated anion gap (above 12): The anion gap is increased if there are unmeasured anions driving the bicarbonate level down. Examples are found in the following table.

> Respiratory alkalosis from hyperventilation compensates for all forms of metabolic acidosis.

Causes of Metabolic Acidosis with an Increased Anion Gap			
	Cause	**Test**	**Treatment**
Lactate	Hypotension or hypoperfusion	Blood lactate level	Correct hypoperfusion
Ketoacids	DKA, starvation	Acetone level	Insulin and fluids
Oxalic acid	Ethylene glycol overdose	Crystals on UA	Fomepizole, dialysis
Formic acid	Methanol overdose	Inflamed retina	Fomepizole, dialysis
Uremia	Renal failure	BUN, creatinine	Dialysis
Salicylates	Aspirin overdose	Aspirin level	Alkalinize urine

Arterial Blood Gas in Metabolic Acidosis

The arterial blood gas (ABG) in metabolic acidosis will always have:

- Decreased pH below 7.4
- Decreased pCO_2 indicating respiratory alkalosis as compensation
- Decreased bicarbonate

▶ **TIP**

You cannot determine the etiology of metabolic acidosis from the ABG.

> Metabolic problems always show compensation.

Metabolic Alkalosis

By definition, **metabolic alkalosis** has an **elevated serum bicarbonate** level. The compensation for metabolic alkalosis is respiratory acidosis. There will be a **relative hypoventilation** that will increase the pCO_2 to compensate for metabolic alkalosis.

ETIOLOGY OF METABOLIC ALKALOSIS

- GI loss: **vomiting** or nasogastric suction
- Increased **aldosterone**: primary hyperaldosteronism, Cushing syndrome, ectopic ACTH, volume contraction, licorice
- **Diuretics**

- Milk-alkali syndrome: high-volume liquid antacids
- Hypokalemia: hydrogen ions move into cells so potassium can be released

Arterial Blood Gas in Metabolic Alkalosis

The ABG in metabolic alkalosis will always have:

- **Increased** pH >7.40
- **Increased** pCO_2 indicating respiratory **acidosis** as compensation
- **Increased** bicarbonate

▶ **TIP**

You cannot determine the etiology of metabolic alkalosis from the ABG.

Respiratory Acidosis and Alkalosis

Respiratory acid/base disturbances are easy to understand because they come down to the single pathway of the effect on minute ventilation.

Minute ventilation = respiratory rate × tidal volume

ETIOLOGY

Causes of Respiratory Acidosis and Alkalosis	
Respiratory alkalosis	**Respiratory acidosis**
Decreased pCO_2	Increased pCO_2
Increased minute ventilation	Decreased minute ventilation
Metabolic acidosis as compensation	Metabolic alkalosis as compensation
<ul><li>Anemia</li><li>Anxiety</li><li>Pain</li><li>Fever</li><li>Interstitial lung disease</li><li>Pulmonary emboli</li></ul>	<ul><li>COPD/emphysema</li><li>Drowning</li><li>Opiate overdose</li><li>Alpha 1-antitrypsin deficiency</li><li>Kyphoscoliosis</li><li>Sleep apnea/morbid obesity</li></ul>

NEPHROLITHIASIS

The most common cause of kidney stones (nephrolithiasis) is **calcium oxalate**, which forms more frequently in an **alkaline urine**. The most common risk factor is the **overexcretion of calcium** in the urine.

CYSTINURIA — HEXAGONAL CRYSTALS | FAM HISTORY OF STONES | CYANIDE NITROPRUSIDE (+)

Sidebar notes:

Metabolic derangements kill patients with cardiac arrhythmia. They also alter potassium levels.

Minute ventilation is more precise than respiratory rate.

Hyperventilation may occur with a tiny tidal volume. This does not increase minute ventilation.

A 46-year-old man comes to the emergency department with excruciating pain in his left flank radiating to the groin. He has some blood in his urine.

What is the most appropriate next step in the management of this patient?

a. Ketorolac
b. X-ray
c. Sonography
d. Urinalysis
e. Serum calcium level

Answer: The correct answer is (A). Ketorolac is an NSAID that is available orally and intravenously. It provides a level of analgesia similar to opiate medications. When the presentation of nephrolithiasis is clear, it is more important to provide relief for this excruciating form of pain than to obtain specific diagnostic tests.

> Crohn disease causes kidney stones because of increased oxalate absorption.

What is the most accurate diagnostic test for nephrolithiasis?

a. CT scan
b. X-ray
c. Sonography
d. Urinalysis
e. Intravenous pyelogram

Answer: The correct answer is (A). The CT scan for nephrolithiasis does not need contrast and is more accurate (sensitive) than an x-ray or sonogram. Intravenous pyelogram (IVP) needs intravenous contrast and takes several hours to perform. Urinalysis and straining the urine may show blood or the passage of a stone, but will not help manage acute renal colic. X-ray has a false negative rate between 10% and 20%. X-rays of the abdomen are useful only in detecting an ileus.

▶ TIP

IVP is always a wrong answer for nephrolithiasis.

TREATMENT

The best initial therapy for acute renal colic is with:

- Analgesics
- Hydration
- Imaging to confirm the location of the stone
- CT and sonography to detect obstruction such as hydronephrosis

> Uric acid stones are not detectable on x-ray but are visualized on CT.

The etiology of the stone is determined with:

- Stone analysis
- Serum calcium, sodium, uric acid, PTH, magnesium, and phosphate levels
- 24-hour urine for volume, calcium, oxalate, citrate, cystine, pH, uric acid, phosphate, and magnesium

> Cystine stones are managed with surgical removal, alkalinizing the urine.

> Fat malabsorption increases stone formation.

A woman with her first episode of renal colic is found to have a 1.8 cm stone in the left renal pelvis. She has no obstruction and her renal function is normal (normal BUN and creatinine).

What is the most appropriate next step in the management of this patient?

a. Wait for it to pass; hydrate and observe
b. Lithotripsy
c. Surgical removal
d. Hydrochlorothiazide
e. Stent placement

Answer: The correct answer is (B). Lithotripsy is used to manage stones between 0.5 and 2 to 3 centimeters. Small stones (less than 5 mm) will spontaneously pass. Stones larger than 2 centimeters are not well-managed with lithotripsy because the fragments will get caught in the ureters. These large stones are best managed surgically. **Stent placement relieves hydronephrosis** from stones caught in the distal ureters. Stones halfway up the ureters are treated with lithotripsy. Those halfway down the ureter are removed from below with a basket.

> Urinary tract infection gives struvite stones (magnesium/ammonium/phosphate). Remove them surgically.

Long-term Management of Nephrolithiasis

50% of those with kidney stones will have a recurrence over the next 5 years.

A man with a calcium oxalate stone is managed with lithotripsy and the stone is destroyed and passes. His urinary calcium level is increased.

Besides increasing hydration, which of the following is most likely to benefit this patient?

a. Calcium restriction
b. Hydrochlorothiazide
c. Furosemide
d. Stent placement
e. Increased dietary oxalate

Answer: The correct answer is (B). **Hydrochlorothiazide removes calcium from the urine** by increasing distal tubular reabsorption of calcium. Furosemide increases calcium excretion into the urine and can make it worse. Calcium restriction actually does not help decrease overexcretion of calcium into the urine. In fact, it can make it more likely to form a stone. This is because calcium binds oxalate in the bowel. When calcium ingestion is low, there is increased oxalate absorption in the gut because there is no calcium to bind it in the gut. Stent placement is done when there is an obstruction in the ureters, especially at the ureteropelvic junction. Hydrochlorothiazide desaturates the urine of calcium. The risk of stone formation is increased if there is a dietary decrease in calcium, increase in oxalate, or decrease in citrate.

Metabolic Acidosis and Stone Formation

Metabolic acidosis removes calcium from bones and increases stone formation. In addition, metabolic acidosis decreases citrate levels. Citrate binds calcium, making it unavailable for stone formation.

Urinary Incontinence		
	Stress incontinence	**Urge incontinence**
Symptoms	Older woman with painless urinary leakage with coughing, laughing, or lifting heavy objects	Sudden pain in the bladder followed immediately by the overwhelming urge to urinate
Test	Have patient stand and cough; observe for leakage	Pressure measurement in half-full bladder; manometry

Treatment	1. Kegel exercises
	2. Local estrogen cream
	3. Surgical tightening of urethra
		1. Bladder training exercises
		2. Local anticholinergic therapy
		  • Oxybutynin
		  • Tolterodine
		  • Solifenacin
		  • Dariferancin
		3. Surgical tightening of urethra

HYPERTENSION

DEFINITION

- **Systolic pressure above 140 mm Hg**
- **Diastolic pressure above 90 mm Hg**

In order to establish the diagnosis of hypertension, blood pressure measurements must be repeated in a calm state over time. The precise interval between measurements over what period of time is not clear.

A **diabetic** patient or someone with chronic renal disease hypertension is **above 130/80 mm Hg**.

Hypertension is:

- The most common disease in the United States
- The most common risk factor for the most common cause of death: myocardial infarction

ETIOLOGY

Ninety-five percent of hypertension has no clear etiology and can be called "essential hypertension." Known causes of hypertension are:

- **Renal artery stenosis**
- Glomerulonephritis
- Coarctation of the aorta
- Acromegaly

- Pheochromocytoma
- Hyperaldosteronism
- Cushing syndrome or any cause of hypercortisolism including therapeutic use of glucocorticoids
- Congenital adrenal hyperplasia

PRESENTATION

The vast majority of cases are found on **routine screening of asymptomatic patients**. When hypertension does have symptoms, they are from end organ damage from atherosclerosis such as:

- Coronary artery disease
- Cerebrovascular disease
- CHF
- Visual disturbance
- Renal insufficiency
- Peripheral artery disease

Presentation of Secondary Hypertension

- Renal artery stenosis: **Bruit is** auscultated at the flank. The bruit is continuous throughout systole and diastole.
- Glomerulonephritis
- Coarctation of the aorta: **upper extremity > lower extremity** blood pressure
- Acromegaly
- Pheochromocytoma: **episodic** hypertension with flushing
- Hyperaldosteronism: weakness from **hypokalemia**

> Hypertension is rarely symptomatic at first presentation.

DIAGNOSTIC TESTS

Repeated in-office measurement or home ambulatory measurements carry equal significance.

Those with hypertension are also tested with:

- EKG
- Urinalysis
- Glucose measurements to exclude concomitant diabetes
- Cholesterol screening

TREATMENT

> Lifestyle modifications are tried for 3 to 6 months before medications are started.

The best initial therapy is with lifestyle management such as:

- **Weight loss** (most effective)
- Sodium restriction

- Dietary modification (less fat and red meat, more fish and vegetables)
- Exercise
- Tobacco cessation does not stop hypertension, but becomes especially important to prevent cardiovascular disease.

Drug Therapy

The best initial drug therapy remains thiazide diuretics.

Seventy percent of patients are controlled by a single medication. If blood pressure is very high on presentation (above 160/100), 2 medications should be used at the outset.

If diuretics do not control blood pressure, the most appropriate next step in management is:

- ACE inhibitor
- Angiotensin receptor blocker (ARB)
- Beta blocker (BB)
- Calcium channel blocker (CCB)

Medications that are not considered first-line or second-line therapy are:

- Central-acting alpha agonists (alpha methyldopa, clonidine)
- Peripheral-acting alpha antagonists (prazosin, terazosin, doxazosin)
- Direct-acting vasodilators (hydralazine, minoxidil)

Compelling Indications for Specific Drugs

If there is another significant disease in the history, you should add a specific drug to lifestyle modifications. In these circumstances you should not start with a thiazide.

Compelling Indications	
If this is in the history...	**This is the best initial therapy...**
Coronary artery disease	BB, ACE, ARB
Diabetes mellitus	ACE, ARB
Benign prostatic hypertrophy	Alpha blockers
Depression and asthma	Avoid BBs
Hyperthyroidism	BB first
Osteoporosis	Thiazides

Hypertensive Crisis

Hypertensive crisis is defined as high blood pressure in association with:

- Confusion
- Blurry vision

> STENT FIBROMUSCULAR DYSPLASIA

> Ninety percent of patients will be controlled by 2 medications.

> THIAZIDE SIDE EFFECTS
> ↑ BG
> ↑ LDL
> ↑ TRIGLYCERIDES
> ↓ Na⁺
> ↓ K⁺
> ↑ Ca²⁺

> Hypertensive crisis is not defined as a specific level of blood pressure. It is defined as **hypertension associated with end-organ damage.**

- Dyspnea
- Chest pain

The best initial therapy for hypertensive crisis is **labetolol or nitroprusside**. Because nitroprusside needs monitoring with an arterial line, this is not usually the first choice.

Equally acceptable forms of therapy for acute hypertensive crises are:

- Enalapril
- CCBs: diltiazem, verapamil
- Esmolol

Any intravenous medication is acceptable. The specific drug available is not as important as giving enough of it to control the blood pressure.

> Do not lower blood pressure in hypertensive crisis to normal, or you may provoke a stroke.

Oncology

11

Breast Cancer

Presentation

Breast cancer is found in **asymptomatic women on screening mammography** or by the **palpation of a mass** by the patient or a physician. When breast cancer presents as a palpable mass, it is hard to the touch. It may also be associated with retraction of the nipple because ligaments in the breast will withdraw and pull the nipple inward.

> Breast cancer is usually painless.

Diagnostic Tests

Biopsy is the best initial test. The different methods of biopsy are:

- **Fine needle aspiration (FNA):** FNA is usually the **best initial biopsy**. The false positive rate is less than 2%. However, because FNA is a small sample, the disadvantages are a **false negative rate of 10%**.

- **Core needle biopsy:** This is a **larger sample** of the breast. It is **more deforming**, but you can test for estrogen receptors (**ER**), progesterone receptors (**PR**), and **HER 2/neu**. Difficulties include greater deformity with the procedure and the possibility that the needle will miss the lesion.

- **Open biopsy:** The "**most accurate diagnostic** test," open biopsy allows for **frozen section** to be done while the patient is in the operating room followed by **immediate resection of cancer**.

> You **cannot** test for **estrogen or progesterone receptors** or HER 2/neu on an FNA.

Mammography

Mammography is indicated to screen for breast cancer in the general population **starting at the age of 50**. IF SEE SOMETHING → DIAGNOSTIC MAMMOGRAPHY

347

A woman finds a hard, nontender breast mass on self-examination. There is no alteration of the mass with menstruation. She is scheduled to undergo a FNA biopsy.

Which of the following is most likely to benefit the patient?

a. Mammography
b. BRCA testing
c. Ultrasound
d. Bone scan
e. PET scan

Answer: The correct answer is (A). If breast biopsy is going to be performed, what is the point in doing a screening test like mammography? The answer is: 5% to 10% of patients have bilateral disease. In addition, there is a huge difference in the management of the patient if there is a single lesion or multiple lesions within the same breast. BRCA testing confirms an extra risk of cancer compared to the general population, but will add nothing to a patient who must already undergo biopsy. Ultrasound is useful in evaluating whether masses that are equivocal by clinical examination are cystic or solid. Bone scan is used after a diagnosis of breast cancer is made to exclude occult metastases. PET scan helps determine the content of abnormal masses within the body or enlarged nodes without biopsy. However, PET scan does not eliminate the need to establish an initial diagnosis with biopsy.

When Is Ultrasound the Answer?

- Clinically **indeterminant mass lesions**. It tells **cysts versus solid lesions**. Answer ultrasound if the lesion:
  - Is **painful**
  - **Varies** in size or pain **with menstruation**

Handwritten margin note: U/S → IF IT IS PAINFUL OR VARIES IN SIZE W/ MENSTRUATION

When Is PET Scan the Answer?

To determine **the content of** abnormal **lymph nodes** that are **not easily accessible to biopsy. Cancer increases uptake on PET scan.**

For example:

- An 80-year-old woman with biopsy-proven breast cancer has no nodes with cancer in the axilla. The primary lesion is small and the woman may not need adjuvant chemotherapy. Chest CT shows an abnormal hilar lymph node.
  - In this case, PET scan is useful to exclude a metastasis and the need for additional chemotherapy.

Margin box: How do you tell the content of an abnormal, inaccessible lesion without biopsy? Try PET scan.

When Is BRCA Testing the Answer?

- **BRCA** is definitely associated with an **increased risk of breast cancer**, particularly within families.
- BRCA is associated with **ovarian cancer**.

Margin box: The precise utility of MRI for breast cancer is not yet clear.

What is not clear is what to do when BRCA is positive. **BRCA has not yet been shown to add mortality benefit to usual management.**

When Is Sentinel Lymph Node Biopsy the Answer?

The first node identified near the operative field of a definitively identified breast cancer is the sentinel node. Contrast or dye is placed into the operative field and the first node identified that it travels to is the sentinel node.

- Sentinel node biopsy is done routinely in all patients at the time of lumpectomy or mastectomy.
- A **negative sentinel node eliminates the need for axillary lymph node dissection.**

When Are Estrogen and Progesterone Receptors Tested?

- Estrogen receptor (ER) and progesterone receptor (PR) testing is routine for all patients.
- Hormone manipulation therapy is done if either test is positive.

▶ **TIP**

With so many methods to lower mortality in breast cancer, USMLE Step 2 CK will not engage in speculation about who should get BRCA testing. It is just not clear.

TREATMENT

Surgery

Lumpectomy with radiation is equal in efficacy to modified radical mastectomy but much less deforming. The addition of radiation to lumpectomy is not a small issue. **Radiation** at the site of the cancer is **indispensible in preventing recurrences at the breast.**

▶ **TIP**

Radical mastectomy is always the wrong answer.

Hormonal Manipulation

All ER or PR positive patients should receive tamoxifen, raloxifene, or one of the aromatase inhibitors (anastrazole, letrozole, exemestane). Aromatase inhibitors seem to have a slight superiority in efficacy. If both are among the answer choices, aromatase inhibitors are the answer to the "most likely to benefit the patient" question.

> Tamoxifen gives endometrial cancer and clots (tamoxifen is a selective ER modifier). Aromatase inhibitors give osteoporosis (aromatase inhibitors inhibit estrogen effect everywhere, even the good effects, like on bone density).

▶ **TIP**

If 2 treatments are very close in efficacy, how can you be tested on them? You will need to understand the differences in their adverse effects.

When Is Trastuzumab the Answer?

- All breast cancers should be tested for Her 2/neu. This is an abnormal estrogen receptor.
- Those who are positive should receive anti-Her 2/neu antibodies known as trastuzumab.
- **Trastuzumab decreases the risk of recurrent disease.**

When Is Adjuvant Chemotherapy the Answer?

"Adjuvant" chemotherapy is not prophylactic, since patients already have the disease. It is not treatment since the term implies there are no clearly identified metastases. **Adjuvant** means an additional therapy to clean up presumed microscopic cancer cells too small in amount to be detected.

Adjuvant chemotherapy is the answer when:

- **Lesions are larger than 1 cm**
- Positive axillary lymph nodes are found

> Use tamoxifen when multiple first-degree relatives have breast cancer. It lowers the risk of breast cancer.

> We do **not** know what to do about BRCA when it is positive.

> Half of men above age 80 have prostate cancer on autopsy.

All of these definitely lower mortality:

- Mammography
- ER/PR testing, then tamoxifen/raloxifene
- Aromatase inhibitors
- Adjuvant **chemotherapy**
- **Lumpectomy and radiation**
- **Modified radical mastectomy**
- **Trastuzumab** (anti-Her 2/neu)
- Prophylaxis with tamoxifen

PROSTATE CANCER

Prostate cancer **presents** with **obstructive symptoms** on voiding similar to benign prostatic hypertrophy or a **palpable lesion** on examination. **Biopsy is the best initial test** and the most accurate test. **Most prostate cancers are asymptomatic.**

TREATMENT

Prostatectomy **may** have a slight benefit over radiation in terms of survival. The most common **complications of prostatectomy** are:

- **Erectile dysfunction**
- **Urinary incontinence**

It is not known whether prostatectomy, external beam radiation, implantable radioactive pellets, or watchful waiting is superior in localized prostate cancer.

You will be expected to know that **surgery is more likely to give erectile dysfunction compared to radiation**.

Adverse effect questions are always clear.

Gleason Grading

Gleason grading is a measure of the **aggressiveness** or **malignant potential** of prostate cancer. A high Gleason grade suggests a greater benefit of surgical removal of the prostate. Get it out before it metastasizes if the Gleason grade is high.

Hormonal Manipulation in Prostate Cancer

Flutamide, GNRH agonists, ketoconazole, and orchiectomy help control the size and progression of metastases once they have occurred. They are not like tamoxifen in breast cancer. They do **not prevent recurrences**; they shrink lesions that are already present.

Management That Is Definitely Not Beneficial in Prostate Cancer

These answers are always wrong:

- **No "screening" imaging study.** Prostate ultrasound is not a screening test. It is used to localize lesions to biopsy when the prostate specific antigen (PSA) is high.
- **No lumpectomy**
- **No chemotherapy** is proven beneficial
- No hormonal manipulation to prevent recurrences

Prostate Specific Antigen (PSA)

PSA is a controversial subject for the following reasons:

- There is **no clear mortality benefit with PSA**.
- PSA is **not** to be routinely **offered** to patients.
- A normal PSA does not exclude the possibility of prostate cancer.

The higher the PSA, the greater the risk of cancer. PSA corresponds to the volume of cancer.

▶ **TIP**

If the question specifically says, "The **patient is requesting PSA** to screen for cancer," then the answer is **do the test**.

Elevated PSA Algorithm

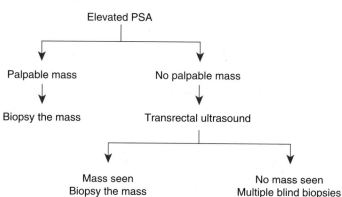

ADENO = NON SMOKER
    PERIPHERAL

S.C.C. →PTH-LIKE SECRETION
        ↑ Ca²⁺

HORNER'S SYNDROME
    ↳ PANCOAST TUMOR

SVC SYNDROME - OBSTRUCTED SVC
    ↳ STEROIDS
        ↳ STENTING

LUNG CANCER

The most important question for lung cancer is who should be treated with surgery?

The size of the lesion is not the most important factor in whether or not the lesion is resectable. If the lesion is large, but is surrounded by normal lung and there is enough remaining lung function post resection, then surgery is still possible.

Surgery is not possible in these cases:

- Bilateral disease
- Malignant pleural effusion
- Heart, carina, aorta, or vena cava is involved

Small cell cancer is considered <u>unresectable</u> in 95% of cases because it is metastatic or spread outside one lung. ↳ CHEMO
SIADH / CENTRAL LESIONS / L-E SYNDROME

ARISE FROM OVARIAN EPITHELIUM
    (USUALLY)

CA-125 > 50
    ↳ USED TO FOLLOW Dx

SEROUS CYSTADENOCARCINOMA IS M.C.

PSAMMOMA BODIES

MEIGS = Ca + ASCITES + ® HYDROTHORAX

KRUKENBERG = OVARIAN Ca FROM
            STOMACH (SIGNET RING)

SERTOLI/LEYDIG TUMOR = ↑ TEST
                    VIRILIZATION

GRANULOSA/THECA TUMOR = ↑ ESTROGEN
                    FEMINIZATION

OVARIAN CANCER

There is no screening test for ovarian cancer.

Look for a woman above the age of 50 with increasing abdominal girth but who is still losing weight. ALSO ASCITES AND SBO AND BLOATING

The initial test is an ultrasound or CT scan. The most accurate diagnostic test is a biopsy.

TREATMENT

Ovarian cancer is the only cancer in which removing large amounts of locally metastatic disease will benefit the patient. Remove all visible tumor and pelvic organs and give chemotherapy.

TESTICULAR CANCER

Testicular cancer presents with a painless lump in the scrotum that does not transilluminate.

DIAGNOSTIC TESTING

Remove the whole testicle with inguinal orchiectomy. **Do not cut the scrotum**, which can spread the disease. Needle biopsy of the testicle is always a **wrong** answer.

Alpha fetoprotein is secreted only by nonseminomatous cancers.

Staging is performed with CT scan of the abdomen, pelvis, and chest. Testicular cancer metastasizes up through the lymphatic channels in the retroperitoneum and moves up into the chest.

TREATMENT

After orchiectomy, **radiation** is used for **local** disease and **chemotherapy** is used for **widespread** disease. Testicular cancer is one of the only malignancies in which chemotherapy can cure widely metastatic disease, including spread into the brain.

CERVICAL CANCER

The management of advanced cervical cancer is clear: Perform a hysterectomy.

IF ALREADY SCC → POST-COITAL BLEEDING IS common

RISK IS HPV FROM SEX

Prevention of Cervical Cancer

- Human papillomavirus (HPV) vaccine is given to all women between ages 11 and 26.
- Pap smear is performed starting at age 21. Repeat the test every 2 to 3 years until the age of 65. Of women with fatal cervical cancer, 85% have never had a Pap smear. *21-65 y.o.*

HPV TYPES 16,18 CAUSE CANCER
6,11 CAUSE WARTS

START AT 21
EVERY 2-3 YRS
EVERY 5 YRS IF CHECK HPV
STOP AT AGE 65

Detection of Cervical Cancer

- Low-grade and high-grade dysplasia on Pap smear is followed up with a colposcopy for a biopsy.
- Atypical squamous cells of undetermined significance (ASCUS) can be a sign of early, preinvasive cancer or an infection, or may simply be a false positive.
- If **ASCUS** is present, perform HPV testing. **If HPV is found, colposcopy is performed.**
- If HPV is not associated with ASCUS, repeat the Pap smear at 6 months.

3 ???

> Pap smear does not lower mortality as much as mammography or colonoscopy.

-LGSIL ≈ CIN I
-HGSIL ≈ CIN II or WORSE

ENDOMETRIAL CANCER

SECTION 2
PREVENTIVE MEDICINE

In terms of preventive medicine, the hardest thing for a medical student to know is which guidelines will be tested. The answer is that the most reliable preventive medicine guidelines, and the standard of care, is the recommendations of the United States Preventive Services Task Force (**USPSTF**). These guidelines are as objective a source as we have. They are not based on the financial incentives of a particular specialty and they are created by those who simply interpret the best available objective data without regard for personal or professional gain. A specialized nonprofit organization like the American Cancer Society or a private professional group like the American Urological Association has a vested interest in increasing detection of certain diseases, even if a given screening test has not clearly been shown to decrease mortality.

▶ **TIP**

Let **mortality benefit** be your guide in choosing which test to do, or "Which of the following is most likely to benefit the patient?"

CANCER SCREENING

The single most important preventive medicine question is:

Which cancer screening method lowers mortality the most? (ie, Which of the following is most likely to benefit the patient?)

a. Pap smear
b. Colonoscopy
c. Prostate-specific antigen (PSA)
d. Mammography above age 40
e. Mammography above age 50

Answer: The correct answer is (E). Controversy may surround the question of how early to begin mammography. Recommendations have recently changed to start mammography at age 50, instead of 40. However, it is not controversial that there is a greater mortality benefit in screening those above age 50. This is because the incidence of breast cancer is greater above age 50. Hence, if you screen 1000 women above age 50, you will detect more cancer than screening 1000 women above age 40.

Breast Cancer

Mammography should be done starting at age 50, because the reduction in mortality is greatest above age 50.

▶ **TIP**

Breast self-examination is a wrong answer. Although it may seem to benefit, there is no proof.

On average, you will detect 10 cases of breast cancer by screening 1000 women above age 50, but you will detect only 2 cancers by screening 1000 women between the ages of 40 and 49. The **MRI, CT**, and **ultrasound** do not yet have a clear place in terms of screening for breast cancer.

> As a screening test only mammography is proven to lower mortality.

Which of the following is most likely to benefit an asymptomatic patient with multiple first-degree relatives with breast cancer?

a. Tamoxifen or raloxifene
b. BRCA testing
c. Aromatase inhibitors (anastrazole, letrazole)
d. Dietary modification (low fat, soy diet)
e. HER-2/neu testing
f. Estrogen and/or progesterone receptor testing

Answer: The correct answer is (A). Both selective estrogen receptor modulators (SERMs), tamoxifen and raloxifene, result in a 50% to 66% reduction in breast cancer when compared with placebo. The benefit is greatest in those with 2 first-degree relatives with breast cancer (mother or sister). SERMs are amazingly underutilized in preventing breast cancer. Aromatase inhibitors are very useful in preventing metastases in those with proven breast cancer, but they are not proven to benefit those who are asymptomatic. Dietary modification is unproven. HER-2/neu testing is useful to guide the use of trastuzumab, which will block this receptor in those with proven cancer, but not as prophylaxis. Estrogen and progesterone receptor testing has no place in managing asymptomatic women. These tests are used in those proven to have cancer.

BRCA Testing

BRCA is associated with increased risk of breast and ovarian cancer. However, this does not mean it is a clearly beneficial screening test. The missing piece is: **What to do** when the patient is positive for BRCA? It is **not clear**. The only truly unambiguous statement about BRCA testing is that a positive test means an increased risk of cancer. **Management remains undetermined.**

► **TIP**

When BRCA is positive, "offer prophylactic bilateral mastectomy" is a wrong answer.

Cervical Cancer Screening

Pap smear definitely lowers mortality. Because there are only 7000 to 10,000 cases of cervical cancer a year, but 185,000 cases of breast cancer, Pap smear is not nearly as beneficial as mammography. It is not clear if Pap smear is done every 2 or every 3 years. Papillomavirus vaccine is routine for all women between the ages of 11 to 26.

> Pap smear is done from 21 to 65 years of age.

► **TIP**

USMLE Step 2 CK will not engage in controversy. The answer must be clear.

Colon Cancer Screening

The lifetime risk of colon cancer for an American is 6% to 8%. Each year, 50,000 people die of colon cancer in the United States. Ninety-five percent of these deaths are preventable with screening.

Which of the following is most likely to benefit the patient?

a. Colonoscopy every 10 years after age 40
b. Colonoscopy every 10 years after age 50
c. Sigmoidoscopy every 3 to 5 years after 50
d. Barium enema after 50
e. Fecal occult blood testing
f. Virtual colonoscopy with CT scanning
g. Capsule endoscopy
h. Digital rectal examination after 50

Answer: The correct answer is (B). Colonoscopy is unquestionably the best of all the colon cancer screening methods. Sigmoidoscopy will miss the 40% of cancers occurring proximal to the sigmoid colon. Barium enema does not allow for biopsy or removal of polyps. Virtual colonoscopy misses cancers in polyps smaller than 0.5 cm. It is inferior to endoscopic colon cancer detection methods. Fecal occult blood testing will detect cancer. If positive, however, it must be followed by colonoscopy.

> Capsule endoscopy detects small bowel bleeding. It is not a cancer screening method.

► **TIP**

Digital rectal exam is not proven to lower mortality in any disease. It is always a wrong choice.

Prostate Cancer Screening

Unfortunately, there is **no clearly beneficial test to lower mortality in prostate cancer** screening. Neither the prostate-specific antigen nor the digital rectal exam has proven sufficiently sensitive or specific to lower mortality. Although PSA does detect prostate cancer, the lesions detected are most often not ones that need treatment. Of patients with prostate cancer, 25% have a normal PSA, and 25% of those with an elevated PSA do not have cancer.

The mortality benefit question for PSA is clear: There is **no** benefit. Whether to do the test is controversial.

▶ **TIP**

If the question asks mortality benefit for PSA, say "No."

If the question says "The patient wants/requests a PSA," say "Yes."

Lung Cancer Screening

There is **no test to lower mortality from lung cancer**. Chest x-ray detects many lesions that turn out to be insignificant and misses many small cancers. High-resolution CT scanning is not proven to lower mortality in lung cancer.

▶ **TIP**

Smoking cessation is always the single most beneficial disease preventive method of any type.

LIPID SCREENING

Cholesterol and LDL measurement is recommended for healthy patients when:

- Men are above age 35
- Women are above age 45

Lipid screening is recommended for all patients with diabetes, hypertension, coronary artery disease, or the equivalents of coronary disease such as:

- Carotid disease
- Peripheral vascular disease
- Aortic disease

HYPERTENSION

Blood pressure testing is indicated for all patients above the age of 18 at every visit. Hypertension screening has never been prospectively evaluated in a meaningful way and probably never will. In order to do the study correctly, you would have to withhold BP measurement and observe for years to detect a mortality difference, which would be unethical. Your answer on the test is still clear: Every adult's BP is tested at every visit.

DIABETES MELLITUS

Screening for diabetes with fasting blood glucose levels (2 measurements over 125) is done when the patient has:

- Hypertension
- Hyperlipidemia

There is no clear recommendation for diabetes mellitus screening in the general asymptomatic public.

VACCINATIONS

For adults, the 2 most beneficial vaccines are:

- Influenza
- Pneumococcus

Influenza and Pneumococcal Vaccine

There is enormous overlap in the groups for which both vaccines are recommended. Both influenza and pneumococcal vaccine are recommended for all patients with:

- Chronic heart, lung, liver, and kidney disease including asthma
- HIV/AIDS
- Steroid users
- Immunocompromised patients in general such as cancer or functional or anatomic asplenia
- Diabetes mellitus

Differences in Indications between Influenza and Pneumococcal Vaccination

The differences in indications for these 2 vaccines are small.

Indications for Influenza and Pneumococcal Vaccination	
Influenza vaccine	**Pneumococcal vaccine**
• Everyone yearly • **Healthcare workers** • Pregnant patients	• Everyone above age 65 • Cochlear implant • CSF leaks • Alcoholics • **One vaccine above 65 only** • Single revaccination after **5 years** if the patient is immunocompromised or the first injection was prior to age 65

Herpes (Varicella) Zoster Vaccine

> Zoster vaccine prevents shingles in adults.

Although varicella vaccination is routinely indicated in all children, there is a higher-dose version of the varicella vaccine that is indicated in all patients above age 60.

Hepatitis A and B Vaccine

> Hepatitis A and B vaccines are most beneficial in those with chronic liver disease.

Both hepatitis A and B vaccines are routinely indicated in children. They are both indicated in adults if there is:

- Chronic liver disease
- Men who have sex with men or multiple sexual partners
- Household contacts with hepatitis A or B
- Injection drug users

Differences in Indication for Hepatitis A and B Vaccine	
Hepatitis A	**Hepatitis B**
• Travelers to countries of high endemicity	• End-stage renal disease (dialysis) • Healthcare workers

Meningococcal Vaccine

Meningococcal vaccine is routinely indicated at the age 11 visit. The vaccine is also indicated for adults with the following circumstances:

- Asplenia
- Terminal complement deficiency
- Military recruits
- Residents of college dormitories
- Travelers to Mecca or Medina in Saudi Arabia for the Hajj (pilgrimage)

Which of the following is the strongest indication for meningococcal vaccination (ie, who will benefit the most)?

a. Asplenia
b. Military recruits
c. Residents of college dormitories
d. Travelers to Mecca or Medina
e. 11-year-old child

*Answer: The correct answer is **(A)**. Asplenia represents a person at high risk for disseminated meningococcal infection. If he or she is exposed to the organism, an asplenic person has the highest risk of dissemination. The other choices represent increased exposure, but not an increased risk of immune compromise leading to dissemination.*

OSTEOPOROSIS

Every woman should be screened with bone densitometry at the age of 65 with a DEXA scan. Hip fracture in an elderly patient carries an extremely high risk of mortality. Preventing fracture with bisphosphonates to increase bone density is potentially more life-saving than beta blockers in coronary disease. In an older woman, a hip fracture is more deadly than a myocardial infarction.

ABDOMINAL AORTIC ANEURYSM

All men above the age of 65 with a smoking history should be screened once with an ultrasound to exclude an aneurysm. Abdominal aortic aneurysm (AAA) should be repaired if they are wider than 5 centimeters.

SMOKING CESSATION

All patients should:

- Be **asked** "Do you smoke?"
- Be **advised** to stop smoking
- **Attempt:** Find out who really wants to stop.
- Be **assisted:** Prescribe a method of aiding nicotine dependence.
- **Arrange** to meet with the patient again to find out if they have set a quit date and have really managed to stop.

INTIMATE PARTNER VIOLENCE (DOMESTIC VIOLENCE)

All patients should be asked about the possibility of intimate partner violence. Patients will most often not volunteer this information. You cannot report this form of injury without the consent of the patient.

ALCOHOLISM (ALCOHOL DEPENDENCE)

Alcoholism is a "self-diagnosed" disease. Alcoholism is not defined as an amount of alcohol used. It is not defined as alcohol use leading to loss of employment. Many alcoholics still maintain their jobs.

Ask:

- **C:** Do they feel the need to **cut down** the amount they are drinking?
- **A:** Do they feel **angry** when asked about their drinking?
- **G:** Do they feel **guilty** about the amount they drink?
- **E:** Do they feel the need for a morning **eye-opener**?

The **CAGE** questions are excellent at helping patients recognize they are alcohol dependent.

ROUTINE SCREENING METHODS THAT ARE ALWAYS INCORRECT

Chest x-ray, EKG, and stress testing are never correct as screening methods in the otherwise healthy general population.

SECTION 3
DERMATOLOGY

CUTANEOUS MALIGNANCIES

All dermal malignances occur more frequently in those with pale skin on more sun-exposed areas. Diagnosis is by biopsy and the treatment is with surgical removal. No form of skin cancer has effective chemotherapy.

Skin Cancer

- More sun, more cancer
- Biopsy
- Remove

Malignant Melanoma

Although melanoma occurs more frequently in sun-exposed areas, it is not exclusive to those areas. Since there are many benign skin lesions, the main question is one of diagnosis. Melanoma is best diagnosed clinically by ABCDE:

A: asymmetry

B: border irregularity

C: color irregularities

D: diameter greater than 6 millimeters

E: evolution (changing in appearance over time)

The diagnosis for any suspicious lesion is by biopsy that includes the entire lesion if possible.

> Worst prognostic significance: growing lesions.

Distinctions between Benign and Malignant Lesions	
Benign	**Malignant**
Round	Asymmetric
Even borders	Borders uneven
Color evenly spread	Color uneven
Diameter constant	Diameter increases

- SUPERFICIAL SPREADING
  ↳ M.C. TYPE

- AMELANOTIC
  ↳ NOT PIGMENTED

- NODULAR
  ↳ BLEED EASILY

- ACRAL LENTIGINOUS
  ↳ HANDS / NAILS / SOLES

Figure 13.1: Benign lesions are characterized by even coloring, with smooth borders and no asymmetry. *Source: Andrew Peredo.*

DIAGNOSTIC TEST

Full thickness biopsy is indispensible in diagnosis. Do not do a shave biopsy.

Treatment/Prognosis

Surgical removal must include a significant removal of normal skin surrounding the lesion. Interferon injection is helpful in widespread disease. Melanoma has a strong tendency to metastasize to the brain.

Squamous Cell Cancer

Besides sunlight, squamous cell cancer is **greatly increased by organ transplant** secondary to the **long-term use of immunosuppressive drug**s. All forms of squamous cell cancer start out by looking like **an ulcer that does not heal or continues to grow**.

Biopsy and remove.

Basal Cell Carcinoma

Basal cell is the most common form of skin cancer. The question will describe a waxy **lesion that is shiny like a pearl**. Unlike melanoma, wide margins are not necessary, and shave biopsy is a fine way to make diagnosis. **Recurrence rates are less than 5%**. Basal cell is a good use of Mohs micrographic surgery.

Mohs Micrographic Surgery

Removal of skin cancer under a dissecting microscope with **immediate frozen section** is one of the most precise methods of treating skin cancer. Mohs allows removal of the skin cancer with the **loss of only the smallest amount of normal tissue**. Under microscopy, very thin slices of skin are removed and examined by frozen section for cancer. You can stop resecting as soon as the margin is cancer-free. In other words, there is **no need to remove a wide margin routinely**.

> Mohs is best for delicate areas like the eyelid or ear.

Figure 13.2: Basal cell carcinoma is very slow to grow and is not hyperpigmented. *Source: Andrew Peredo.*

Kaposi Sarcoma

In the past, Kaposi sarcoma (KS) was seen in older men of Mediterranean origin. The **most common cause now is AIDS**. KS is from **human herpes virus 8**, which is oncogenic. The lesion is more reddish/purplish because it is more vascular than other forms of skin cancer. KS is **also found in the GI tract and in the lung**. Only AIDS acquired through sexual contact is associated with KS; AIDS from injection drug use is rarely associated with KS.

Figure 13.3: Kaposi sarcoma occurs in patients with AIDS and fewer than 100 CD4 cells per μl. *Source: Andrew Peredo.*

[Handwritten margin notes:]
ERYTHEMA NODOSUM — RED PAINFUL SUB Q NODULES
POST STREP
DRUGS
SARCOID
IBD

LICHEN PLANUS
P's
HIV/HCV
STEROIDS (TOPICAL/ORAL)
ORAL RETINOIDS

TREATMENT

Unlike other skin cancers, **KS is not routinely treated with surgical removal**.

1. **Treat the AIDS with antiretrovirals** and the majority of KS will disappear as the CD4 count improves.
2. Intralesional injections of vincristine or interferon are very successful.
3. If these fail, use chemotherapy with liposomal doxorubicin.

Actinic Keratoses

These are **premalignant** skin lesions from high-intensity sun exposure in fair-skinned people. They have a very small **risk of squamous** cell cancer for each individual lesion. Since many actinic keratoses can occur in a single person, the risk is cumulative and significant (like the relationship between cervical dysplasia and the risk of cervical cancer). They are **slow to progress**, but must be removed with curettage, cryotherapy, laser, or topical 5-fluorocuracil before they transform. The local immunostimulant imiquimod is also effective. Imiquimod is used for molluscum contagiosum and condyloma acuminatum as well.

Seborrheic Keratoses

These lesions are extremely common in the elderly. They are hyperpigmented lesions commonly referred to as liver spots. They give a "stuck on" appearance. Although they may look like melanoma to some people, seborrheic keratoses have no premalignant potential. They do not transform into melanoma. They are removed with cryotherapy, surgery, or laser for cosmetic reasons.

ATOPIC DERMATITIS (ECZEMA)

Atopic dermatitis is a common skin disorder associated with **overactivity of mast cells and the immune system**. Look for a history of:

- **Asthma**
- **Allergic rhinitis**
- Family history of atopic disorders
- Onset before age 5, very **rare to start after age 30**

PRESENTATION

Because of premature and idiosyncratic release of transmitters such as histamine, **pruritus and scratching is the most common presentation**. Scratching leads to **scaly rough areas of thickened skin** on the face, neck, and skin folds of the popliteal area behind the knee.

> Skin that has thickened because of scratching and drying is described as **lichenified.**

Itching leads to scratching. Scratching leads to more itching. **Superficial skin infections from *Staphylococcus* are common** because microorganisms are driven under the epidermis by scratching. This, in turn, leads to more itching.

> Food allergies do not exacerbate atopic dermatitis.

TREATMENT

Skin Care

1. **Stay moisturized:** Dry skin is more itchy. Use a humidifier, especially in the winter. Use skin moisturizers frequently. Less itching = less scratching = less itching.
2. **Avoid bathing, soap, and washcloths.** The skin in atopic dermatitis is hyperirritable. Brushes, washcloths, hot water, and anything that rubs on the skin, even if minimal, can make it worse.
3. **Cotton is less irritating** to skin than wool.

> IgE levels are elevated in atopic dermatitis.

Medical Therapy

1. **Topical corticosteroids** are used in flares of disease. Oral steroids are used only in the most severe acute flares of disease.
2. **Tacrolimus and pimecrolimus** are T cell–inhibiting agents that provide longer-term control and **help get the patient off steroids**. They are used systemically in organ transplant recipients to prevent organ rejection and keep patients off steroids. They are used topically for atopic dermatitis because this disorder is a form of immune system hyperactivity.
3. **Antihistamines:**
   - Mild disease: nonsedating drugs (cetirizine, fexofenadine, loratadine)
   - Severe disease: hydroxyzine, diphenhydramine, **doxepine**
4. **Antibiotics** such as cephalexin, mupirocin, repatamulin **when impetigo occurs**
5. Ultraviolet light (phototherapy) for severe recalcitrant disease

> Tacrolimus and pimecrolimus are rarely associated with developing lymphoma.

▶ TIP

Atopic dermatitis and psoriasis are the only two dermatologic diseases with complex knowledge bases. Everything else in dermatology is about two sentences long.

PSORIASIS

Psoriasis is incredibly common, with nearly 2 million patients in the United States.

PRESENTATION

Psoriasis is characterized by **silvery, scaly plaques** that **are not itchy most of the time**. Less than 10% have arthritis. Extensive disease is associated with depression.

Figure 13.4: Psoriasis is characterized by silvery, scaly plaques. *Source: Andrew Peredo.*

TREATMENT

Local Disease

1. Topical high-potency steroids: fluocinonide, amcinolone, betamethasone, clobetasol
2. Vitamin A and vitamin D ointment help get the patient off steroids. The vitamin D agent is calcipotriene. Steroids cause skin atrophy.
3. **Coal tar** preparation
4. **Pimecrolimus and tacrolimus** are used on more delicate areas such as the face and penis. They are an alternative to steroids and are less potentially deforming.

Extensive Disease

1. **Ultraviolet light**
2. **Antitumor necrosis factor (TNF) inhibitors** (etanercept, adalimumab, infliximab). These agents can be miraculous in efficacy for severe disease.
3. **Methotrexate:** used last because of adverse effects on the liver and lung. It is a drug of last resort except for psoriatic arthritis.

> Steroids cause atrophy because they inhibit collagen formation and growth. Steroids try to convert all amino acids into glucose for gluconeogenesis.

> TNF inhibitors can reactivate tuberculosis. Screen with a PPD prior to using them.

PITYRIASIS ROSEA

Pityriasis rosea is an idiopathic, transient dermatitis that **starts out with a single lesion** (herald patch) and then disseminates. It can look like secondary syphilis but it spares the palms and soles. It is transient, but if symptomatic it is treated with steroids or ultraviolet light.

Figure 13.5: Note the diffuse erythematous, largely macular lesions. *Source: Andrew Peredo.*

SEBORRHEIC DERMATITIS (DANDRUFF)

Seborrheic dermatitis is a **hypersensitivity reaction to a dermal infection** with noninvasive dermatophyte organisms. This is why both topical steroids (hydrocortisone, alclometasone) and antifungal agents (ketoconazole) are useful.

It is increased in:

- AIDS
- Parkinson disease

▶ **TIP**

The term **seborrheic** is synonymous with **benign**.

BLISTERING DISEASES

Pemphigus Vulgaris — ANTI-DESMOSOME

Pemphigus vulgaris has both an idiopathic autoimmune form and a drug-induced form.

Pemphigus, although idiopathic, is associated with:

- **ACE inhibitors**
- Penicillamine
- Phenobarbital
- Penicillin

Autoantibodies split the epidermis, resulting in:

- **Bullae that easily rupture** because they are thin walled
- **Involvement of the mouth**
- **Fluid loss and infection** if widespread; they act like a burn

WARFARIN - INDUCED SKIN NECROSIS

The most characteristic finding is the **Nikolsky sign**. This is the loss or **"denuding" of skin from just mild pressure**. The Nikolsky sign is the removal of the superficial layer of skin in a single sheet while pulling on it with a finger's worth of pressure.

The most **accurate diagnostic test is a biopsy** showing autoantibodies on immunofluorescent studies.

> Without treatment, pemphigus is a fatal disease.

Treatment

1. Systemic steroids (prednisone)
2. **Azathioprine or mycophenolate to wean the patient off steroids**
3. Rituximab (anti-CD20 antibodies) or IVIG in refractory cases

Bullous Pemphigoid   *ANTI - BASEMENT MEMBRANE*
This is a much **milder disease than pemphigus** because:

- **Bullae stay intact** and there is **less loss of fluid and infection**.
- Mouth involvement is uncommon.

Biopsy with immunofluorescent stains is the most accurate test and the best **initial therapy is prednisone**. To get patients off steroids, use azathioprine, cyclophosphamide, or mycophenolate.

> Nikolsky sign is absent in bullous pemphigoid.

Mild bullous pemphigoid responds to erythromycin, **dapsone, and nicotinamide (not niacin)**.

Porphyria Cutanea Tarda
Porphyria cutanea tarda (PCT) is a blistering skin disease of sun-exposed areas in those with a history of: *BACK OF HANDS & FACE*

> Look for involvement of the backs of the **hands** and the face.

- Liver disease (**hepatitis C**, alcoholism)
- Estrogen use
- **Iron overload** (hemochromatosis)

▶ **TIP**

Hepatitis C is the most frequently tested association with PCT.

Diagnostic Tests/Treatment

The most accurate diagnostic test is **increased uroporphyrins in a 24-hour urine collection**.

> PCT is a **hypersensitivity** of the skin **to abnormal porphyrins** when they are exposed to light.

It is a deficiency of uroporphyrin decarboxylase activity. Correct the underlying cause (**stop alcohol**, **stop estrogens**) and remove iron with **phlebotomy**.

SKIN INFECTIONS

Impetigo

Impetigo is the most **superficial** of the bacterial skin infections. *Staphylococcus* and *Streptococcus* invade the epidermis, resulting in **weeping, crusting, oozing, and draining** of the skin.

TREATMENT

Mild disease with topical agents:

- **Mupirocin**
- Bacitracin
- Repatamulin

Severe disease with oral agents:

- Dicloxacillin or cephalexin

Community-acquired MRSA with:

- Doxycycline
- **Clindamycin**
- **Trimethoprim/sulfamethoxazole (TMP/SMZ)**

Erysipelas

Erysipelas is a much **more severe disease** than impetigo because it occurs at a deeper level in the skin. Erysipelas is much more often **from *Streptococcus*** than *Staphylococcus*. Erysipelas invades dermal lymphatics and causes bacteremia, leukocytosis, fever, and chills. Untreated disease can be fatal.

> Skin infections with group A beta hemolytic *Streptococcus* can cause glomerulonephritis, but not rheumatic fever.

PRESENTATION

Look for a bright, red, hot swollen lesion on the face. **Leukocytosis** can occur because it is more often a systemic disease.

TREATMENT

Although erysipelas is more often from streptococci, you must treat for *Staphylococcus* as well unless you have a definitive diagnostic test such as blood cultures.

▶ **TIP**

The treatment of all skin infections is similar. The following answers are the same answers as for cellulitis, folliculitis, furuncles, and carbuncles.

Cross reaction between penicillins and cephalosporins is unusual (less than 5%).

USMLE Step 2 CK tests **route of administration (oral vs. intravenous).**

Antistaphylococcal penicillins **OX*CLOX*DICLOX*NAF**

Skin infection is caused by *Staphylococcus aureus*, **not *S. epidermidis*. *S. epidermidis* lives on skin as part of normal flora.

Mild disease: Use **oral** medications:

- Dicloxacillin, cephalexin, cefadroxyl
- Penicillin allergic: erythromycin, clarithromycin, or clindamycin
- MRSA: doxycycline, **clindamycin, trimethoprim/sulfamethoxazole**

Severe disease (fever present): Use **intravenous** medications:

- Oxacillin, nafcillin, cefazolin
- Penicillin allergic: clindamycin, vancomycin
- MRSA: vancomycin, linezolid, daptomycin, tigecycline

Cellulitis

Cellulitis is an infection of the soft tissue of the skin. It extends from the dermis into the subcutaneous tissue. The skin is warm, red, swollen, and tender. Cellulitis involves the legs more often than the arms. Cellulitis does not have collections of walled-off infection; that is an abscess. Cellulitis is not only at the hair follicle; that is folliculitis, furuncles, and carbuncles.

DIAGNOSTIC TESTS

No diagnostic testing is needed to establish a diagnosis of cellulitis. The most accurate test is to inject sterile saline into the skin and aspirate it for culture. The yield is only 20%. *Staphylococcus* is much more common than *Streptococcus*.

▶ **TIP**

UMSLE Step 2 does **not test dosing** of antibiotics.

TREATMENT

See previous section on erysipelas.

Topical antibiotics will not cover cellulitis. The infection is below the dermal/epidermal junction and topical antibiotics will not reach it.

Folliculitis, Furuncles, Carbuncles

These infections originate around hair follicles. The different terms do not have precise definitions, and there is no cutoff point in size that distinguishes them from one another.

Severe disease = fever, chills, bacteremia

Size of the Infection

Folliculitis is the earliest and mildest. A furuncle is a **small abscess** or collection of infected material. A carbuncle is a collection of furuncles. Treat as previously described.

Folliculitis < Furuncle < Carbuncle

Figure 13.6: Cellulitis is often bright red, warm, and tender. There is no weeping of purulent material as occurs in impetigo. *Source: Farshad Baheri, MD.*

Figure 13.7: A furuncle is like a small skin abscess. Note the small area of folliculitis above it on the neck. *Source: Andrew Peredo.*

Penicillin Allergy

If the reaction to penicillin is a **rash, use cephalosporins**.

If the reaction is **anaphylaxis**:

- **Mild** infection: **macrolides, clindamycin, doxycycline, or TMP/SMZ**
- **Severe** infection: **vancomycin, linezolid**, daptomycin, or tigecycline

Other Antistaphylococcal Medications

See the list of drugs described in the section on erysipelas.

Medications that **cover *Staphylococcus*** but are **not specific for skin infections** are:

- Second-generation cephalosporins (cefoxitin, cefotetan, cefuroxime)
- Beta-lactam/beta-lactamase combinations
    - Amoxicillin/clavulanate
    - Ticarcillin/clavulanate
    - Ampicillin/sulbactam
    - Piperacillin/tazobactam
- Carbapenems (imipenem, meropenem)

These agents cover additional Gram-negative organisms.

These medications would **not** be used as first-line agents for skin infections because they would be considered excessive in terms of spectrum. They all cover more than is necessary. However, if the patient is already on one of these medications, you do not need to add anything to cover skin infection.

Fungal Infections

DEFINITION

Dermatophyte = superficial fungal infection = tinea

The proper term for superficial fungal infections is *tinea*, followed by the name of the body part in Latin. For example:

Tinea corporis = body
Tinea manus = hand
Tinea pedis = foot
Tinea cruris = groin ("jock itch")

▶ **TIP**

We prepare for USMLE Step 2 CK by extracting the questions from each disease. ("What is the best initial test?" "What is the most accurate test?" "What is the best initial therapy?") The answer to these questions is the same for all forms of tinea, so we do not learn them separately.

DIAGNOSTIC TESTS/TREATMENT

- The best initial test is a KOH (potassium hydroxide) preparation. KOH will dissolve epidermal skin cells and leave the fungi intact so they can be visualized.
- The most **accurate** test is a fungal **culture**.
- The best initial therapy is a topical antifungal agent if no hair or nails are involved.
- The best initial therapy for hair (tinea capitis) and nail (tinea unguium) infections is terbinafine. Itraconazole is close in efficacy.

▶ **TIP**

Remember that "What is the most accurate test?" and "What will you **do**?" are often **not** the same answer. Fungal culture may be "the most accurate **test**" for tinea cruris, but it is not "what you will **do** next?" In most cases, tinea cruris is treated without a specific diagnostic test. A KOH aided scraping is often useful for immediate diagnosis, and if positive no culture is necessary.

Topical antifungal agents:

- Clotrimazole
- Ketoconazole
- Econazole
- Miconazole
- Nystatin (effective only in yeast infections, not other common fungal infections)
- Ciclopirox

Oral and Vaginal Candidiasis

For the sake of preparing for USMLE Step 2 CK, these two infections are the **same disease**. KOH is the best initial test and fungal culture the most accurate test. However, **with a clear presentation** of the disease, **what you will do next is treat with a topical antifungal** from the previous list.

Ketoconazole is antiandrogenic. **Oral** ketoconazole causes gynecomastia.

Griseofulvin has less efficacy compared to terbinafine or itraconazole.

DRUG REACTIONS

Hypersensitivity reactions to medications vary in severity. When the severity of the reaction changes, the name of the reaction changes.

The drugs that commonly cause hypersensitivity reactions are:

- Penicillins
- Sulfa drugs (including thiazides, furosemide, and sulfonylureas)
- Allopurinol
- Phenytoin
- Lamotrigine
- NSAIDs

The drugs that cause hypersensitivity reactions of the skin are the same that cause hemolysis, interstitial nephritis, and often drug-induced thrombocytopenia (except heparin).

Morbilliform rash < Erythema Multiforme < Stevens-Johnson < Toxic Epidermal Necrolysis

Morbilliform rash: mildest reaction. Skin stays intact without mucous membrane involvement. **No specific therapy**.

Erythema multiforme: widespread, small "target" lesions; most are on the trunk. No mucous membrane involvement. May also be from herpes or mycoplasma. Prednisone may benefit some patients.

Stevens-Johnson syndrome: very severe. Involves the mucous membranes. Sloughs off respiratory epithelium and may lead to respiratory failure. **Steroids not clearly beneficial. Use intravenous immunoglobulins (IVIG)**.

Toxic epidermal necrolysis (TEN): rash with mucous membrane involvement and adds Nikolsky sign. **Steroids definitely do not help**. Treat with IVIG.

Figure 13.8: Erythema multiforme is characterized by multiple small target-shaped lesions that can be confluent, as in this case. *Source: Andrew Peredo.*

Figure 13.9: The skin comes off in a sheet in TEN, simulating a burn. *Source: Conrad Fischer, MD.*

STAPHYLOCOCCAL SCALDED SKIN SYNDROME AND TOXIC SHOCK SYNDROME

Staphylococcal scalded skin syndrome (SSSS) and toxic shock syndrome (TSS) are different severities of the same event: a reaction to a toxin in the surface of *Staphylococcus*.

SSSS looks similar to TEN, including Nikolsky sign. TSS has the same skin involvement as well as life-threatening multiorgan involvement such as:

- Hypotension
- Renal dysfunction (elevated BUN and creatinine)
- Liver dysfunction
- CNS involvement (delirium)

Both are treated with supportive care and the antistaphylococcal medications previously described. In the absence of penicillin allergy and with a sensitive organism, **oxacillin** or **nafcillin** are the most effective medications. Cefazolin is interchangeable to treat *Staphylococcus*. **Antibiotics do not reverse the disease**, but they kill the *Staphylococcus* that is producing the toxin.

ACNE → IF SCARRING → GIVE ISOTRETINOIN!!!

BENZOYL
↓
TOPICAL ABX
↓
TOPICAL VIT A
↓
ORAL ABX
↓
ORAL VIT A

TREATMENT

Mild acne: Use topical antibacterials such as **benzoyl peroxide**. If this is ineffective, add topical antibiotics such as **clindamycin** or **erythromycin**.

Moderate acne: Add **topical vitamin A derivatives** such as **tretinoin, adapalene**, or **tazarotene** to topical antibiotics. If there is no response to topical vitamin A derivatives and antibiotics, use **oral antibiotics** such as **minocycline** or **doxycycline**.

Vitamin A derivatives are extremely **teratogenic**. Do a pregnancy test. Only treat patients on suitable hormonal and barrier birth control.

Severe acne: Add **oral vitamin A, isotretinoin** to oral antibiotics. Isotretinoin causes hyperlipidemia. | 2 FORMS OF B.C. | HEPATOTOXICITY DEPRESSION SCREENING

NEC FASC - LIKE CELLULITIS, BUT PAIN BEYOND REDNESS
IMMEDIATE SURGICAL DEBRIDEMENT
ABX ⟹ STREP

DRY GANGRENE
AUTO AMPUTATION | ANGIOGRAPHY | AMPUTATION

WET GANGRENE
DEBRIDEMENT | AMPUTATION → BIGGER AMPUTATION | ABX

STOP

A = Airway

The primary step in any trauma is to assess and secure the airway.

- **Orotracheal tubes** are the best way to maintain an airway in patients **with no facial trauma**.
- Patients with **facial trauma** require a **cricothyroidotomy**.
- Patients with **cervical spine injury** still need an **orotracheal tube** intubation. This should be performed with **flexible bronchoscopy** to reduce risk of further cervical spine injury.

B = Breathing

Proper ventilation is necessary to maintain oxygen saturation. The routine goal in management is to keep oxygen saturation above 90%.

C = Circulation

Insert 2 large-bore IVs into the patient and begin aggressive fluid resuscitation to prevent hypovolemic shock.

A 43-year-old woman was texting while driving when she lost control of the car and ran into a tree. She is complaining of chest pain; physical examination reveals pallor and cool extremities with a heart rate of 120 beats per minute and JVD. Blood pressure is 80/40. Chest x-ray reveals 3 broken ribs over the left side of the chest.

Which of the following is the most likely type of shock?

a. Hypovolemic shock
b. Cardiogenic shock
c. Neurogenic shock
d. Septic shock

*Answer: The correct answer is (B). Cardiogenic shock is most likely secondary to pericardial tamponade. The patient's car injury caused blood to collect in the pericardial sac, leading to right ventricular diastolic collapse and impaired filling. The broken ribs are the source of injury to the pericardium. Hypovolemic shock is **unlikely**, as the patient cannot lose that much volume into her pericardium. Neurogenic shock would have hyperreflexia, and upgoing toes. Septic shock is unlikely as there is no fever and chills.*

Shock

Shock occurs when the tissues in the body do not receive enough oxygen and nutrients to allow the cells to function. Shock is more than just tachycardia and hypotension. You will see:

- Brain: confusion
- Kidney: increased BUN/creatinine ratio
- Liver: elevated AST and ALT
- Heart: chest pain and shortness of breath

Four Kinds of Shock							
	Signs and symptoms	**CVP**	**SVR**	**HR**	**CO**	**LVEDP or PCWP**	**Treatment**
Hypovolemic shock	Pale and cool	Decrease	Increase	Increase	Decrease	Decrease	Fluids and pressors
Cardiogenic shock	Pale and cool	Increase	Increase	Increase	Decrease	Increase	Treat cardiac problem
Neurogenic shock	Warm	Decrease	Decrease	Increase	Decrease	Decrease	Fluids and pressors
Septic shock	Warm and faint	Decrease	Decrease	Increase	Increase	No change	Fluids, antibiotics, and pressors

CVP central venous pressure; SVR = Systemic vascular resistance, HR = heat rate

> The **most common** cause of **cardiogenic shock** is myocardial infarction. The **most common** organisms associated with **septic shock** are *E. coli* and *Staphylococcus aureus*. The **most common** cause of **neurogenic shock** is spinal cord injury in the cervical or thoracic region. The **most common** cause of **hypovolemic shock** is massive hemorrhage.

Abdominal Trauma

A 27-year-old man presents with severe abdominal pain that radiates to his back and began after his car was hit by another car. He says his abdomen hurts after colliding with the steering wheel. He is admitted, and after 2 days in the hospital a large ecchymosis is seen on the right flank.

What is the most likely diagnosis?

a. Hemorrhagic pancreatitis
b. Pseudocyst
c. Renal trauma
d. Aortic dissection

Answer: The correct answer is (A). The patient's history of blunt abdominal trauma leads to the diagnosis of pancreatitis. The bruising in the flank shows a hemorrhage. This location suggests a retroperitoneal hemorrhage. This is where blood collections occur in the setting of pancreatitis. Pseudocysts develop 6 to 8 weeks postpancreatitis, and in this patient, the timing would be too soon. Renal trauma does not present with ecchymosis, and aortic dissection does not have bruising. Aortic dissection will present in a patient with extremely elevated blood pressure, and tearing pain in the midepigastrum that radiates sharply into the back.

Signs Associated with Abdominal Trauma		
Sign	**What is it?**	**Cause(s)**
Cullen sign	Bruising around the umbilicus	Hemorrhagic pancreatitis, ruptured abdominal aortic aneurysm
Grey Turner sign	Bruising in the flank	Retroperitoneal hemorrhage
Kehr sign	Pain in the left shoulder	Splenic rupture
Balance sign	Dull percussion on the left and shifting dullness on the right	Splenic rupture
Seatbelt sign	Bruising where a seatbelt was	Deceleration injury

Figure 14.1: Between 10% and 50% of patients with acute pancreatitis will have bruising in the flanks. *Source: Niket Sonpal, MD.*

> Upright chest x-ray is the best initial test for the evaluation of free air under the diaphragm. Free air under the diaphragm indicates a perforation of the bowel.

> The abdominal x-ray is also useful for evaluating ileus, which is a nonmechanical etiology for lack of peristalsis in the GI tract.

Thoracic Trauma

A 29-year-old woman presents to the ED with a sudden onset of left-sided chest pain and difficulty breathing. She states her only medication is birth control pills. She has smoked 1 pack of cigarettes per day for 10 years. She is tachypneic, with a rate of 24 breaths per minute, and her heart rate is 120 beats per minute. Physical examination reveals diminished breath sounds on the left and the trachea is deviated to the right.

What is the most likely diagnosis?

a. Pericardial tamponade
b. Pulmonary embolus (PE)
c. Tension pneumothorax
d. Hemothorax

Answer: The correct answer is (C). Tension pneumothorax presents with decreased breath sound on one side and tracheal deviation. PE does not give tracheal deviation, it does have chest pain and tachycardia. Muffled heart sounds are seen typically in pericardial tamponade. This patient's risk for pneumothorax is that she is a smoker. It is likely she has a pleural bleb that burst due to her smoking history.

Thoracic Abnormalities Secondary to Trauma				
	Etiology	**Signs and symptoms**	**Diagnostic tests**	**Treatment**
Pericardial tamponade	Trauma with penetration to the pericardium; secondary to broken ribs, knives, or bullet wounds	JVD, hypotension, muffled heart sounds, and electrical alternans on EKG	Cardiac echocardiogram	Pericardiocentesis is the most effective therapy.
Pneumothorax	Air in the pleural space	Chest pain, hyperresonance, and decreased breath sounds	Chest x-ray	Chest tube placement
Tension pneumothorax	Air in the pleural space through a one-way leak	Chest pain, hyperresonance and decreased breath sounds, and tracheal deviation away from the involved lung	Chest x-ray	Immediate needle decompression followed by chest tube placement
Hemothorax	Blood in the pleural space	Absent breath sounds and dull to percussion	Blunting of costophrenic angle on chest x-ray and CT scan	Chest tube drainage and possible thoracotomy

Tension pneumothorax **pushes** the trachea **away** from the involved lung, and atelectasis **pulls** the trachea **toward** the involved lung.

Figure 14.2: Pneumothorax on chest x-ray is characterized by absent vascular patterns and lack of x-ray absorption leading to a "blackout" of the affected lung. *Source: Niket Sonpal, MD.*

An 18-year-old boy is hit by a car while riding his bicycle. He presents to the ED with severe groin pain after falling on the central bar of the bike. Physical examination reveals blood at the urethral meatus and a high-riding prostate.

What is the most appropriate next step in the management of this patient?

a. Place a Foley
b. Get a retrograde urethrogram
c. Empiric antibiotics
d. CBC and electrolytes
e. Discharge the patient with reassurance

Answer: The correct answer is (B). The patient has a urethral disruption that needs to be evaluated. A kidney, ureters, and bladder (KUB) x-ray followed by a retrograde urethrogram must be conducted prior to any other tests. Placing a Foley catheter without such an imaging modality can lead to further urethral damage. The step after urethrogram is a Foley catheter placement to aid in urination. There is no role for antibiotics for trauma without evidence of infection.

THE ABDOMEN
Abdominal Pain

A 75-year-old man with a history of atrial fibrillation, coronary artery disease (CAD), and dyslipidemia presents with severe abdominal pain that is worsened with eating. He states the pain is 10/10 but no peritoneal signs are present. Laboratory analysis shows a white count of $15 \times 10^3/uL$ with increased neutrophils and decreased bicarbonate.

What is the most appropriate next step in management of this patient?

a. CT scan of the abdomen
b. Angiography
c. Liver function tests
d. Colonoscopy
e. Oral antibiotics

Answer: The correct answer is (B). Angiography is the most appropriate next step in a patient suffering from acute mesenteric ischemia. The patient will present with complaints of abdominal pain that is severe and out of proportion to physical findings. This patient could also be a surgical candidate, but that was not an answer choice. Angiography is done prior to surgery as quickly as possible to avoid perforation; colonoscopy may lead to perforation.

Ischemic Bowel Disease
Ischemic bowel disease is due to a lack of blood flow to the mesentery of the bowel. It is a progressive disease that begins with mild ischemia and progresses to full occlusion of blood flow.

> **Severe abdominal pain** that is out of proportion to physical findings = 10/10 pain, with no guarding, soft abdomen, and no rebound tenderness.

Figure 14.3: A lack of blood flow causes ischemia to the bowel wall and sloughing of the mucosa.
Source: Niket Sonpal, MD.

Ischemia of the bowel is analogous to angina. The pain occurs shortly after eating as the muscular contraction of the bowel increases the oxygen requirements of the bowel.

The most common symptoms are:

• Abdominal pain after eating
• Bloody diarrhea

DIAGNOSTIC TESTS/TREATMENT

The best initial test is a CT scan of the abdomen. The most accurate test is angiography. Colonoscopy with biopsy can also show ischemic mucosa, but it takes time for pathology to come back.

Treatment is IV normal saline followed by surgical intervention to remove necrotic bowel.

Mesenteric Ischemia

Atrial fibrillation can send emboli to the vasculature of the GI tract, causing ischemia of the small and large bowel. The most common vessel affected is the superior mesenteric artery. Surgical resection is the most effective therapy for mesenteric ischemia.

MI, GERD, lower lobe pneumonias, and acute porphyria are causes of abdominal pain that do not require surgery.

The most common locations for infarction are the 2 watershed areas: splenic and hepatic flexures.

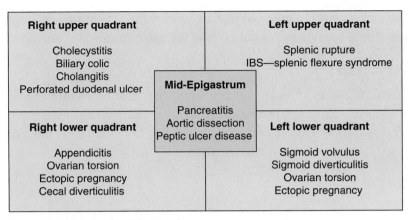

Right upper quadrant	Mid-Epigastrum	Left upper quadrant
Cholecystitis Biliary colic Cholangitis Perforated duodenal ulcer	Pancreatitis Aortic dissection Peptic ulcer disease	Splenic rupture IBS—splenic flexure syndrome
Right lower quadrant Appendicitis Ovarian torsion Ectopic pregnancy Cecal diverticulitis		**Left lower quadrant** Sigmoid volvulus Sigmoid diverticulitis Ovarian torsion Ectopic pregnancy

Figure 14.4: Causes of Pain by Location

A 65-year-old homeless woman presents to the ED with substernal chest pain that began shortly after vomiting. The patient has a history of alcoholism and has just finished a 3-day binge of vodka. Physical examination reveals a "snap, crackle, and pop" upon palpation around the clavicles.

What is the most likely diagnosis?

a. Boerhaave syndrome
b. Pancreatitis
c. Biliary colic
d. Volvulus
e. Mycocardial infarction

*Answer: The correct answer is **(A)**. **Boerhaave syndrome** is a full thickness tear of the esophagus secondary to retching. The patient will have a history of severe incessant vomiting, often due to alcoholism. The other choices **do not have** substernal chest pain except for MI, and MI is unlikely in this patient given the subcutaneous emphysema. Pancreatitis will present with abdominal pain that radiates to the back in the setting of alcohol intake, but **would not** present with air in the subcutaneous space. Biliary colic has postprandial RUQ pain. Volvulus is malrotation of the colon.*

Esophageal Perforation

Esophageal perforation is due to the rapid increase in intraesophageal pressure combined with negative intrathoracic pressure caused by vomiting.

Perforation of the esophagus can present with:

- Severe and acute onset of excruciating retrosternal chest pain
- Odynophagia
- Positive **Hamman sign**, a crunching heard upon palpation of the thorax due to subcutaneous emphysema
- Pain that can radiate to the left shoulder

Boerhaave syndrome is a **full thickness** tear secondary to extreme retching and vomiting. It is most commonly tested in the setting of an alcoholic. The most common location is at the left posterolateral aspect of the distal esophagus.

> The most common cause of **esophageal perforation is iatrogenic**. The most common procedure that causes an esophageal perforation is upper **endoscopy**. Boerhaave syndrome carries 25% mortality, even with surgery.

Mallory-Weiss syndrome is a **mucosal** tear and is also due to vomiting. It is not a perforation. The most common location is at the gastroesophageal junction.

DIAGNOSTIC TEST

The most accurate test is an **esophogram** using diatrizoate meglumine and diatrizoate sodium solution (**Gastrografin**; Bracco Diagnostics, Princeton, New Jersey); it will show leakage of contrast outside of the esophagus. Barium cannot be used because it is caustic to the tissues.

TREATMENT

Surgical exploration with debridement of the mediastinum and closure of the perforation is an absolute emergency. **Mediastinitis** is a complication that carries a very high mortality rate.

A 53-year-old obese man presents with sudden onset of abdominal pain that radiates to his right shoulder. The patient also says he has vomited blood earlier in the day. The patient has a full bottle of esomeprazole in his pocket and says he uses those for his heartburn. Physical examination reveals rebound tenderness in the midepigastrum. Upright chest x-ray shows air under the diaphragm.

What is the most likely diagnosis?

a. Gastric perforation
b. Hemorrhagic ulcer
c. Cholecystitis
d. Ischemic colitis

Answer: The correct answer is (A). This is gastric perforation in the setting of peptic ulcer disease. The patient's bottle filled with PPIs is due to his history of ulcers. The fact that it is a full bottle implies the patient is noncompliant with his medication. Hemorrhagic ulcers will present with hematemesis, specifically coffee ground emesis. Cholecystitis would have right upper quadrant pain that is colicky in nature. Ischemic colitis would have an abdominal pain that is out of proportion to physical findings.

Gastric Perforation

ETIOLOGY

Gastric **perforation** is most commonly seen **secondary to ulcer disease**. Risk factors include *Helicobacter pylori* infections, NSAID abuse, burns, head injury, trauma, and cancer. They either diminish the stomach's barrier against acid, or create increased levels of gastric acid. Alcohol and smoking prevent ulcer healing. The ulcer, once it erodes deep enough into the stomach, allows for the leakage of gastric acid into the abdominal cavity and causes peritonitis. The gastric acid has also been shown to cause pancreatitis if the ulcer is in the posterior part of the stomach. The acid leaks out the back of the stomach and literally fries the pancreas.

The patient will present with:

- Acute, progressive worsening abdominal pain that radiates to the right shoulder due to acid irritation of the phrenic nerve
- Likely signs of peritonitis by the time the patient comes to the ED, including:
  - Guarding
  - Rebound tenderness
  - Abdominal rigidity

DIAGNOSTIC TESTS

The best initial test is an upright chest x-ray which shows free air under the diaphragm. The most accurate test is a CT scan.

4-Step Treatment Process

1. Make the patient stop eating and drinking (NPO) to prevent food and water escaping into the peritoneum.
2. Place an NG tube to suction the 4 liters of gastric juices produced.
3. Start IV normal saline and broad-spectrum antibiotics.
4. Surgically repair the perforation.

A 9-year-old boy comes with decreased appetite and abdominal pain around his umbilicus. His parents think he doesn't want to go to school, and while in math class he begins to have sharp pain in his right lower abdomen. He is rushed to the ED and laboratory analysis shows a WBC of 12,500.

What is the most likely diagnosis?

a. Acute appendicitis
b. Acute diverticulitis
c. Cholecystitis
d. Acute pancreatitis

Answer: The correct answer is (A). Acute appendicitis presents with pain that originates in the umbilical region and later begins to localize to the right lower quadrant. The patient will then develop signs of peritonitis. This patient is too young for diverticulitis. Diverticultitis also gives pain in the left lower quadrant. Cholecystitis would present with right upper quadrant pain. Pancreatitis would have midepigastric pain that radiates to the back with high amylase and lipase levels. The number one consideration is the location of the pain. It gives away 95% of the diagnosis.

If the RLQ pain was in a female patient of childbearing age, ectopic pregnancy, cysts, and torsion must be considered. Get a beta-HCG and pelvic sonogram. Remember, avoid radiation imaging tests (CT and x-rays) in a patient who may be pregnant. If the sonogram shows an ectopic pregnancy, emergent surgery must be performed.

A 76-year-old woman with no significant past medical history presents with severe left lower quadrant pain, fever, and anorexia of one day in duration. The patient's daughter says her only medical history is that she is usually constipated and takes stool softeners every day to help her bowel movements. Physical exam shows guarding and rigidity.

What is the most likely diagnosis?

a. Acute appendicitis
b. Acute diverticulitis
c. Ectopic pregnancy
d. Cholecystitis
e. Acute pancreatitis

> Barium enema and colonoscopy are **contraindicated** in diverticulitis due to an increased incidence of perforation.

*Answer: The correct answer is (**B**). Acute diverticulitis has an acute onset of severe abdominal pain that is most likely located in the lower left quadrant. Patients with the first bout of diverticulitis are treated medically if there are no complications warranting surgery. However, recurrent diverticulitis will need resection of the affected loop of bowel. The most common complication after diverticulitis is abscess formation. Appendicitis gives pain in the right lower quadrant. Diverticulosis can occur anywhere in the colon, but in elderly patients, the sigmoid region is most involved, making it the most likely location for inflammation. Diverticulitis is highly associated with constipation. Pregnancy is implausible in this age group. Cholecystitis would have right upper quadrant pain. Pancreatitis would have pain that radiates to the back.*

Abdominal Abscess

Abscesses occur after invasive procedures, inflammatory conditions, and traumatic events. They are diagnosed by CT scan and incision and drainage is the only therapy. Percutaneous drainage can be done by CT or ultrasound guidance. Antibiotics must also be given to prevent bacteremia.

A 40-year-old obese woman with 5 children presents with a "gnawing" pain that recently has become severe. She notes the pain right after she finishes a meal and states that it radiates to her right shoulder. Physical exam reveals a cessation of inspiration upon palpation of the right upper quadrant and rebound tenderness. Laboratory analysis shows white cell count of 15,000 and a left shift.

What is the most likely diagnosis?

a. Acute appendicitis
b. Acute diverticulitis
c. Ectopic pregnancy
d. Cholecystitis
e. Acute pancreatitis

> Abdominal pain that radiates to the back has 2 emergent conditions: pancreatitis and aortic dissection.

*Answer: The correct answer is (**D**). Acute cholecystitis is a common inflammatory condition that occurs often in obese, women in their 40s. A gallstone occludes the lumen of the cystic duct. Patients have peritoneal signs and a positive Murphy sign. A sonographic Murphy sign is the ultrasound probe causing a cessation of breathing when it presses against the abdominal wall. On ultrasound, cholecystitis is characterized by pericholecystic fluid and a thickened gallbladder wall. Diverticulitis would be lower left or right quadrant pain in an elderly person with a history of constipation. Pancreatitis* would have deep epigastric pain radiating to the back. Appendicitis would typically present with right lower quadrant pain. An ectopic pregnancy would have pain in the LLQ or RLQ.

Inflammatory Abdominal Conditions					
	Etiology	**Signs and symptoms**	**Diagnostic tests**	**Treatment**	**Complications**
Appendicitis	Fecolith obstructing the appendiceal orifice, causing inflammation	Anorexia, fever, periumbilical pain with RLQ tenderness. Elevated white count with left shift.	CT scan is most accurate test.	Laparoscopic surgery	Abscess formation and gangrenous perforation
Acute pancreatitis	Alcohol or gallstone obstruction of the duct, causing inflammation	Fever, severe midabdominal pain radiating to the back, nausea and vomiting	CT scan is the best test. Amylase is sensitive and lipase is specific.	Aggressive IV fluids and NPO until symptoms resolve	Hemorrhagic pancreatitis and pseudocyst formation
Diverticulitis	Fecal impaction into pseudodiverticula, causing inflammation	Fever, nausea, most commonly LLQ pain, and peritonitis	CT scan is the best and most accurate test.	Antibiotics for the first attack; surgical resection if it recurs or perforates	Abscess formation. No endoscopy due to risk of perforation.
Cholecystitis	Gallstones occluding the lumen of the cystic duct, causing inflammation of the gallbladder	Fever, severe RUQ tenderness, Murphy sign; pain on inspiration causing a cessation of breathing, nausea, and vomiting	Ultrasound will reveal pericholecystic fluid, gallbladder wall thickening, and stones in the gallbladder. HIDA scan is the most accurate test.	Laparoscopic surgery, or open surgery if there is perforation of the gallbladder	Perforation of the gallbladder

Signs of Appendicitis

Rovsing sign: palpation of the left lower quadrant causes pain in the right lower quadrant

Psoas sign: pain with extension of the hip

Obturator sign: pain with internal rotation of the right thigh

HIDA scan will show delayed emptying of the gallbladder in acute cholecystitis by failure to visualize the gallbladder from isotope accumulation.

A 63-year-old woman presents to the ED with nausea, vomiting, and severe abdominal pain that has gradually been increasing in intensity. The patient also states she has not had a bowel movement in 3 days and cannot remember the last time she passed gas. Her past medical history is significant for an abdominal hysterectomy. Physical exam reveals a temperature of 101.5 and hyperactive bowel sounds, and the medical student thought he heard a tinkling sound. Laboratory results show a white blood cell count of 15,000.

What is the most likely diagnosis?

a. Acute appendicitis
b. Acute diverticulitis
c. Small bowel obstruction
d. Cholecystitis
e. Acute pancreatitis

*Answer: The correct answer is **(C)**. Small bowel obstruction is characterized by a failure to pass stool, flatus, and a complete absence of bowel sounds. Nausea, vomiting, and abdominal pain with hyperactive bowel sounds are hallmark signs. A history of abdominal surgery is a very significant risk factor as adhesions can form from surgery. The other choices have focal abdominal pain localized to one quadrant, whereas with obstruction, diffuse unlocalized pain is seen.*

Bowel Obstruction

Bowel obstruction is a mechanical or functional obstruction of the intestines due to various causes. Upon occlusion of the lumen, gas and fluid build up proximal to the site. This gas leads to severe increase in pressure from within the lumen that leads to decreased perfusion of the bowel and necrosis. The most common cause of small bowel obstruction is previous abdominal surgeries. There are 2 main types of obstruction:

1. Partial: A small amount of GI contents can pass.
2. Complete: No GI contents can pass.

Signs and Symptoms
- Severe waves of intermittent crampy abdominal pain
- Nausea and vomiting
- Fever
- Hyperactive bowel sounds
- High-pitched "tinkling" sounds indicate that the intestinal fluid and air are under high pressure in the bowel.
- Hypovolemia due to third spacing

Causes of Bowel Obstruction

- Adhesions from previous abdominal surgery
- Hernias
- Crohn disease
- Neoplasms
- Intussusception
- Volvulus
- Foreign bodies
- Intestinal atresia
- Carcinoid

DIAGNOSTIC TESTS

- An elevated white count is sensitive but not specific.
- An elevated lactate with marked acidosis is a hallmark sign.
- The best initial test is abdominal x-ray, which will show multiple air-fluid levels with dilated loops of small bowel.
- The most accurate test is a CT scan of the abdomen. It will show a transition zone from dilated loops of bowel with contrast to an area of bowel with no contrast.

TREATMENT

1. Make the patient NPO.
2. Place an NG tube to help decompress the bowel.
3. IV fluid hydration as volume is lost to third spacing.
4. Transport to the operation room for emergent surgical resection.

ORTHOPEDICS

Fractures are always diagnosed with an x-ray. In terms of therapy, general rules are:

- **Closed reduction:** mild fractures without displacement
- **Open reduction and internal fixation:** severe fractures with displacement or misalignment of bone pieces
- **Open fractures:** skin must be closed and the bone must be set in the operating room with debridement

Fractures

There are 5 main types of fractures, all of which present with pain, swelling, and deformity.

1. **Comminuted fractures:** a fracture in which the bone gets broken into multiple pieces
   - Most commonly caused by crush injuries

2. **Stress fractures:** a complete fracture from repetitive insults to the bone in question
   - Most common stress fracture is of the metatarsals.
   - On the USMLE Step 2 CK, vignettes may describe an athlete with persistent pain.
   - X-ray does not show evidence, so a CT or MRI must be conducted in order for diagnosis.
   - Treatment is with rehabilitation, reduced physical activity, and casting. If persistent, surgery is indicated.

3. **Compression fractures:** a specific fracture of the vertebra in the setting of osteoporosis
   - Approximately one-third of osteoporotic vertebral injuries are lumbar, one-third are thoracolumbar, and one-third are thoracic in origin.

4. **Pathologic fracture:** a fracture that occurs from minimal trauma to bone that is weakened by disease
   - Metastatic carcinoma (eg, breast or colon), multiple myeloma, and Paget disease are a few examples of diseases that cause brittle bones.
   - On the USMLE Step 2 CK, look for a vignette in which an older person fractures a rib from coughing.
   - Treatment is surgical realignment of the bone and treatment of the underlying disease.

5. **Open fracture:** a fracture when injury causes a broken bone to pierce the skin
   - An open fracture is associated with high rates of bacterial infection to the surrounding tissue
   - **Surgery is always the right answer.**

Shoulder Injuries				
	Etiology	**Signs and symptoms**	**Diagnosis**	**Treatment**
Anterior shoulder dislocation	Any injury that causes strain on the glenohumoral ligaments. **Most common type**, more than 95%.	Arm held to the side with externally rotated forearm with severe pain	X-ray is the best initial test and MRI is the most accurate test.	Shoulder relocation and immobilization
Posterior shoulder dislocation	Seizure or electrical burn	Arm is medially rotated and held to the side	X-ray is the best initial test and MRI is the most accurate test.	Traction and surgery if pulses or sensation are diminished during physical exam
Clavicular fracture	Trauma	Pain over location	X-ray is the best test.	Simple arm sling
Scaphoid fracture	Falling on an outstretched hand	Persistent pain in the anatomical "snuffbox"	X-ray won't show results for 3 weeks.	Thumb spica cast

A 39-year-old woman awoke from a nap with severe pain in her index finger and found it to be flexed while all other fingers were extended. When she tried to pull it free she heard a loud popping sound and the pain subsided. The following day she comes to her doctor's office concerned about the sound and pain.

What is the most appropriate next stop in the management of this patient?

a. Amputate the finger
b. Steroid injection
c. Rehabilitation
d. Admit to the hospital
e. NSAID therapy

For clavicular fractures, figure 8 slings are no longer used, as their outcomes have not been shown to be any better than a simple arm sling.

Answer: The correct answer is (B). Trigger finger is an acutely flexed and painful finger. Steroid injections have been shown to decrease pain and recurrence of trigger finger. It is the most cost-effective treatment, and studies have shown a trial of steroids should be attempted prior to surgery. Trigger finger is caused by a stenosis of the tendon sheath leading to the finger in question. If steroids fail, surgery to cut the sheath that is restricting the tendon is the definitive treatment.

Do not confuse trigger finger with **Dupuytren contracture, a condition more common in men over the age of 40.** Dupuytren contracture is when the palmar fascia becomes constricted and the hand can no longer be properly extended open. **Surgery** is the only effective therapy.

A 19-year-old woman broke her femur 3 days ago during a college soccer tryout. This morning her mother brought her to the ED because she was short of breath. Physical examination reveals a confused patient who is awake but not alert or oriented and a splotchy magenta rash around the base of the neck and back. ABG reveals a P02 under 60 mm Hg.

What is the most likely diagnosis?

a. Fat embolism
b. Myocardial infarction
c. Pancreatitis
d. Rhabdomyolysis

Answer: The correct answer is (A). Fat embolism syndrome is characterized by a combination of confusion, petechial rash, and dyspnea. It is caused by fracture of long bones. Myocardial infarction may have shortness of breath, but is unlikely in a 19-year-old woman. Pancreatitis would present with severe abdominal pain. Rhabdomyolysis has high CPK from muscle breakdown with a urine analysis and dipstick that shows positive blood with fewer than 5 RBCs.

Fat Embolism

Fracture of the long bone allows for fat to escape as little vesicles and cause occlusion of vasculature throughout the body. The most common bone is the femur. Onset of symptoms is within 5 days of the fracture. The patient will present with:

- Confusion
- Petechial rash on the upper extremity and trunk
- Shortness of breath and tachypnea with dyspnea

DIAGNOSTIC TESTS

- ABG will show P02 under 60 mm Hg.
- Chest x-ray will show infiltrates.
- Urine analysis may show fat droplets.

TREATMENT

Treatment for fat embolism requires oxygen to keep P02 over 95%. If the patient becomes severely hypoxic, intubation followed by mechanical ventilation is necessary.

Compartment Syndrome

Compartment syndrome is due to the compression of nerves, blood vessels, and muscle inside a closed space. This can also be within a cast after setting a fracture. The 6 signs of compartment syndrome are:

1. Pain: most commonly the first symptom
2. Pallor: lack of blood flow causes pale skin

3. Paresthesia: "pins and needles" sensation
4. Paralysis: inability to move the limb
5. Pulselessness: lack of distal pulses
6. Poikilothermia: cold to the touch

This is a medical emergency and immediate fasciotomy must be completed in order to relieve pressure before necrosis occurs.

A 19-year-old man takes a hard blow from the oncoming defense during his second college football game. He complains of severe progressive pain in his knee and has difficulty ambulating. He is seen by the team doctor, who tells him to ice the knee. A week later the pain and swelling are still present. His family doctor orders an MRI that shows a torn ACL.

What is the best therapy?

a. Total knee replacement
b. Rehabilitation
c. NSAIDs
d. Arthroscopic repair
e. Reassurance

*Answer: The correct answer is **(D)**. Arthroscopic repair is the most definitive therapy, followed by rehabilitation. The risk factor that should be considered is that he had direct trauma to the front of his knee. The mechanism of injury can give some insight into the type of problem that may subsequently arise.*

Figure 14.5: A torn ACL seen during arthroscopic repair. In the U.S. alone more than 100,000 people are affected by ACL injuries. *Source: Niket Sonpal, MD.*

Knee Injuries				
	Etiology	**Signs and symptoms**	**Diagnosis**	**Treatment**
Medial and lateral collateral ligament injury	Trauma to the opposite side of the injury	Pain	MRI	Surgical repair
Anterior cruciate ligament	Direct trauma to the knee	Pain and positive anterior drawer sign	MRI	Arthroscopic repair
Posterior cruciate ligament	Direct trauma to the knee	Pain and positive posterior drawer sign	MRI	Arthroscopic repair
Meniscal injury	Traumatic injury of the knee	Popping sound upon flexion and extension	MRI	Arthroscopic repair

▶ **TIP**

Anterior cruciate ligament (ACL) injury is the most common knee ligament injury.

The unhappy triad of knee injury in the setting of sports trauma involves 3 structures:

1. The anterior cruciate ligament

2. The medial collateral ligament

3. The meniscus

A 41-year-old man presents to the ED after acute onset of lower back pain that began after he tried to lift an engine block at his job. He says he feels like lightning bolts are shooting down his legs and he is unable to move. Physical exam reveals a positive straight leg raise test and positive anal wink.

What is the most appropriate next diagnostic step?

a. X-ray of the cervical spine
b. MRI of the spine
c. CBC
d. ESR
e. Lumbar puncture

Answer: The correct answer is (B). A patient who presents with acute onset of back pain and is under the age of 50 should have an MRI to rule out spinal cord compression due to a slipped disc or lumbar disc herniation. If asked for the most appropriate next step in management, antiinflammatory agents would be the answer. The most common sites of lumbar disc herniation are L4-L5 and L5-S1. The other choices are applicable but the most appropriate next step is an MRI. Lumbar puncture, however, has no role in the treatment of slipped disc.

VASCULAR

A third-year medical student is examining a patient who has acute onset of abdominal pain. The patient is a 65-year-old smoker with HTN and DM who has had dull abdominal pain gradually building for the last 12 hours. It is not related to food nor relieved by taking famotidine. On physical examination, auscultation reveals a bruit. Palpation shows a pulsatile mass. While lightly palpating the epigastrum, the patient suddenly becomes hypotensive and passes out.

What is the most likely diagnosis?

a. Ruptured abdominal aortic aneurysm
b. Ruptured peptic ulcer
c. Hemorrhagic gastritis
d. Narcolepsy

Answer: The correct answer is (A). A bruit and pulsatile abdominal mass are hallmark signs of an abdominal aortic aneurysm (AAA). The fact that the medical student was palpating the area and the patient passed out was a coincidence; however, syncope in the setting of the AAA is rupture until proven otherwise. Ruptured peptic ulcer would have more severe and sharp abdominal pain. Hemorrhagic gastritis could cause syncope, but the bleeding would cause emesis, and the patient is supine, so orthostasis is not of concern. Narcolepsy would not have hypotension. This patient's abdominal pain was from the AAA beginning to rupture and was dull and gradual in onset.

Abdominal Aortic Aneurysm

An AAA occurs when the portion of the aorta in the abdomen grows to 1.5 times its normal size or exceeds the normal diameter by more than 50 percent through dilation. It is a true aneurysm, since it involves all layers of the arterial wall.

DIAGNOSTIC TESTS

- CT or MRI will give information regarding the relationship of the AAA to the surrounding vessels.
- Ultrasound **must** be done because it gives information on size and can be used as a cost-effective and safe means to monitor the AAA over time.
- Surgery is indicated when the AAA reaches 5 cm.

POSTOPERATIVE CARE

A 57-year-old woman who underwent emergent cholecystectomy for a perforated gallbladder 3 days prior now has a fever of 103°F and is complaining of chills. The patient has not been ambulating and says she is in a great deal of pain at her incision.

What is the most likely cause of her fever?

a. Atelectasis

b. UTI

c. Wound infection

d. DVT

e. Abscess

*Answer: The correct answer is **(B)**. This is what it is **most likely**; however, **all of the choices are possible**. In this patient with a complicated surgery and obvious risk factors for other possibilities, you must use your clinical acumen to judge the most likely source of infection, but the other choices are still on your mind for consideration.*

Postoperative Fever Assessment				
	Mnemonic	**Possible cause**	**Diagnostic test**	**Therapy**
POD 1–2	Wind	Atelectasis or postoperative pneumonia	Chest x-ray followed by sputum cultures	Prevention by incentive spirometry; vancomycin and tazobactam-pipercillin for hospital-acquired pneumonia
POD 3–5	Water	Urinary tract infection	Urine analysis showing positive nitrates and leukocyte esterase. Urine culture for species and sensitivity.	Antibiotics appropriate for the organism
POD 5–7	Walking	Deep vein thrombosis or thrombophlebitis of the IV access lines. Must also consider pulmonary embolism for new-onset tachycardia and chest pain.	Doppler ultrasound of the extremities. Changing of IV access lines and culture of the IV tips.	Heparin for 5 days as a bridge to coumadin for 3–6 months
POD 7	Wound	Wound infections and cellulitis	Physical exam of the wound for erythema, purulent discharge, and/or swelling	Incision and drainage if abscess or fluid followed by antibiotics
POD 8–15	Wonder	Drug fever or deep abscess	CT scan for examination of a deep fluid collection	CT guided percutaneous guided drainage of the abscess; otherwise surgery

POD = Postoperative Day

Postoperative Complications

Postoperative Confusion

It is likely that a confused patient is hypoxic or septic. You must get an ABG, chest x-ray, blood cultures, urine culture, and CBC, and then treat the appropriate organism. If the patient is hypoxic, consider pulmonary embolism, atelectasis, or pneumonia as a cause.

Adult Respiratory Distress Syndrome

This will be seen postoperatively with severe hypoxia, tachypnea, accessory muscle use for ventilation, and hypercapnia. Diagnose with a chest x-ray that will show bilateral pulmonary infiltrates without JVD (rule out CHF) and treat with positive end expiratory pressure.

Pulmonary Embolism

PE presents as an acute onset of chest pain with clear lung exam. The best initial diagnostic test is an EKG, which will show sinus tachycardia without evidence of ST segment changes. You can confirm noncardiac chest pain with troponins and cardiac enzymes. Then follow with a CT angiogram of the chest. Treat with heparin as a bridge to coumadin therapy. If the patient has a second PE while on coumadin, then you must place an IVC filter via inguinal catheterization.

2yrs - 12 yes kid should gain 5 lbs/yr : 2 inches/year

4 mos - 2x birth wt
12 mos - 3x
2 year - 4x

6 mos - stranger anxiety
9 - 15 mos - seperation anxiety

12 mos - 2 block tower
18 mos - 4 block   walks well
24 mos - 6 blocks   running   3-word sentence
3 yrs - 9 blocks
4 yrs -

6 mos - all infatile reflexes should be gone

0 - 2 yrs   back car seat
2 - 4   front face
4 - 8   booster
8 +   normal belt

breast milk = 20 kcal/ounce   100-120 kcal/kg/day   needed

if ↓ umbilical artery → need renal u/s

oral thrush in newborn → oral nystatin

delayed fontanelle closure → not closed by 2 yrs → Downs | rickets | achondroplasia

ping pong ball occiput = rickets

↓ weight with no ↓ height = under norished | malabsorption → assess intake | stool studies | sweat chloride

↓ height with no ↓ weight = hormonal | excess cortisol → GH via IGF | TSH | 24 hr cortisol | bone age

↓ weight AND ↓ height = systemic | cardiac | inflamm | genetic → CRP/ESR | LFT's / electrolytes | bone age

bone age → genetic predisposition = actual bone age = chronologic age
          → constitutional delay = bone age delayed vs chronological age

breast feeding contraindications → HIV | CMV | substance abuse | some drugs

SECTION 5
PEDIATRICS

by Niket Sonpal, MD

ROUTINE MANAGEMENT OF THE NEWBORN

Pediatric medicine begins just after the birth with routine management of the newborn, which involves a physical examination, Apgar scoring, eye care, and routine disease prevention and screening.

A 28-year-old G_1P_0 woman delivers a 3.9 kg male infant whose Apgar scores are 9 and 10 at 1 and 5 minutes respectively. The delivery was uncomplicated and both mother and child are in no acute distress.

What is the most appropriate next step in management of this patient?

a. Intubate the child
b. Send cord blood for arterial blood gas (ABG)
c. Suction the mouth and nose
d. Nasogastric tube (NGT) placement
e. Give prophylactic antibiotics

Answer: The correct answer is (C). Once the child is delivered, the mouth and nose are suctioned, followed by clamping and cutting of the umbilical cord. The newborn is then dried, wrapped in clean towels, and placed under a warmer as he has just descended from an environment of 98.6° F to approximately 65° F. Gentle rubbing or stimulating the heels of the newborn helps to stimulate crying and breathing. Intubation and ABG analysis of the child are indicated only if the newborn is not breathing or is in respiratory distress. Nasogastric tube placement is indicated when GI decompression is needed. Antibiotics are indicated for sepsis.

> **Late preterm** neonate: between 34 and 37 weeks
> **Term** neonate: gestational age 38 weeks or more

Normal Vital Signs in a Newborn

Respiratory rate (RR) of <u>40 to 60 breaths</u> per minute (BrPM)

Heart rate (HR) of **120 to 160 beats** per minute (BPM)

403

Apgar Score: Newborn Assessment

The Apgar score delineates a quantifiable measurement for the need and effectiveness of resuscitation. The Apgar score does not predict mortality.

- **One-minute score** evaluates conditions **during labor and delivery**.
- **Five-minute score** evaluates the **response to resuscitative efforts**.

▶ **TIP**

A low score on the Apgar is **not** associated with future cerebral palsy.

Criteria of the Apgar Score				
Acronym		**0 points**	**1 point**	**2 points**
Appearance	Skin color/ complexion	Blue all over	Normal except extremities	Normal all over
Pulse	Pulse rate	<60 bpm or asystole	>60 bpm but <100 bpm	>100 bpm
Grimace	Reflex irritability	No response	Grimace/ feeble cry	Sneeze/ cough
Activity	Muscle tone	None	Some flexion	Active movement
Respiration	Breathing	Absent	Weak or irregular	Strong

Eye Care

A 3.9 kg male infant whose Apgar scores were 9 and 10 at 1 and 5 minutes, respectively, after delivery is brought in by his parents because his eyes are red. The delivery was without any complications and both mother and child are in no acute distress.

What is the most likely diagnosis at 1 day, at 2 to 7 days, and at greater than 7 days?

a. Chemical irritation   1 DAY
b. Neisseria gonorrhoeae   1 WEEK
c. Chlamydia trachomatis   2 WEEKS
d. Herpes simplex   3 WEEKS
e. All of the above

Answer: The correct answer is (E). To diagnose the cause of conjunctivitis in the newborn, you must consider when the redness and irritation begins.

- **At 1 day**, the most likely cause of the conjunctivitis is **chemical irritation**.
- From **days 2 to 7**, the most likely cause of the conjunctivitis is *Neisseria gonorrhoeae*.

- Conjunctivitis after **more than 7 days** post delivery is most likely due to *Chlamydia trachomatis.*
- Conjunctivitis after **3 weeks or more** is most likely due to herpes infection.

TREATMENT

In the delivery room, all newborns must be given 2 types of antibiotic drops in each eye to prevent **ophthalmia neonatorum**. This condition can be attributed most commonly to *Neisseria gonorrhoeae* or *Chlamydia trachomatis.* Use:

- Erythromycin ointment or tetracycline ointment
- Silver nitrate solution

Vitamin K Deficient Bleeding

DEFINITION

As the neonate's colonic flora has not adequately colonized, *E. coli* is not present in sufficient quantities to make enough **vitamin K** to produce clotting **factors II, VII, IX, and X and proteins C and S**. Without such factors, the newborn is more likely to have bleeding from the GI tract, belly button, and urinary tract.

Prophylactic Treatment

To prevent vitamin K deficient bleeding (VKDB, formerly known as **hemorrhagic disease of the newborn**), a single intramuscular **dose of vitamin K is recommended** and has been shown to decrease the incidence of VKDB.

▶ **TIP**

Anything that decreases mortality is most likely to be tested on the USMLE Step 2 CK.

▶ **TIP**

Only nationally recommended guidelines can appear on your examination.

Screening Tests

All children must be screened for these diseases **prior** to discharge:

- PKU
- congenital adrenal hyperplasia (CAH)
- Biotinidase
- Beta thalassemia
- Galactosemia
- Hypothyroidism
- Homocysteinuria

Most Commonly Tested Disorders in Newborns

- **G6PD Deficiency:** X-linked recessive disease characterized by hemolytic crises. Treatment involves reducing oxidative stress and specialized diets.
- **Phenylketonuria (PKU):** autosomal recessive genetic disorder characterized by a deficiency in the enzyme phenylalanine hydroxylase (PAH) that leads to mental retardation. Treatment involves patients adhering to a **special diet low in phenylalanine** for at least the first 16 years of their lives.
- **Galactosemia:** a rare genetic disorder that precludes the ability to properly metabolize galactose. Treatment is to cut out all lactose-containing products.
- **Congenital adrenal hyperplasia:** any of several autosomal recessive diseases resulting in errors in steroidogenesis. Treatment is to replace mineralocorticoids and glucocorticoid deficiencies and possible genital reconstructive surgery.
- **Congenital hypothyroidism:** a condition affecting 1 in 4000 infants that can result in **cretinism.**
- **Hearing test:** excludes congenital sensory-neural hearing loss. Necessary for early detection to maintain speech patterns and assess the need for cochlear implantation.

Hepatitis B Vaccination

Every child gets a hepatitis B vaccination, but only those with HBsAg-positive mothers should receive hepatitis B immunoglobulin (HBIG) in addition to the vaccine.

TRANSIENT CONDITIONS OF THE NEWBORN

Transient Polycythemia of the Newborn

Hypoxia during delivery **stimulates erythropoeitin** and causes an increase in circulating red blood cells. The newborn's **first breath** will **increase O$_2$** and cause a drop in erythropoeitin, which in turn will lead to normalization of hemoglobin.

Splenomegaly is a **normal** finding in newborns.

Transient Tachypnea of the Newborn

Compression of the rib cage by passing through the mother's vaginal canal helps to remove fluid from the lungs. Newborns who are delivered via cesarean birth may have excess fluid in the lungs and therefore be hypoxic. If **tachypnea lasts more than 4 hours**, it is considered sepsis and must be evaluated with

[handwritten margin notes:]
R.D.S. → Not enough surfactant
→ usually premies
→ L:S > 2:1 = in the clear
  ↳ any less = ↑ chance of RDS
→ give surfactant
→ xray = ground glass

[handwritten note in text:] most common problem is resp from thick blood

[handwritten note at bottom:] ↳ x-ray ↑ lung volumes / sunburst pattern

blood and urine cultures. Lumbar puncture with CSF analysis and culture is done when the newborn displays neurological signs such as irritability, lethargy, temperature irregularity, and feeding problems.

Transient Hyperbilirubinemia

Over **60%** of all newborn infants are jaundiced. This is due to the infant's spleen removing excess red blood cells that carry Hgb F. This excess breakdown of RBCs leads to a physiological release of hemoglobin and in turn a rise in bilirubin.

DELIVERY-ASSOCIATED INJURY IN THE NEWBORN

Subconjunctival Hemorrhage

Minute hemorrhages may be present in the eyes of the infant due to a rapid rise in intrathoracic pressure as the chest is compressed while passing through the birth canal. No treatment is indicated.

Skull Fractures

There are 3 major types of skull fractures in the newborn:

1. Linear: **most common**
2. Depressed: can cause further cortical damage without surgical intervention
3. Basilar: **most fatal**

Scalp Injuries

Caput succedaneum is a swelling of the soft tissues of the scalp **that does cross** suture lines. Cephalohematoma is a subperiosteal hemorrhage that **does not cross** suture lines. Diagnosis is made clinically and improvement occurs gradually without treatment over a few weeks to months.

Brachial Palsy

ETIOLOGY

Brachial plexus injuries are secondary to births with traction in the event of shoulder dystocia. Brachial palsy is **most commonly seen in macrosomic** infants of diabetic mothers and has 2 major forms.

Duchenne-Erb Paralysis: C5–C6

- "Waiter's tip" appearance; secondary to shoulder dystocia
- The infant is **unable** to **abduct** the shoulder or **externally rotate** and **supinate** the arm.

Diagnosis is made clinically and immobilization is the best treatment.

> Shoulder dystocia occurs when, after delivery of the fetal head, the baby's anterior shoulder gets stuck behind the mother's pubic bone.

Klumpke Paralysis: C7–C8+/– T1
- "Claw hand" due to a lack of grasp reflex
- **Paralyzed hand** with Horner syndrome (ptosis, miosis, and anhydrosis)

Diagnosis is made clinically and immobilization is the best treatment.

Clavicular Fracture

This is the most common newborn fracture as a result of shoulder dystocia. X-ray is the best diagnostic test, and the fracture is treated with immobilization, splinting, and physical therapy. → DO NOTHING

Facial Nerve Palsy

Facial nerve palsy is paralysis of structures innervated by the facial nerve, caused by trauma secondary to forcep use in delivery. Diagnosis is made clinically and improvement occurs gradually over a few weeks to months. However, if no recovery is seen, then surgical nerve repair is necessary.

Amniotic Fluid Abnormalities and Associated Manifestations

- In amniotic fluid, 80% is a filtrate of the mother's plasma.
- The baby produces the remaining 20% by swallowing, absorbing, filtering, and urinating.

Polyhydramnios: Too Much Fluid Secondary to Fetus Not Swallowing

Causes are:

- Neurological: Werdnig-Hoffmann
  - Infant unable to swallow

- GI
  - Intestinal atresias

Oligohydramnios: Too Little Fluid Because Fetus Cannot Urinate

Causes are:

- Prune belly: lack of abdominal muscles, so unable to bear down and urinate
  - Treatment is with serial Foley catheter placements, but carries high risk of UTI

- Renal agenesis: incompatible with life
  - Associated with Potter syndrome

- Flat facies due to high atmospheric pressure causing compression of the fetus that is normally buffered by the amniotic fluid

A premature infant born at 28 weeks is in respiratory distress, with grunting, nasal flaring, and the use of accessory muscles. Bowel sounds are heard upon ausculta-tion of the back and chest x-ray shows air fluid levels are seen in the chest.

Which of the following is the most likely diagnosis?

a. Hydrocele
b. Gastroschisis
c. Diaphragmatic hernia
d. Hiatal hernia
e. Omphalocele

*Answer: The correct answer is **(C)**. A hernia in the diaphragm will allow for bowel con-tents to move into the chest and impair ventilation. Hydrocele is a urinary defect and is not seen on x-ray. It cannot be gastroschisis or omphalocele, as those are defined as an extrusion of abdominal contents outside of the body. Hiatal hernia is a benign finding most commonly seen in elderly or obese patients.*

No MECONIVM

HIRSCHSPUNGS → NO MECONVM & NO STOOL IN RECTUM

CF

MATERNAL DRUG ABUSE

Figure 15.1: Multiple air fluid levels are seen during obstruction and can be a clue to guiding the clinician. *Source: Niket Sonpal, MD.*

Abnormal Abdominal Findings

Diaphragmatic Hernia

Diaphragmatic hernia is a hole in the diaphragm that allows the abdominal contents to move into the thorax.

- Bowel sound in the chest can be heard.

- Air fluid levels are seen on chest x-ray.

→ CXR

→ INTUBATE → SURGERY

- Two types:

  - **Morgagni:** Defect is **midline**

  - **Bochdalek:** Defect can be **bilateral**

Omphalocele (ASSOCIATED WITH TRI 18 — "SEALED ELECTION VOTES")

An **omphalocele** is a wall defect in which **intestines and organs** form beyond the abdominal wall with **a sac covering.** This is due to a defect in the development of abdominal wall musculature.

Screening is conducted by maternal alpha fetoprotein (AFP) levels and ultrasound. Surgical reintroduction of contents is needed. Omphalocele is highly associated with Edwards syndrome (trisomy 18).

> High AFP levels indicate both neural tube defects and abdominal wall defects.

▶ TIP

The most common cause for elevated AFP is incorrect dating.

Umbilical Hernia

3. y.a IS CUT-OFF FOR SPONTANEOUS RESOLUTION → SURGERY @ 4

With umbilical hernia there is a congenital weakness of the rectus abdominis muscle which allows for protrusion of vessels and bowel. It is highly associated with congenital hypothyroidism. Ninety percent close spontaneously by age 3. After the age of 4, surgical intervention is indicated to prevent bowel strangulation and subsequent necrosis.

Gastroschisis

Gastroschisis is a wall defect **lateral to midline** with intestines and organs forming beyond the abdominal wall with **no sac covering.** In many cases multiple intestinal atresias can occur. Treatment calls for immediate surgical intervention with gradual introduction of bowel and silo formation. Overly agressive surgical reintroduction of the bowel will lead to third spacing and bowel infarction.

Wilms Tumor

PRESENTATION

> Wilms tumor is the most common abdominal mass in children.

With Wilms tumor, a large palpable abdominal mass is felt. It is caused by hemihypertrophy of one kidney due to its increased vascular demands. Aniridia is highly associated with this malignancy and is usually the clinician's most valuable clue. An affected child will show signs of constipation and complain of abdominal pain that is accompanied by nausea and vomiting.

DIAGNOSTIC TESTS

Wilms tumor is diagnosed with abdominal ultrasonography, which is the **best initial** imaging study. Contrast-enhanced computed tomography (CT) is **the most accurate test.**

TREATMENT

> Wilms tumor, aniridia, genitourinary malformations, and mental retardation is referred to as WAGR syndrome. The syndrome results from a deletion on chromosome 11.

Total nephrectomy with **chemotherapy and radiation** may be indicated based upon staging. If bilateral kidney involvement is seen, partial nephrectomy is indicated.

Neuroblastoma

Neuroblastoma is an adrenal medulla tumor **similar to a pheochromocytoma** but with fewer cardiac manifestations. The percentage of cases presenting with metastases ranges from 50% to 60%. Look for two highly tested findings:

- Hypsarrythmia (dancing eyes) and opsoclonus (dancing feet) are hallmark signs.
- Increased vanillyl mandelic acid (VMA) and metanephrines on urine collection are diagnostic.

> Neuroblastoma are statistically the most common cancers in infancy and the most common extracranial solid malignancy.

Abnormal Genitourinary Findings

Hydrocele

Hydrocele is a painless, swollen fluid-filled sac along the spermatic cords within the scrotum that transilluminates upon inspection.

- Remnant of tunica vaginalis
- Usually will resolve within 6 months
- Must differentiate from inguinal hernia

Cryptorchidism

Cryptorchidism is an **absence of one testicle** in the scrotum, and is usually found within the inguinal canal.

- Ninety percent of cases can be felt in the inguinal canal.
- **Orchipexy** is indicated to bring the testicle down into the scrotum after the age of 1 to avoid sterility.

> Cryptorchidism is associated with an increased risk of malignancy regardless of surgical intervention.

Hypospadias

With **hypospadias**, the opening of the urethra is found on the **ventral surface** of the penis.

- High association with cryptorchidism and inguinal hernias
- Needs surgical correction
- Circumcision contraindicated due to difficulties in surgical correction of the hypospadias

Epispadias

With **epispadias**, the opening to the urethra is found on the **dorsal surface**.

- High association with urinary incontinence
- Must evaluate for concomitant bladder exstrophy
- Needs surgical correction

POSTERIOR URETHRAL VALVES

- *MALE PTS*
- *VALVE IN URETHRA*
- *OLIGURIA*
- *ENLARGED BLADDER*
- *UTI*
- *→ VCUG*
- *→ TRANSURETHRAL ABLATION OF VALVES*
- *→ FOLEY IS OK.*

DEVELOPMENTAL ACHIEVEMENTS

Reflexes

1. Sucking reflex: Baby will automatically suck on a nipplelike object.
2. Grasping reflex

3. Babinski reflex: toe extension
4. Rooting reflex: If you touch a baby's cheek, the baby will turn to that side.
5. Moro reflex: Arms spread symmetrically when the baby is scared.
6. Stepping reflex: walking-like maneuvers when toes touch the ground
7. Superman reflex: When held facing the floor, arms go out.

CARDIOLOGY

Cyanotic Lesions

A 5-year-old boy is seen for routine examination by his doctor, but his parents have stated that lately he becomes short of breath while playing with his friends, and has a bluish hue to his lips when coming back from playing. The boy's teacher also says he finds the boy squatting while playing outside during recess.

Which of the following is the most likely diagnosis?

a. Atrial septal defect
b. Patent foramen ovale
c. Hypertrophic obstructive cardiomyopathy
d. Tetralogy of Fallot
e. Restrictive cardiomyopathy

*Answer: The correct answer is **(D)**. The history of exercise intolerance and squatting while playing outside (tet spells) is pathonomonic for tetralogy of Fallot. The remainder of choices do not present with tet spells such as squatting during exertion.*

Tetralogy of Fallot

▶ TIP

Tetralogy of Fallot is the most common cyanotic heart defect in children.

DEFINITION/ETIOLOGY

Tetralogy of Fallot (TOF) is a condition characterized by:

- Overriding aorta
- Pulmonary stenosis
- Right ventricular hypertrophy
- Ventricular septal defect (VSD)

Its cause is thought to be due to genetic factors and environmental factors. It is associated with **chromosome 22 deletions**.

PRESENTATION

- Cyanosis of the lips and extremities
- **Holosystolic murmur** best heard at the left lower sternal border
- **Squatting** after exertive activities

- Causes an increased preload and increased systemic vascular resistance. This decreases the right-to-left shunting, leading to increased pulmonary blood flow, and increased blood oxygen saturation.

DIAGNOSTIC TESTS/TREATMENT

- Chest x-ray showing a **boot-shaped heart**
- Decreased pulmonary vascular marking

Surgical intervention is the only definitive therapy.

> ▶ **TIP**
>
> There are only 3 holosystolic murmurs:
>
> 1. Mitral regurgitation
> 2. Tricuspid regurgitation
> 3. Ventricular septal defect

MITRAL REGURG (MR)
TRICUSPID REGURG (TR)
VSD

> VSDs are common in **Down** (trisomy 21), **Edwards** (trisomy 18), and **Patau** (trisomy 13).

Transposition of the Great Vessels

DEFINITION

This condition is characterized by an aorta that originates from the right ventricle and pulmonary artery that comes from the left ventricle. **No** oxygenation of blood can occur **without** a patent ductus arteriosus (PDA), atrial septal defect (ASD), or VSD.

PRESENTATION/DIAGNOSTIC TESTS

Early and severe cyanosis is seen. A single S2 is heard. Chest x-ray will show an "egg on a string."

TREATMENT

Neonates must have an open ductus arteriosus (PDA). They require prostaglandin E1 to keep the ductus open, and NSAIDs (especially indomethacin) are contraindicated because they will cause closure of the ductus.

Two separate surgeries are necessary; however, each surgery carries a 50% mortality rate. Therefore, only 1 in 4 will survive the surgeries.

> Tetralogy of Fallot is the most common cyanotic condition in children after the neonatal period. Transposition of the great vessels (TOGV) is the most common cyanotic lesion during the neonatal period.

Pulses

STRONG thought to be as result of in starling preload emptying by of incomplete previous systole

- ◉ Pulsus alternans: sign of left ventricular systolic dysfunction → *STRONG THEN WEAK PULSE*
- ◉ Pulsus bigeminus: sign of hypertrophic obstructive cardiomyopathy (HOCM)
- ◉ Pulsus bisferiens: in aortic regurgitation *AR 2 PULSES FOR EACH HEART BEAT*
- ◉ Pulsus tardus et parvus: aortic stenosis *AS WEAK & SMALL*
- Pulsus paradoxus: cardiac tamponade and tension pneumothorax
- Irregularly irregular: atrial fibrillation

Hypoplastic Left Heart Syndrome

This is a syndrome consisting of left ventricular hypoplasia, mitral valve atresia, and aortic valve lesions.

PRESENTATION

- Absent pulses with a single S2
- Increased right ventricular impulse
- **Gray** rather than bluish cyanosis

[handwritten margin: Ø PULSE SINGLE S2]

[handwritten note: JUST SINGLE S2 = TRANSPOSITION / S+ S2 + MURMUR = TA]

DIAGNOSTIC TESTS/TREATMENT

Chest x-ray will show a **globular-shaped heart** with pulmonary edema. Echocardiogram is the most accurate diagnostic test.

The only therapy is 3 separate surgeries or a heart transplant. Each surgery carries an extremely high mortality.

Truncus Arteriosus

Truncus arteriosus (TA) occurs when a single trunk emerges from both right and left ventricles and gives rise to all major circulations.

PRESENTATION

Symptoms occur within the first few days of life and are characterized by:

- Severe dyspnea
- Early and frequent respiratory infections

[handwritten margin: SINGLE S2 MURMUR PULM HTN]

Single S2 is heard as there is only one semilunar valve and a systolic ejection murmur is heard because these valve leaflets are usually abnormal in functionality. Peripheral pulses are bounding.

DIAGNOSTIC TESTS

Chest x-ray will show cardiomegaly with increased pulmonary markings.

TREATMENT

The most severe sequela of this condition is pulmonary hypertension, which will develop within 4 months. **Surgery must be completed early to prevent pulmonary hypertension.**

Total Anomalous Pulmonary Venous Return

In total anomalous pulmonary venous return (TAPVR), a congenital condition in which there is **no venous return between pulmonary veins and the left atrium**, oxygenated blood instead returns to the superior vena cava. There are 2 forms: with or without obstruction of the venous return. Obstruction refers to the angle at which the veins enter the sinus.

[handwritten note: → TRICUSPID ATRESIA = LEFT AXIS DEVIATION]

TAPVR with and without Obstruction			
	Signs/Symptoms	**Diagnostic tests**	**Treatment**
TAPVR <u>with</u> obstruction	Early in life with respiratory distress and severe cyanosis	CXR shows pulmonary edema. Echocardiography is definitive.	Surgery is the definitive choice for treatment.
TAPVR <u>without</u> obstruction	Age 1–2 years with right heart failure and tachypnea	CXR shows snowman or figure 8 sign. Most accurate diagnostic test is an echocardiogram. Diagnosed with echocardiogram and not by x-ray.	Surgical intervention to restore proper blood flow

Acyanotic Lesions → MOST COMMONLY PRESENT AS HEART FAILURE

A 3-month-old female infant is brought in because her parents say she will not eat anymore. Upon physical examination, a loud pansystolic murmur is appreciated. The child also appears small for her age, but her records show no maternal or delivery complications.

Which of the following is the most likely finding on EKG?

a. Right ventricular hypertrophy
b. Right bundle branch block
c. ST segment elevation
d. QT interval elongation
e. P wave inversion

*Answer: The correct answer is (A). The key to this case is understanding that a child who was otherwise healthy but presents with a holosystolic murmur and symptoms of failure to thrive most likely has a VSD. Right ventricular hypertrophy occurs from blood shunting from the high pressure left system to the low pressure right system. This could later lead to **Eisenmenger syndrome** (ES). ES is defined as the process in which a left-to-right shunt caused by a VSD reverses into a right-to-left shunt due to hypertrophy of the right ventricle.*

Ventricular Septal Defect

VSD is the most common congenital heart lesion.

PRESENTATION

- Dyspnea with respiratory distress
- High-pitched holosystolic murmur over lower left sternal border —HARSH
- Loud pulmonic S2

415

DIAGNOSTIC TESTS

- Chest x-ray shows increased vascular markings.
- Echocardiogram is diagnostic and cardiac catheterization is definitive.

TREATMENT

Smaller lesions usually close in the first 1 to 2 years while larger or more symptomatic lesions require surgical intervention. **Diuretics and digoxin** can be used for more conservative treatment. If left untreated, complications can lead to congestive heart failure (CHF), endocarditis, and pulmonary hypertension.

EISENMENGER'S SYNDROME

▶ **TIP**

Pansystolic = holosystolic = throughout systole

PRESENTS LIKE VSD

AV CANAL — DOWN'S SURGERY BY PULM HTN SETS IN

A 17-year-old boy who just flew from Australia and landed in New York presents in the ED with facial drooping, altered mental status, and left side paralysis. He took some diphenhydramine to get through the flight. Physical exam reveals a swollen left calf muscle.

Which of the following is the most likely process underlying this patient's stroke?

a. Emboli from his carotid artery
b. Emboli from his middle cerebral artery
c. Trauma brain injury
d. Paradoxical emboli from deep leg veins
e. Medication side effect

Answer: The correct answer is (D). The patient most likely has thrown a clot to his brain. The clot was formed in the setting of venous stasis and was able to travel to his brain via a patent ASD. Without the ASD, this clot would have embolized to the pulmonary circulation. Choices (A) and (B) are incorrect because he is too young for such advanced vascular disease; (C) is incorrect because there is no history of trauma; diphenhydramine does not cause emboli, ruling out choice (E).

Atrial Septal Defect

ASD is a hole in the septum between both atria that is twice as common in women as in men.

There are 3 major types of ASD:

1. Primum defect: concomitant mitral valve abnormalities *→ SURGERY*
2. Secundum defect: most common and located in the center of the atrial septum
3. Sinus venosus defect: least common *→ SURGERY*

PRESENTATION/DIAGNOSTIC TESTS

Patients are usually asymptomatic except for a **fixed wide splitting of S2.**

The most definitive test is cardiac catheterization. However, echocardiography is less invasive and can be just as effective.

Chest x-ray (CXR) shows increased vascular markings and cardiomegaly.

TREATMENT

- Vast majority close spontaneously
- Surgery or transcatheter closure is indicated for all symptomatic patients
- **Dysrhythmias** and possible **paradoxical emboli** from DVTs later in life

Patent Ductus Arteriosus (PDA)

PDA is defined as the failure of spontaneous closure of the ductus. It usually closes when PO_2 rises above 50 mm Hg. Low PO_2 can be caused by pulmonary compromise due to prematurity. Areas of high altitude have an increased occurrence of PDA due to low levels of atmospheric oxygen.

MORE COMMON IN GIRLS | MOMS w/ RUBELLA | PREMIES

▶ **TIP**

PDA is a **normal finding** in the first **12** hours of life. After **24** hours it is considered **pathologic**.

PRESENTATION

- "Machinery"-like murmur with
- Wide pulse pressure
- Bounding pulses
- A high occurrence of respiratory infections and infective endocarditis is the most common complication later in the child's life.

DIAGNOSTIC TESTS

Echocardiography is the **best initial test**, while **cardiac catheterization** is the **most accurate test**.

EKG may show LVH secondary to high systemic resistance.

TREATMENT

Give indomethacin (NSAID inhibits prostaglandins) to close the PDA unless it is needed to live in concurrent conditions such as TOF.

▶ **TIP**

Give **prostaglandins to pop** open a **PDA**.

Give **indomethacin to inhibit** popping.

▶ **TIP**

Mitral lesions radiate to the axilla.

Tricuspid and pulmonary lesions radiate to the back.

Aortic lesions radiate to the neck.

> **Cardiac X-Ray Findings**
>
> - Pear-shaped; pericardial effusion
> - Boot-shaped heart: tetralogy of Fallot
> - Jug handle appearance: primary pulmonary artery hypertension
> - "3"-like appearance: coarctation of the aorta
> - Rib notching—coarcation of the aorta

Coarctation of the Aorta

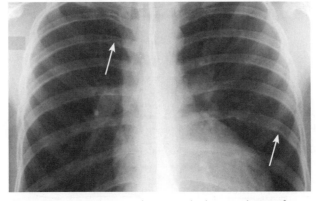

Figure 15.2: Due to increased pressure in the vasculature of the subcostal vessels, the ribs become eroded, leading to the notched appearance seen here. *Source: Niket Sonpal, MD.*

▶ **TIP**

If the exam question mentions a short girl with webbed neck, shield chest, streak gonads, horseshoe kidneys, or shortened fourth metacarpal, think coarctation of the aorta.

DEFINITION

Coarctation of the aorta is a congenital malformation where a narrowing at the aorta is found in the area of ductus arteriosus. It has a frequent association with Turner syndrome.

PRESENTATION

- Severe CHF and respiratory distress within the first few months of life
- Differential pressures and pulses between the upper and lower extremities
- Reduced pulses in the lower extremities and hypertension in the upper extremities due to narrowing

DIAGNOSTIC TESTS

- Rib notching and a "3" sign are seen on chest x-ray.
- Cardiac catheterization is the most accurate test.

TREATMENT

Primary treatment is surgical resection of the narrowed segment and then balloon dilation if recurrent stenosis occurs.

GASTROENTEROLOGY

Pathologic Jaundice (Hyperbilirubinemia) in the Newborn

Hyperbilirubinemia is considered pathological when:

- It appears on the first day of life.
- Bilirubin rises more than 5 mg/dL /day.
- Bilirubin rises above 19.5 mg/dL in a term child.
- Direct bilirubin rises above 2 mg/dL at any time.
- Hyperbilirubinemia persists after the second week of life.

The most serious complication is the deposition of bilirubin in the basal ganglia called **kernicterus**. Kernicterus presents with **hypotonia**, **seizures**, **choreoathetosis**, and **hearing loss**.

DIAGNOSTIC TESTS

- Direct and indirect bilirubin levels.
- Blood type of the infant and mother must be checked for ABO and Rh incompatibility.
- Peripheral blood smear and reticulocyte count must be analyzed for hemolysis.

TREATMENT

Phototherapy with blue-green light helps to break down bilirubin into excretable components; otherwise, exchange transfusion is considered if bilirubin rises to 20 to 25 mg/dL.

1-day-old child is given her first feeding, at which time she begins to choke and milk bubbles appear to be coming out of her nose. The child then appears to be in significant respiratory distress. CXR reveals an air bubble in the upper esophagus and a lack of gas pattern in the remainder of the GI tract. A coiled NGT is also seen.

What is the most common complication of this condition?

a. Meningitis
b. Pneumonia
c. Dental caries
d. Dyspepsia
e. Belching

[Handwritten margin notes:]
↑ INDIRECT COOMBS (−)
High Hgb CAUSES — Polycythemia — Twin-Twin — Mat-Fetal Transfsn — IUGR — IODM
Low Hgb — Spherocytosis — Elliptocytosis — G6PD — Pyruvate Kinase
COOMBS (+) ABO/Rh THALASSEMIA minor
→ COOMBS TEST → U/A & Blood Cx for Sepsis
↑ DIRECT — Sepsis — TORCHs — TPN — Hypothyroid — Galactosemia — CF — Choledochal cyst

419

Answer: The correct answer is (B). The signs described both on physical exam and radiological exam point towards an esophageal atresia with a tracheoesophageal fistula. Aspiration pneumonia is a severe and common complication of this condition as food contents are aspirated via the fistula in the respiratory system. Aspiration leads to abscess formation from anaerobic proliferation. Dental caries cannot form because the child is only 1 day old and therefore does not have teeth. Food cannot reach the stomach, so there is no possibility for either dyspepsia or belching.

Esophageal Atresia

In esophageal atresia, the esophagus ends blindly. In nearly 90% of cases it communicates with the trachea through a fistula known as a tracheoesophageal fistula (TEF).

PRESENTATION

The child will typically exhibit "**vomiting with first feeding**" or choking/coughing and cyanosis due to the **TEF**. There will be a history of possible **polyhydramnios**.

Recurrent aspiration pneumonia is due to food and secretions traveling into lungs via the TEF.

DIAGNOSTIC TESTS

- A gastric air bubble and esophageal air bubble can be seen on chest X-ray (CXR).
- Coiling of the NG tube seen on CXR and an inability to pass it into the stomach are diagnostic.
- CT or esophagram can also be used.

TREATMENT

- Surgical repair must be done in 2 steps to correct the congenital anomaly.
- Antibiotic coverage for anaerobes must also be considered due to high risk of lung abscess formation secondary to aspiration.
- Fluid resuscitation before surgery must be done to prevent dehydration of the infant.

1-month-old child is fed, after which he has vomitus that is forceful and winds up across the nursery. The vomitus is nonbloody and nonbilious. Physical examination reveals a palpable mass in the abdomen. An upper GI series is ordered.

Which of the following is the most likely finding on this radiologic exam?

a. String sign
b. Doughnut sign
c. Bird's beak sign
d. Steeple sign
e. Murphy sign

Answer: The correct answer is (A). Projectile vomiting and palpable abdominal mass is characteristic of pyloric stenosis. String sign is seen on upper GI series (barium is swallowed and its passage is watched under fluoroscopy). Doughnut sign is seen during intussusceptions. Bird's beak is seen in achalasia, steeple sign is seen during croup, and the Murphy sign is not ever a radiological sign, but rather a physical exam sign with right upper quadrant tenderness that causes cessation of breathing.

Pyloric Stenosis

A hypertrophic pyloric sphincter prevents proper passage of GI contents from the stomach into the duodenum. The most common cause is idiopathic.

PRESENTATION

Hypertrophy of the **pylorus** is not commonly found at birth but rather becomes most pronounced by the **first month of life**. It can present as late as 6 months after birth.

Auscultation will reveal a succussion splash, which is the sound of stomach contents slapping into the pylorus like waves on a beach.

Nonbilious projectile vomiting is the hallmark feature. Metabolic imbalance demonstrates a **hypochloremic, hypokalemic metabolic alkalosis** due to the vast loss of hydrogen ions in the vomitus. The potassium loss also worsens from **aldosterone** release in response to hypovolemia. Aldosterone increases urinary excretion of potassium.

Olive sign, which delineates a palpable mass the size of an olive felt in the epigastric region, is highly associated with this condition.

▶**TIP**

Olive sign is frequently tested on the USMLE Step 2 CK.

DIAGNOSTIC TESTS

The best initial test is an abdominal ultrasound that will show a thickened pyloric sphincter.

The most accurate test is an upper GI series, which will show 4 signs:

1. String sign: **thin column** of barium leaking through the tightened muscle
2. Shoulder sign: filling defect in the antrum due to prolapse of muscle inward
3. Mushroom sign: **hypertrophic pylorus** against the duodenum
4. Railroad track sign: **excess mucosa** in the pyloric lumen resulting in 2 columns of barium

TREATMENT

Replace lost volume with IV fluids; replace lost electrolytes, specifically potassium, as the closure of the anion gap is crucial. NGT must be used to decompress the bowel. Surgical myotomy must follow.

Choanal Atresia

In choanal atresia, the infant is born with a membrane between the nostrils and pharyngeal space that prevents breathing during feeding. This condition is associated with CHARGE syndrome.

CHARGE syndrome is a set of congenital defects seen in conjunction.

C: coloboma of the eye, central nervous system anomalies

H: heart defects

A: atresia of the choanae

R: retardation of growth and/or development

G: genital and/or urinary defects (hypogonadism)

E: ear anomalies and/or deafness

PRESENTATION

Child will **turn blue when feeding** and then **pink when crying**. This recurrent series of events is clinically diagnostic.

DIAGNOSTIC TESTS/TREATMENT

Diagnosis is confirmed by **CT scan**.

The only definitive treatment is **surgical intervention** to perforate the membrane and reconnect the pharynx to the nostrils.

Hirschsprung Disease

Hirschsprung disease is a congenital lack of innervation of the distal bowel by the Auerbach plexus. This lack causes a constant contracture of muscle tone. There is frequent association with Down syndrome and it is more common in boys than in girls (approximately 4:1).

PRESENTATION

[handwritten: ⌐ ALSO SEEN IN CF]

- Of unaffected infants, 90% pass first meconium within 24 hours, whereas children with Hirschsprung **do not pass** meconium for over **48** hours or fail to pass meconium at all.
- Extreme constipation is followed by **large bowel obstruction**.
- Rectal exam shows an extremely tight sphincter; an **inability to pass flatus** is also common.

DIAGNOSTIC TESTS/TREATMENT

- Plain x-rays show **distended bowel loops** with a lack of air in the rectum. Contrast enemas will show retention of barium for greater than 24 hours.

- Manometry will show **high pressures** in the anal sphincter.
- The mainstay of diagnosis is a **full thickness biopsy** that reveals a lack of ganglionic cells in the submucosa.

A 3-stage surgery procedure is curative.

Imperforate Anus

With imperforate anus, the **opening** to the **anus** is **missing** and the rectum ends in a blind pouch with conservation of the sphincter. The cause is unknown but has a high association with **Down syndrome**.

Figure 15.3: Imperforate anus is a clinical diagnosis from extreme constipation and lack of anal orifice on physical exam. *Source: Niket Sonpal, MD.*

Imperforate anus is one of the components of VACTERL syndrome.

V: vertebral anomalies

A: anal atresia

C: cardiovascular anomalies

T: tracheoesophageal fistula

E: esophageal atresia

R: renal anomalies

L: limb anomalies

PRESENTATION/DIAGNOSTIC TESTS/TREATMENT

Complete failure to pass meconium is diagnostic. A physical exam will reveal no anus. Surgery is curative.

1-day-old child is given her first feeding, at which time she begins to have very dark green vomiting. On physical examination, the child has oblique eye fissures with epicanthic skin folds and a single palmar crease. A holosystolic murmur is also heard. CXR reveals a double bubble sign.

Which of the following is the most likely diagnosis?

a. Biliary atresia
b. Duodenal atresia
c. Volvulus
d. Intussusception
e. Pyloric stenosis

Answer: The correct answer is (B). The child's bilious vomiting on the first day of life is the prototypic finding in children with this condition. Furthermore, the description of Down syndrome-like characteristics such as eye shape, simian crease, and congenital murmur also points to duodenal atresia. Volvulus and intussusception would present with symptoms of obstruction such as distension and failure to pass flatus and stool, and do not have vomiting as a presenting symptom. Biliary atresia would not have any bilious vomiting, nor would pyloric stenosis. Pyloric stenosis has a projectile vomitus.

Duodenal Atresia

Duodenal atresia (DA) is a **lack or absence of apoptosis** (programmed cell death) that leads to improper canalization of the lumen of the duodenum.

Duodenal atresia is associated with an annular pancreas and Down syndrome.

PRESENTATION/DIAGNOSTIC TESTS

Duodenal atresia is typically characterized by the onset of bilious vomiting within 12 hours of birth.

Chest x-ray will show a classic double bubble sign.

TREATMENT

Replace lost volume with IV fluids, taking special care to replace lost electrolytes. Potassium is often low from vomiting. NGT must be used to decompress the bowel. Surgical duodenostomy is the most common surgical procedure and definitive treatment

Volvulus

A volvulus is a bowel obstruction in which a loop of bowel has twisted on itself abnormally.

In children, volvulus occurs in the midgut, with the majority being in the ileum.

PRESENTATION/DIAGNOSTIC TESTS

The signs are nonspecific and include vomiting and colicky abdominal pain. Multiple air fluid levels can be seen and on upper GI series a "bird beak" appearance is typically seen at the site of rotation.

Figure 15.4: A sign seen during acute episodes of volvulus showing a malrotated segment. *Source: Niket Sonpal, MD.*

TREATMENT

Surgical or endoscopic untwisting is emergently needed; bowel necrosis with perforation can lead to life-threatening sepsis.

The best initial therapy is endoscopic decompression and the most effective therapy (and if the endoscopy fails) is surgical decompression.

A 1-year-old child is having his diaper changed when his father notices the stool looks like a purple jelly. He quickly rushes to the ED and reports that the previous night, the child was very irritable, complained of pain, and had an episode of vomiting. On physical exam the child seems lethargic and a firm sausage-shaped mass is palpated.

Which of the following is the most likely diagnosis?

a. Biliary atresia
b. Duodenal atresia
c. Volvulus
d. Intussusception
e. Pyloric stenosis

*Answer: The correct answer is **(D)**. Intussusception presents with currant jelly stool, sausage-shaped mass, neurologic signs, and abdominal pains. The remaining choices do not fit this description.*

Intussusception

Intussusception is a condition in which part of the bowel telescopes into another segment of bowel distal to it. It can be caused by a polyp, hard stool, or lymphoma, or even have a viral origin. Most often, however, there is no clear etiology.

▶ **TIP**

Currant jelly can be seen with *Klebsiella* pneumonia in the lungs as sputum, or as stool in the setting of intussusception.

PRESENTATION

Intussusception presents with **colicky abdominal pain**, **bilious vomiting**, and **currant jelly stool**. A right quadrant sausage-shaped mass can be palpated.

▶ **TIP**

Currant jelly is a frequently tested item on USMLE Step 2 CK.

DIAGNOSTIC TESTS

Ultrasound is the **best initial test** and will show a doughnut sign or target sign, which is generated by concentric alternating echogenic (mucosa) and hypoechogenic (submucosa) bands.

AIR or Barium enema is **both diagnostic and therapeutic** and therefore the most accurate test. However, it is contraindicated if the child has signs of peritonitis, shock, or perforation.

TREATMENT

Fluid resuscitation and balancing of electrolytes (K^+, Ca^{+2}, Mg^{+2}) are the **most important initial steps** followed by NGT decompression of the bowel.

Barium enema also acts as curative therapy. The child must be carefully observed, as approximately 10% recur within 24 hours.

If barium enema is not curative, then emergent surgical intervention is necessary to prevent bowel necrosis.

Meckel's Diverticulum

Meckel's diverticulum is the only true congenital diverticulum in which the vitelline duct remains and persists in the small intestinal tract. It has been known to contain ectopic gastric tissue.

Rule of 2s

1. Affects 2% of the population
2. Occurs 2 feet from the ileocecal valve
3. Affects 2 types of ectopic tissue (gastric and pancreatic)
4. Male patients 2 times more affected
5. Patient under the age of 2 years
6. Only 2% of patients symptomatic
7. About 2 inches long

PRESENTATION

The classic presentation is with **painless rectal bleeding**. Massive frank bright red blood per rectum is due to gastric acid secretion by the ectopic tissue causing searing of the nearby small bowel tissue.

DIAGNOSTIC TESTS/TREATMENT

The most accurate test for Meckel's diverticulum is a technetium 99m scan. It is so accurate that it has been dubbed a **Meckel scan**. **Surgical removal** of the diverticulum is the only curative therapy.

An 11-month-old girl is brought from daycare to the ED for severe diarrhea and a fever of 103°F. The parents are still not present, but the daycare provider states that the girl has been lethargic, has not been eating, and has had several episodes of diarrhea. The last episode was bloody and contained mucus. Physical exam reveals a child who is listless and drowsy. Her skin shows signs of tenting. Laboratory findings show marked leuokocytosis, elevated BUN and creatinine, and markedly decreased bicarbonate and elevated hematocrit.

Which of the following is the most appropriate next step in management of this patient?

a. CT of the abdomen and pelvis
b. Discharge home
c. Fluid resuscitation
d. Stool ova and parasite (O&P) analysis
e. Empiric antibiotic delivery

*Answer: The correct answer is **(C)**. The child is severely dehydrated as demonstrated by acute renal failure secondary to hypovolemia, skin tenting, and hemoconcentration. The most appropriate next step is aggressive IV fluid rehydration and electrolyte replenishment. At this time, no other test or therapy is important; this child is unstable and could be on the brink of hypovolemeic shock. Radiologic imaging delays the administration of fluids and discharging the child home could result in fatal consequences. Antibiotic coverage is not the most appropriate next step because antibiotics can take 12 to 24 hours to become effective. Antibiotics are needed, but fluids work faster and are needed more urgently at this time.*

Diarrhea and Gastroenteritis

Acute diarrhea—the acute loss of fluids and electrolytes in the stool due to underlying pathologic process—is the **second most common cause of infant death worldwide**. Gastroenteritis is the inflammation of the GI tract secondary to microbiologic infiltrate and spread.

PRESENTATION

- Inflammatory diarrhea will have fever, abdominal pain, and possible bloody diarrhea.
- Noninflammatory diarrhea will have vomiting, crampy abdominal pain, and watery diarrhea.

DIAGNOSTIC TESTS

- Send stool for blood and leukocyte count to detect the presence of invasive toxins.
- Stool cultures with O&P for identifying the causative agent
- Possible sigmoidoscopy to examine for pseudomembranes in the setting of *C. difficile*

TREATMENT

The most important next step is rehydration.

- **Mild** cases: **oral** fluids
- **Severe** cases: **IV** fluids

▶ TIP

Antidiarrheal compounds such as **loperamide** are always the **wrong** answer.

Necrotizing Enterocolitis

Necrotizing enterocolitis (NE) is a condition seen in premature infants where the bowel undergoes necrosis and bacteria invade the intestinal wall. The condition carries a mortality of up to 30%.

PRESENTATION

- Child born severely premature with low birth weight
- Vomiting and abdominal distension
- Fever

DIAGNOSTIC TESTS

- **Abdominal x-ray** will reveal the pathognomonic "**pneumatosis intestinalis**" or air within the bowel wall and CT will reveal air in the portal vein, dilated bowel loops, and pneumoperitoneum if a perforation has occurred.
- **Frank** or **occult blood** can be seen in stool.

→ MECONIUM PLUGS → LOWER COLON OBSTRUCTION

↳ IODM | HIRSCHSPRUNG | CF | MAT DRUG USE

→ MECONIUM ILEUS → ILEUS OBSTRUCTION

↳ CF

AB X-RAY

FOR ILEUS → GASTROGRAFIN ENEMA

Figure 15.5: Due to the necrosis of bowel, gas is seen building up in the intestinal wall. *Source: Niket Sonpal, MD.*

TREATMENT

1. Feeding must be discontinued for bowel rest.
2. **IV fluids** must be started immediately.
3. NGT must be placed for bowel decompression.
4. If medical management does not lead to resolution, then **surgery** is indicated to remove the affected bowel.

ENDOCRINOLOGY

Infants of Diabetic Mothers (IDM)

A 10.5-pound infant is born to a mother with Type I diabetes. Upon examination of the newborn, he is shaking and a holosystolic murmur is heard over the precordium. The baby's right arm is adducted and internally rotated. His lab findings show elevated bilirubin.

Which of the following is the most appropriate next step in management?

a. IV insulin
b. Blood sugar level
c. Serum calcium levels
d. Serums TSH
e. CT head and neck

*Answer: The correct answer is (B). Infants of diabetic mothers (IDMs) are born macrosomic, with plethora, and can be very jittery. The newborn usually has dramatically high circulating levels of glucose, but upon delivery, maternal glucose is no longer available. This child is still producing high levels of insulin, and thus his blood sugar levels have dropped. Cardiac anomalies are common, as in this child, who most likely has a VSD. When we think of diabetes, our first thought is insulin treatment. This is the most common **wrong** answer, since it would further exacerbate these newborns' problems.*

Findings in IDM

Macrosomia

With macrosomia, all organs are enlarged except for the brain. An increased output from the bone marrow leads to polycythemia and hyperviscosity. Possible shoulder dystocia and brachial plexus palsy can also be in the history.

Small Left Colon Syndrome

A congenitally smaller descending colon leads to distension from constipation. It can be diagnosed by a barium study and treated with smaller and more frequent feeds.

Cardiac Abnormalities

The major cardiac change in IDM is asymmetric septal hypertrophy due to obliteration of the left ventricular lumen, leading to decreased cardiac output. It is diagnosed with EKG and echocardiography and treated with beta blockers and IV fluids.

Renal Vein Thrombosis

- Flank mass and possible bruit can be appreciated
- Hematuria and thrombocytopenia

Metabolic Findings and Effects

- Hypoglycemia: seizures
- Hypocalcemia: tetany, lethargy
- Hypomagnesemia: hypocalcaemia and PTH decrease
- Hyperbilirubinemia: icterus and kernicterus

> In congenital adrenal hyperplasia, 90% or more of cases are due to 21-hydroxylase deficiency.

Congenital Adrenal Hyperplasia (CAH)

CAH is an inherited defect of steroid synthesis that has 3 forms:

1. 21-hydroxylase
2. 17 hydroxylase
3. 11-beta-hydroxylase

PRESENTATION

- The most common presentation is a hypotensive child with severe electrolyte abnormalities.
- Genitalia are ambiguous in girls; boys do not initially exhibit any abnormalities, but begin to lose their defining sexual features as they age. Inappropriate facial hair, virilization, and menstrual abnormalities are also seen.
- Hyponatremia, hypochloremia, hypoglycemia, and hyperkalemia are seen as a result of decreased aldosterone and cortisol production. This also results in acidosis due to hydrogen ion retention.

DIAGNOSTIC TESTS

CAH is diagnosed at birth by serum electrolytes and increased 17-OH progesterone levels.

TREATMENT

- Fluid and electrolyte replacement along with lifelong steroids to maintain adequate levels of mineralo/glucocorticoid levels
- Specific psychiatric counseling to aid with gender identity issues

A 2-year-old girl who has grown up in England is brought in for a routine visit. The parents seem anxious and state that they are worried because their daughter appears to walk abnormally and falls a great deal when she tries to play with her older brother. The child's delivery was unremarkable, and physical exam reveals a very unsteady gait and bowing of the tibia. The parents state that the child does not like milk and withdrew from both breastfeeding and cow's milk quite early on. X-ray reveals a beading of the ribs and genu varum.

What is the most likely diagnosis?

a. Rickets
b. Kartagener syndrome
c. Coarctation of the aorta
d. Traumatic fracture
e. Cerebellar injury

*Answer: The correct answer is **(A)**. Vitamin D-deficient rickets is a disorder due to a lack of vitamin D and calcium. This child's risk factors include living in a sunless environment and low milk intake. The child displays classic signs including a "rachitic rosary" of the ribs on CXR and bowing of tibia. Kartagener syndrome is characterized by infertility and situs inversus. Coarctation has rib notching on the CXR; traumatic injury would show a clearer break of the tibia; and cerebellar injury would present with ataxia rather than simply an unsteady gait.*

Rickets

Rickets is a disorder caused by a lack of vitamin D, calcium, or phosphate. It leads to softening and weakening of the bones, making them more susceptible to fractures.

Children 6 to 24 months are at highest risk because their bones are rapidly growing.

There are 3 main etiologies of rickets:

1. Vitamin D-**deficient** rickets caused by a **lack of enough vitamin D** in the child's diet.
2. Vitamin D-**dependent** rickets is the **inability to convert** 25-OH to $1,25(OH)_2$ and therefore the infant is dependent on vitamin D supplementation.
3. X-linked **hypophosphatemic** rickets occurs when an innate kidney defect results in the **inability to retain phosphate**. Without phosphate, adequate bone mineralization cannot take place and bones are weakened.

PRESENTATION

Child will present with ulnar/radial bowing and a waddling gait due to tibial/femoral bowing.

Figure 15.6: Bowlegs are a common physical finding in deficient rickets. *Source: Niket Sonpal, MD.*

DIAGNOSTIC TESTS

- **Rachitic rosary**-like appearance on CXR of the costochondral joints with cupping and fraying of the epiphyses
- Bowlegs is a characteristic sign.

TREATMENT

Replacement of phosphate, calcium, and vitamin D in the form of ergocalciferol or 1,25(OH)$_2$, calcitrol and annual blood vitamin D monitoring.

The American Academy of Pediatrics recommends that infants who are exclusively breastfed be given vitamin D supplements beginning at 2 months of age.

Chemical Consequences of Vitamin D Disorders				
Type	Calcium	Phosphate	1,25(OH)$_2$ Vit. D	25(OH) Vit. D
Vitamin D-deficient	Normal or decreased	Decreased	Decreased	Decreased
Vitamin D-dependent	Decreased	Normal	Decreased	Normal
X-linked hypophosphatemia	Normal	Decreased	Normal	Normal

INFECTIOUS DISEASE

A 6-month-old infant is brought in by his mother after what she describes as a seizure. The mother says the child has had a fever of 103°F for the last 3 days and has been very irritable lately. The child appears unresponsive but is breathing. Physical examination reveals a markedly delayed capillary refill and a blood pressure of 80/20.

What is the most likely diagnosis?

a. Febrile seizure
b. Absence seizure
c. Dog bite
d. Cocaine withdrawal
e. Epilepsy

Answer: The correct answer is (A): febrile seizure secondary to sepsis. The real take-home message with this case is to evaluate the child for the underlying cause of the sepsis. Understanding he has had a febrile seizure is only the surface of the case. A full sepsis evaluation must be ordered, which includes **CBC with differential blood** *and* **urine cultures, urinalysis, chest x-ray,** *and* **lumbar puncture** *(if irritability or lethargy is mentioned = meningitis). Dog bites do not present with seizures. Cocaine withdrawal does not have seizures.*

Neonatal Sepsis

Sepsis	
Most common causes	Pneumonia #(Meningitis
Most common organisms	Group B strep E. coli S. aureus Listeria monocytogenes
Diagnostic tests	Blood cultures and urine cultures Chest x-ray
Treatment	Ampicillin and gentamicin

↳ IF SUSPECT MENINGITIS → AMP & CEFTA2

T: toxoplasmosis

O: other infections such as *Syphilis*

R: rubella

C: cytomegalovirus

H: herpes simplex virus

ORBITAL CELLULITIS VS PRESEPTAL   *ORBITAL = (+) OPHTHALMOPLEGIA*
                                                   (+) VISION CHANGE   *> NOT FOUND*
                                                   (+) PROPTOSIS   *IN PRESEPTAL*

TORCH Infections

Type	Presentation	Diagnostic tests	Treatment
Toxoplasmosis	Chorioretinitis, hydrocephalus, and multiple ring-enhancing lesions on CT caused by *Toxoplasma gondii*	Best initial test is elevated IgM to toxoplasma; most accurate test is PCR for toxoplasmosis.	Pyrimethamine and sulfadiazine
Syphilis	Rash on the palms and soles, snuffles, frontal bossing, Hutchinson eighth nerve palsy, and saddle nose	Best initial test is VDRL or RPR; most accurate test is FTA ABS or dark field microscopy.	Penicillin
Rubella	PDA, cataracts, deafness, ~~TRIAD~~ hepatosplenomegaly, thrombocytopenia, blueberry muffin rash, and hyperbilirubinemia	Maternal IgM status along with clinical diagnosis. Each disease manifestation must be individually addressed.	Supportive
CMV	Periventricular calcifications with microencephaly, chorioretinitis, hearing loss, and petechiae	Best initial test is urine or saliva viral titers; most accurate test is urine or saliva PCR for viral DNA.	Ganciclovir with signs of end organ damage
Herpes	Week 1: shock and DIC Week 2: vesicular skin lesions Week 3: encephalitis	Best initial test is Tzanck smear; most accurate test is PCR.	Acyclovir and supportive care

(handwritten notes:) SCARLET FEVER (STREP PYOGENES) — SANDPAPER RASH → TRUNK → SPREAD / STRAWBERRY TONGUE / RAPID STREP — TENDER
COXSACKIE — ORAL VESICLES | HANDS | FEET — CLINICAL — SUPPORTIVE

Viral Childhood Illnesses

Virus	Etiology	Presentation	Diagnostic tests	Treatment
Varicella	Varicella zoster virus	Multiple highly pruritic vesicular rash that begins on the face; possible fever and malaise	Best initial test is Tzanck smear showing multinucleated giant cells; most accurate test is viral culture	Supportive treatment with topical ointments
Rubeola or measles	Paramyxovirus	The 3 C's: cough, coryza, and conjunctivitis with a Koplik spot (grayish macule on buccal surface)	Clinical diagnosis; most accurate is measles IgM antibodies	Supportive treatment *(handwritten: VITAMIN A ??)*
Fifth disease or erythema infectiosum	Parvovirus B19	Starts with fever and URI and progresses to rash with "slapped cheek" appearance	Clinical diagnosis	Supportive
Roseola	Herpesvirus types 6 and 7	Fever and URI progressing to diffuse rash *(handwritten: FEVER THEN RASH)*	Clinical diagnosis	Supportive
Mumps	Paramyxovirus	Fever precedes classic parotid gland swelling with possible orchitis.	Clinical diagnosis	Supportive

(handwritten right margin:) MOST PROB → LIKELY CAUSE FE SEIZURE

(handwritten bottom notes:) RUBELLA | LYMPHADENOPATHY RASH — SUBOCCIPUT / POST CERV — RASH STARTS AT FACE! — DOES NOT DARKEN — POLY ARTHRITIS

[handwritten notes at top:]
ACUTE BILATERAL LYMPHADENITIS — VIRUSES / STREP / ~~nut~~ / CMV
ACUTE UNILATERAL — STAPH / GROUP A / GBS
CHRONIC unilateral — BARTONELLA / TOXO / TB
→ KAWASAKI / HODGKINS LYMPHOMA

PULMONARY DISEASE

[handwritten:] → X-RAY (ABG / CULTURES)
→ O₂ (CPAP / ABx)

[handwritten right margin:]
A
B RONCHIOLITIS
C ROUP
D
E PIGLOTTITIS
F OREIGN BODIES

A 2-year-old child is brought in by her daycare provider for a severe cough, fever, and runny nose. The child's cough sounds like a bark and she is in obvious respiratory distress. Upon physical examination, the child refuses to lie flat. CXR shows a positive steeple sign.

What is the most appropriate next step in management?

a. Intubate
b. Racemic epinephrine
c. Empiric antibiotics
d. Acetaminophen
e. CT neck

Answer: The correct answer is (B). This child presents with classic signs of croup, an inflammation that is quite literally choking off the child's upper airway. The seallike barking cough with URI-like symptoms gives it away. This is a medical emergency. To prevent asphyxiation and probable tracheostomy, you must administer racemic epinephrine to decrease swelling and monitor the child. Do not waste time with radiology. There is no medical evidence suggesting that intubation, antibiotics, or antipyretics decrease mortality.

Croup

Croup is an infectious upper airway condition characterized by severe inflammation. It is most commonly caused by parainfluenza virus types 1 and 2. Respiratory syncytial virus (RSV) is the second most common cause.

PRESENTATION

Classic triad of:

- **Barking cough**
- **Coryza**
- **Inspiratory stridor**

The child will have more difficulty breathing when lying down and may show signs of **hypoxia** such as peripheral cyanosis and accessory muscle use.

Chest x-ray will show the classic **steeple sign**, a **narrowing** of the air column in the **trachea**. However, x-ray is rarely done and is always the wrong answer to the most appropriate next step.

DIAGNOSTIC TESTS/TREATMENT

The diagnosis is made clinically and can be aided by radiology if the symptoms are mild. Hypoxia aids in differentiating croup from epiglottitis. For mild symptoms, give steroids. For moderate and severe symptoms, give racemic epinephrine.

> Croup = hypoxia on presentation
> Epiglottitis = hypoxia imminent

435

FOREIGN BODIES

- STRIDOR
- No CONSTITUTIONAL Sx

BRONCHIOLITIS

- RSV
- CRACKLES
  - RETRACTIONS
  - GRUNTING

- SUCTIONING NOSE
- ALBUTEROL ??
- RACEMIC EPI ??
- STEROIDS DON'T HELP

A 4-year-old child is brought in by his daycare provider because the child is extremely irritable and refuses to eat. The child refuses to lean back, speaks in muffled words, looks extremely ill, and is drooling. CXR shows a positive thumb-print sign.

What is the most appropriate next step in management?

a. Intubate
b. Racemic epinephrine
c. Empiric antibiotics
d. Physical examination
e. CT neck

*Answer: The correct answer is **(A)**. This child presents with classic signs of epiglottitis, the truest of medical emergencies in pediatrics. Do not waste time with anything else, including a full physical examination, as his airway may close off any minute. In this case, a thumbprint sign is mentioned to aid your studies, but CXR is rarely done with such a convincing presentation. This child must be ushered into the operating room and intubated. Purists even say to avoid startling the child, as it may precipitate closure. The remaining choices are not indicated until airway management is conducted. Remember your ABCs.*

Epiglottitis

Epiglottitis is a severe, life-threatening swelling of the epiglottis and arytenoids due to haemophilus influenza type B.

PRESENTATION

Look for a child with a history of vaccination delinquency with:

- **"Hot potato" voice**
- **Fever**
- **Drooling in the tripod position**
- **Refusal to lie flat**

Physical examination will reveal an extremely hot cherry-red epiglottis.

DIAGNOSTIC TESTS/TREATMENT

Diagnosis is made clinically but x-ray may reveal a classic "thumbprint sign."

To treat:

- **Intubate** the child in the operating room (OR). The OR is the preferred setting in case unsuccessful intubation makes tracheostomy necessary.
- Administer **ceftriaxone** for 7 to 10 days.
- **Rifampin** must be given to all close contacts.

Whooping Cough

Whooping cough is a form of bronchitis caused by *Bordetella pertussis*.

PRESENTATION

- **Catarrhal stage:** severe congestion and rhinorrhea—14 days in duration
- **Paroxysmal stage:** severe coughing episodes with extreme gasp for air (inspiratory whoop) followed by vomiting—14 to 30 days in duration
- **Convalescent stage:** decrease of frequency of coughing—14 days in duration

DIAGNOSTIC TESTS

- Clinically made diagnosis with **whooping inspiration**, vomiting, and burst blood vessels in eyes
- "Butterfly pattern" on chest x-ray
- PCR of nasal secretions or *Bordetella pertussis* toxin ELISA

TREATMENT

- Erythromycin or azithromycin aids only in the catarrhal stage, not in the paroxysmal stage.
- Isolate the child, and macrolides must be given for all close contacts.
- DTaP vaccine has decreased incidence.

Upper and Lower Airway Diseases				
Disease	**Etiology**	**Presentation**	**Diagnosis**	**Treatment**
Bronchitis	Various bacteria and viruses causing inflammation of the airways	Productive cough lasting 7–10 days with fever	Clinical	Supportive
Pharyngitis	Inflammation of the pharynx and adjacent structures caused by group A beta hemolytic strep	Cervical adenopathy, petechiae, fever above 104°F, and other URI symptoms; acute rheumatic fever and glomerulonephritis	Rapid DNAse antigen detection test	Oral penicillin for 10 days or macrolides for penicillin allergy
Diptheria	Membranous inflammation of the pharynx due to bacterial invasion by *Corynebacterium diphtheriae*	Gray highly vascular pseudomembranous plaques on the pharyngeal wall. **Do not scrape.**	Culture of a small portion of superficial membrane	Antitoxin: remember, antibiotics do not work

CLINICAL

CLUBFOOT
(TALIPES EQUINOVARUS)   NEONATE   EQUINUS & VARUS   X-RAY
                                   CALCANEUS & TALUS

IMMEDIATE
STRETCHING / MANIPULATION /
CASTING

Musculoskeletal Diseases

Disease	Age	Presentation	Diagnosis	Treatment
Congenital hip dysplasia	Infants FEMALE 1ST BORN BREECH	Usually found on screening during the first few newborn exams	Ortolani and Barlow maneuver; "click" or (more precisely) "clunk" in the hip is present. → U/S	Pavlik harness WEARING TWO DIAPERS
Legg-Calvé-Perthes disease	Avascular necrosis of the the femoral head; ages 2–8	Presents with painful limp	X-rays show joint effusions and widening	Rest and NSAIDs; follow with surgery on both hips, because if one necroses, then the other will eventually as well. BOTH IF HYPOTHYROID?
Slipped capital femoral epiphysis	Displacement of the femoral epiphysis, commonly found in obese adolescents	Painful limp and externally rotated leg	X-ray shows widening of the joint space ICE CREAM CONE SLIP	Internal fixation with pinning

UTI → NEED VCUG IF → 2 MOS – 2 YEARS OLD
                &
         RENAL → MALE
          U/S
              → FEMALE < 3 YO

      POOR VCUG ←→ MORE THAN 1 UTI OR FEBRILE

REFLUX CAUSES UTI'S ; PYELO → CAUSES SCARRING

SECTION 6
OBSTETRICS AND GYNECOLOGY

TERATOGENS

- COUMADIN
- FLOUROQUINOLONES
- AMINOGLYCOSIDES - DEAFNESS
- DIAZEPAM

- MARIJUANA → SMALLER HEAD???

OBSTETRICS

By Elizabeth V. August, MD

The most common first symptom of pregnancy in women with regular menstruation is amenorrhea. However, in patients who have irregular menses, amenorrhea may be missed. Other symptoms include breast tenderness, nausea, and vomiting. Pregnant women experience a surge in estrogen, progesterone, and beta-human chorionic gonadotropin (beta-HCG) that leads to these symptoms.

A 27-year-old woman presents with nausea and vomiting for the past 2 weeks. Symptoms are worse in the morning, but can occur at any time during the day. She has a decrease in appetite. Her last menstrual period (LMP) was 6 weeks ago. Physical examination is unremarkable.

Which of the following is the best next step in the management of this patient?

a. Complete blood count
b. Beta-HCG
c. HIDA scan
d. Comprehensive metabolic panel
e. Urinanaylsis

Answer: The correct answer is (B). A pregnancy test should be done first in all symptomatic women of childbearing age. Her LMP occurred 6 weeks ago and the patient is experiencing "morning sickness." Morning sickness is caused by an increase in beta-HCG produced by the placenta. This can occur until the 12th to 14th week of pregnancy. A complete blood count (CBC), comprehensive metabolic panel (CMP), and urinalysis are used to evaluate the severity of dehydration, not the etiology. A HIDA scan is done in patients with suspected cholecystitis.

DEFINITIONS

Embryo: fertilization to eight weeks

Fetus: eight weeks to birth

Infant: birth to one year old

DATING METHODS

Developmental age (DA): number of days since fertilization *38 weeks*

Gestational age (GA): number of days/weeks since the last menstrual period (usually 2 weeks longer than DA) *40 weeks*

Nägele rule: estimation of the day of delivery by taking the last menstrual period, subtracting 3 months, and adding 7 days. For example, a woman with an LMP of July 1, 2010 will have an estimated delivery date of April 8, 2011.

> Nägele rule: LMP – 3 months + 7 days = estimated day of delivery

TRIMESTER BREAKDOWN

First trimester: fertilization until 12 weeks (DA) or 14 weeks (GA)

Second trimester: 12(DA)/14(GA) weeks until the 24 week (DA) or 26 week (GA)

Third trimester: 24(DA)/26(GA) weeks until delivery

TERM LENGTHS

Pre-viable: fetus born before 24 weeks

Preterm: fetus born between 25 and 37 weeks

Term: fetus born between 37 and 42 weeks

Postterm: fetus born after 42 weeks

GRAVIDITY/PARITY

Gravidity is the number of times a patient has been pregnant. **Parity** is what happens to the pregnancy. This is broken down into 4 numbers:

1. Full-term births
2. Preterm births
3. Abortions (both spontaneous and induced)
4. Living children (if a patient has a multiple gestation pregnancy, one birth results in 2 living children)

For example, a 35-year-old woman presents to the office for her sixth pregnancy. She has had 2 abortions, 2 children born at term, and a set of twins born preterm. This patient's gravidity and parity are: $G_6 P_{2124}$.

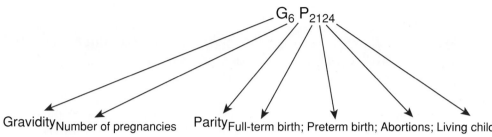

G = Gravidity, or the number of pregnancies (in this example, G = 6).
P = Parity, which is made up of four numbers:

- the number of full-term births (eg, 2)
- the number of preterm births (eg, 1)
- the number of abortions (eg, 2)
- the number of living children (eg, 4)

Figure 16.1: Explanation of Gravidity/Parity

▶ **TIP**

Full-term birth (F); Preterm birth (P); Abortions (A); Living Children (L) = F-PAL

SIGNS OF PREGNANCY

A 20-year-old woman presents to the office because she believes that she is pregnant. Her sexual partner usually pulls out, but did not do so 2 weeks ago. She is now 4 weeks late for her menstruation.

Which of the following is one of the first signs of pregnancy found on physical exam?

a. Quickening
b. Goodell sign
c. Ladin sign
d. Linea nigra
e. Chloasma

Answer: The correct answer is (B). One of the first signs of pregnancy that is seen on physical exam is the Goodell sign, softening of the cervix that is felt first at 4 weeks. Quickening is the first time the mother feels fetal movement.

Signs of Pregnancy		
Sign	**Physical finding**	**Time from conception**
Goodell sign	Softening of the cervix	4 weeks (first trimester)
Ladin sign	Softening of the midline of the uterus	6 weeks (first trimester)
Chadwick sign	Blue discoloration of vagina and cervix	6–8 weeks (first trimester)
Telangiectasias/ palmar erythema	Small blood vessels/reddening of the palms	First trimester
Chloasma	The "mask of pregnancy" is a hyperpigmentation of the face most commonly on forehead, nose, and cheeks; it can worsen with sun exposure.	16 weeks (second trimester)
Linea nigra	A line of hyperpigmentation that can extend from xiphoid process to pubic symphysis	Second trimester

DIAGNOSTIC EVALUATION

> The best initial test when suspecting pregnancy is a beta-HCG.

Both urine and serum testing are based on the beta-HCG, which is produced by the placenta. Beta-HCG is produced rapidly in the first trimester, doubling every 48 hours for the first 4 weeks. At 10 weeks of gestation, the beta-HCG peaks, and levels will typically drop in the second trimester. In the third trimester, the levels will increase slowly again to a level of 20,000 to 30,000 IU/mL. Beta-HCG tests are all highly sensitive. **Ultrasound is used to confirm an intrauterine pregnancy.** At 5 weeks or a beta-HCG of 1000 to 1500 IU/mL, a gestational sac should be seen on ultrasound.

PHYSIOLOGIC CHANGES IN PREGNANCY

> Beta-HCG of 1000 to 1500 or 5 weeks = gestational sac on ultrasound

There are many physiologic changes in pregnancy; however, only a few are tested.

Cardiology

- Increase in cardiac output (results in increased heart rate) 40% ↑   ↑HR
- Slightly lower blood pressure (lowest point occurs at 24 to 28 weeks)

SYSTOLIC MURMUR

↓ PCO_2

Gastrointestinal

- **Morning sickness:** Nausea and vomiting occur anytime throughout the day and are **caused by an increase in estrogen**, **progesterone**, and HCG made by the placenta.
- Gastroesophageal reflux: Lower esophageal sphincter has decreased tone.
- **Constipation:** Motility in the large intestine is decreased.

Handwritten margin note:

NORMAL PREG LABS
↑ ESR
↑ T4 & TBG (NML FREE T4)
↑ Hgb } ↑ VOLUME = ↓ Hct
↓ BUN/CREAT B/C OF ↑ GFR
↑ ALK PHOS

Renal

- Increase in the size of kidney and ureters increases the risk of pyelonephritis from compression of the ureters by the uterus. *(handwritten: ⓇR > ⓁL)*
- **Increase in GFR** (secondary to a 50% increase in plasma volume)
  - Decrease in BUN/creatinine

Hematology

- **Anemia** from an increase in plasma volume by 50% *(handwritten: WITHOUT ↑ RED CELLS → TREAT IF < 11 g/dL)*
- **Hypercoagulable state**
  - No increase in PT, PTT, or INR
  - Increase in fibrinogen
  - Virchow triad elements occur *(handwritten: → STASIS, HYPERCOAG, ENDOTHELIAL INJURY)*
    - Venous stasis

PRENATAL CARE

First Trimester

In the first trimester, patients should be seen every 4 to 6 weeks. Between 11 and 14 weeks, ultrasound can be done to confirm gestational age and check for nuchal translucency. Fetal heart sounds can be heard at the end of the first trimester.

> A thickened or enlarged nuchal translucency is an indication of Down syndrome.

A 17-year-old woman presents for a routine prenatal checkup at 12 weeks.

Which of the following is the most accurate method to establish gestational age?

a. Ultrasound
b. Beta-HCG
c. Pelvic exam
d. Fundal height
e. LMP

↑ AFP → SPINAL DEFECTS
      → DATING ERROR
      → AB WALL DEFECT (GASTROSCHISIS)

↓ AFP → DOWN SYNDROME

*Answer: The correct answer is (A). Ultrasound is the most accurate way of establishing gestational age at 11 to 14 weeks. Beta-HCG is unreliable in confirming dates, as the levels can be increased in twins or decreased in early abortions. Pelvic exam and fundal height are **not** the most accurate methods to confirm dates because they may change with multiple gestations. **A patient's account of LMP is often unreliable** because histories are inaccurately remembered.*

Second Trimester

Visits in the second trimester are used to screen for genetic and congenital problems. At 15 to 20 weeks, perform a "triple" or a "quad."

A triple screen includes maternal serum alpha fetoprotein (MSAFP), beta-HCG, and estriol. The quad screen **adds inhibin A** to the triple screen.

An increase in MSAFP may indicate a dating error, neural tube defect, or abdominal wall defect. The addition of beta-HCG, estriol, and inhibin A helps increase the sensitivity of the MSAFP test. The following are also done in the second trimester:

- Auscultation of fetal heart rate
- 16 to 20 weeks: quickening (feeling fetal movement for the first time)
  - Multiparous women feel the quickening earlier than primiparous women.
- 18 to 20 weeks: routine ultrasound for fetal malformation

> Triple screen: maternal serum alpha fetoprotein, beta-HCG, estriol
> Quad screen: maternal serum alpha fetoprotein, beta-HCG, estriol, **and inhibin A**
> Triple or quad screen is done at a visit at 15 to 20 weeks.

Third Trimester

In the third trimester, visits are every 2 to 3 weeks until 36 weeks. **After 36 weeks, there is a visit every week.**

Braxton-Hicks Contractions

Braxton-Hicks contractions occur during the third trimester. They are sporadic and do not cause cervical dilation. If they become regular, the cervix should be checked to rule out preterm labor before 37 weeks. Preterm labor opens the cervix, but Braxton-Hicks do not. Beginning at 37 weeks, the cervix should be examined at every visit.

> Continued Braxton-Hicks contractions means you should **check the cervix.**

Third Trimester Testing		
Week	**Test**	**Action**
27	Complete blood count	If hemoglobin <11, replace iron orally
26–28	Glucose **load**	If glucose >140 at one hour, perform **oral glucose tolerance test** 3 HOUR
36	Cervical cultures for *Chlamydia* and gonorrhea	Treatment if positive
	Rectovaginal culture for group B *Streptococcus*	Prophylactic antibiotics during labor

10-12 WEEKS DATING   *15 WEEKS TRIPLE SCREEN*   *20 WEEKS ANATOMY*

▶ **TIP**

Glucose **load** test: fasting or nonfasting ingestion of **50 g** of glucose, and serum glucose check **1 hour** later.

Glucose **tolerance** test: fasting serum glucose, ingestion of **100 g** of glucose, serum glucose checks at **1, 2, and 3 hours.** Elevated glucose during any two of these tests is gestational diabetes.

> Don't forget to give stool softeners with the iron supplements, as the iron will increase constipation.

Other Screening Tests

Chorionic Villus Sampling   *BEFORE 15 WEEKS   1 in 150 Loss*

- Done at 9 to 12 weeks **in advanced maternal age** or known genetic disease in parent
- Obtains fetal karyotype
- Catheter into intrauterine cavity to aspirate chorionic villi from placenta (can be done transabdominally or transvaginally)

Amniocentesis   *AFTER 15 WEEKS   1 in 200 Loss*

- Done after 15 weeks for advanced maternal age or known genetic disease in parent

ALSO USED TO CHECK L:S RATIO FOR LUNG MATURITY

- Obtains fetal karyotype (advanced maternal age) | *AFP*
- Needle transabdominally into the amniotic sac and withdraw amniotic fluid

Fetal Blood Sampling   *1 in 30 Loss*

- Percutaneous umbilical blood sample
- Done in patients with Rh isoimmunization and when a fetal CBC is needed
- Needle transabdominally into the uterus to get blood from the umbilical cord

COMPLICATIONS IN EARLY PREGNANCY

A 29-year-old woman with a past medical history of chlamydia presents with left lower quadrant abdominal pain for the past eight hours. She also states that she has some abnormal vaginal bleeding. Her LMP was 6 weeks ago. On physical exam the patient's temperature is 99°F, heart rate is 100 bpm, blood pressure is 130/80 mm Hg, and respiratory rate is 13 per minute.

Which of the following is the most likely diagnosis?

a. Ectopic pregnancy
b. Menstrual cramps
c. Diverticulitis
d. Ovarian torsion
e. Ovarian cyst

Answer: The correct answer is (A). See the following section on ectopic pregnancy. Diverticulitis causes left lower quadrant abdominal pain and rectal bleeding, not vaginal bleeding. The age range of the patients has almost no overlap between ectopic pregnancy and diverticulitis. Ovarian torsion and ovarian cysts do not cause vaginal bleeding. Menstrual cramps are not associated with an altered menstrual pattern.

Ectopic Pregnancy

Ectopic pregnancy is a pregnancy that implants in an area outside the uterus. This most commonly occurs in the ampulla of the fallopian tube.

Risk Factors

- Pelvic inflammatory disease (**PID**)
- Intrauterine devices (**IUD**)
- Previous ectopic pregnancies (strongest risk factor)

PRESENTATION

- Unilateral lower abdominal or **pelvic pain**
- Vaginal **bleeding**
- If **ruptured**, can be **hypotensive** with peritoneal irritation

DIAGNOSTIC TESTS

- **Beta-HCG:** done to confirm the presence of a pregnancy *NOT RISING ENOUGH*
- **Ultrasound:** to locate the site of implantation of the ectopic pregnancy *1500 IN UTERUS*
- **Laparoscopy:** invasive test and treatment to visualize the ectopic pregnancy

TREATMENT

Unstable patients (low BP, high HR) should be given fluids and sent to surgery immediately.

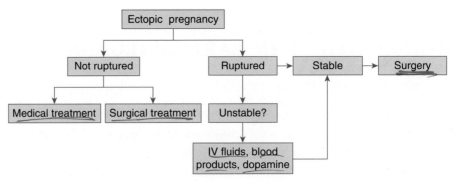

Figure 16.2: Ectopic Pregnancy Algorithm

Medical treatment should begin with baseline exams such as:

- CBC to monitor for anemia
- Transaminases to detect changes indicating hepatotoxicity from the medications (eg, methotrexate)
- Beta-HCG to assess for success of treatment via a decrease in beta-HCG

After these are obtained, methotrexate, a folate receptor antagonist, may be given. The patient's beta-HCG is followed to see if there is a 15% decrease in 4 to 7 days. If there is no decrease in the beta-HCG, a second dose of methotrexate may be given. If the patient's beta-HCG is still not decreasing after the second dose, surgery should be done.

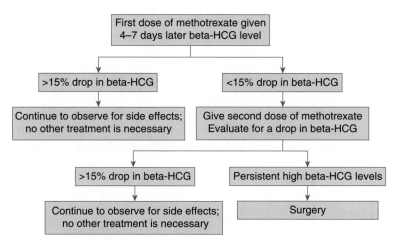

Figure 16.3: Ectopic Pregnancy Treatment Algorithm

★ *Exclusion Criteria for Methotrexate*

- Patients who have **completed their families.**
- **Immunodeficiency:** Avoid methotrexate, which is an immunosuppressive drug.
- **Noncompliant** patients: Who knows if they will follow up? Patients need to return for evaluation to know if the treatment worked and if they need a second dose or surgery.
- Liver disease: **Hepatotoxicity** is a serious side effect of methotrexate. Baseline liver disease increases the risk of subsequent toxicity.
- **Ectopic is 3.5 cm or larger:** The larger the ectopic, the greater the risk of treatment failure with methotrexate.
- Fetal heartbeat auscultated: A pregnancy developed enough to have a heartbeat detectable by auscultation has an increased risk of failure with methotrexate.

Surgery is done to try and preserve the fallopian tube **by cutting a hole in it via salpingostomy.** However, **removal of the whole fallopian tube via**

-ostomy = cut
-ectomy = removal

salpingectomy may be necessary. Mothers who are Rh negative should receive anti-D Rh immunoglobulin (RhoGAM) so that subsequent pregnancies will not be affected by hemolytic disease.

Abortion

A 20-year-old woman presents to the emergency department for vaginal bleeding and lower abdominal pain for one day. She states that she is 15 weeks pregnant. Vital signs include temperature 99.0°F, heart rate 100 bpm, blood pressure 110/75 mm Hg, and respiratory rate 12 per minute. On pelvic exam, there is blood present in the vault. Ultrasound shows intrauterine bleeding, products of conception, and a dilated cervix.

Which of the following is the most likely diagnosis in this patient?

a. Complete abortion
b. Incomplete abortion
c. Inevitable abortion
d. Threatened abortion
e. Septic abortion

*Answer: The correct answer is (**C**). An inevitable abortion is characterized by intrauterine bleeding with a dilated cervix. (See table "Types of Abortions" for explanation of other answer choices.)*

DEFINITION

Abortion is defined as a pregnancy that ends before 20 weeks gestation. Almost 80% of spontaneous abortions occur prior to 12 weeks gestation.

ETIOLOGY

Chromosomal abnormalities in the fetus account for 60% to 80% of spontaneous abortions. However, maternal factors that increase risk of abortion include:

- Anatomic abnormalities
- Infections (STDs)
- Immunological factors (Rh isoimmunization)
- Endocrinological factors (uncontrolled hyperthyroidism or diabetes)
- Malnutrition
- Trauma

PRESENTATION

- Cramping abdominal **pain**
- Vaginal **bleeding**
- May be stable or unstable, depending on the amount of blood loss

DIAGNOSTIC TESTS

- **CBC** to evaluate blood loss and need for transfusion
- **Blood type** and Rh screen: should blood need to be transfused, and evaluation of need for anti-D Rh immunoglobulin
- **Ultrasound** to distinguish between the types of abortions

> You cannot answer the "most likely diagnosis" question about abortion without an ultrasound.

	Types of Abortions	
Type of abortion	**Ultrasound finding/ answer to "most likely diagnosis" question**	**Treatment**
Complete abortion	No products of conception found	Follow up in office
Incomplete abortion	Some products of conception found	Dilation and curettage (D&C)
Inevitable abortion	Products of conception intact, but intrauterine bleeding present and dilation of cervix	D&C
Threatened abortion	Products of conception intact, intrauterine bleeding, **no** dilation of cervix	Bed rest, pelvic rest
Missed abortion	Death of fetus, but all products of conception present in the uterus	D&C
Septic abortion	Infection of the uterus and the surrounding areas	D&C and IV antibiotics, such as levofloxacin and metronidazole

▶ **TIP**

Mothers who are Rh negative should also receive anti-D Rh immunoglobulin at this time.

> Fertility drugs increase multiple gestations.

Multiple Gestations

PRESENTATION

- Exponential growth of uterus
- Rapid weight gain by mother
- Elevated beta-HCG and MSAFP (levels higher than expected for estimated gestational age is the first clue to multiple gestation)

ANY MONO = IDENTICAL TWINS

MONOZYGOTIC TIMING OF SPLIT

0-3 DAYS → DICHORIO DIAMNIO

4-8 DAYS → MONO CHORIO DIAMNIO

9-12 DAYS → MONO CHORIO MONO AMNIO

>12 DAYS → CONJOINED

TWIN-TWIN TRANSFUSION w/ MONOCHORIONIC

ORDER OF DIVISION
↓
ZYGOTE
↓
CHORION
↓
AMNION

DIAGNOSTIC TESTS

An ultrasound is done to visualize the fetuses.

Types of Twins		
Types	**Fertilization**	**Characteristics**
Monozygotic	1 egg and 1 sperm that splits	identical twins: same gender, same physical characteristics, same blood type, fingerprints differ
Dizygotic	2 eggs and 2 sperm	fraternal twins: different or same sex; they resemble each other, as any siblings would

Complications

- Spontaneous abortion of one fetus
- Premature labor and delivery
- Placenta previa
- Anemia
- Post partum hemorrhage

LATE PREGNANCY COMPLICATIONS

A 28-year-old woman in her 28th week of pregnancy presents for severe lower back pain. She complains that the pain is cyclical and that it seems to be increasing in intensity. On physical examination, she seems to be in pain. Her temperature is 98.9°F, HR 104 bpm, BP 135/80 mm Hg, RR 15 per minute. On pelvic examination, her cervix is 3 cm dilated.

Which of the following is the most likely diagnosis?

a. Premature rupture of membranes
b. Preterm labor
c. Cervical incompetence
d. Preterm contractions

Answer: The correct answer is (B). Preterm labor is diagnosed when there is a combination of contractions with cervical dilation. A premature rupture of membranes patient would have a history of a "gush of fluid" from the vagina. Patients with cervical incompetence do not have a history of contractions, but there is painless dilation of the cervix. Preterm contractions do not lead to cervical dilation.

Preterm Labor

Risk Factors

- Premature rupture of membranes
- Multiple gestation
- Previous history of preterm labor
- Placental abruption

- Maternal factors
  - Uterine anatomical abnormalities
  - Infections (chorioamnionitis)
  - Preeclampsia
  - Intraabdominal surgery

PRESENTATION

- Contractions (abdominal pain, lower back pain, or pelvic pain)
- Dilation of the cervix
- Occurs between <u>20 and 37</u> weeks

Evaluation

The fetus should be evaluated for weight, gestational age, and the presenting part (cephalic versus breech). Circumstances in which preterm labor should **not** be stopped with tocolytics and delivery should occur are:

- Maternal severe hypertension (preeclampsia/eclampsia) →DELIVER
- Maternal cardiac disease → DELIVER
- Maternal cervical dilation of more than 4 cm → DELIVER
- Maternal hemorrhage (abruptio placenta, DIC) → DELIVER
- Fetal death → DELIVER
- Chorioamnionitis → DELIVER

▶ TIP

When any of these is present, answer delivery.

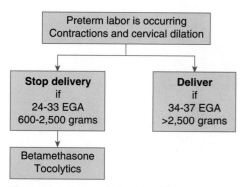

Figure 16.4: Preterm Labor Algorithm

Corticosteroids

Patient should be given betamethasone, a corticosteroid used to mature the fetus' lungs. The effects begin within 24 hours, <u>peak at 48 hours</u>, and persist for 7 days. Corticosteroids decrease the risk of respiratory distress syndrome and neonatal mortality.

> "Mature the fetus' lungs" means increase surfactant.

Magnesium toxicity can lead to respiratory depression and cardiac arrest, so check deep tendon reflexes often.

Tocolytics

When steroids are administered, a tocolytic should follow to allow time for steroids to work. Tocolytics slow the progression of cervical dilation by decreasing uterine contractions.

Magnesium sulfate is the most **commonly used tocolytic**. It decreases uterine tone and contractions. Side effects include flushing, headaches, diplopia, and fatigue.

Calcium channel blockers can also be used as a tocolytic. Side effects include headache, flushing, and dizziness.

▶ TIP

Although indomethacin can be used as a tocolytic, it is **always** the wrong answer in obstetrics. Use it to close a patent ductus arteriosus.

Premature Rupture of Membranes

Premature rupture of membranes presents with a history of a **gush of fluid** from the vagina.

DIAGNOSTIC TEST

Sterile speculum examination should confirm the fluid as amniotic fluid:

- Fluid is present in posterior fornix.
- Fluid turns nitrazine paper blue.
- When placed on slide and allowed to air dry, fluid has ferning pattern.

Figure 16.5: Ferning. *Source: Elizabeth August, MD.*

Premature rupture of the membranes (PROM) can happen at any time throughout pregnancy. It becomes the biggest problem when the fetus is preterm or with **prolonged** rupture of membranes. "**Prolonged**" means that labor starts more than 24 hours before delivery. Premature rupture of membranes leads to:

- Preterm labor
- Cord prolapse

Chorioamnionitis is dangerous.
PROM = do fewer exams = decrease chorioamnionitis.

- Placental abruption
- Chorioamnionitis

TREATMENT

Treatment of PROM depends on the fetus' gestational age and the presence of chorioamnionitis.

Chorioamnionitis = delivery now.

If the fetus is at term and there is no chorioamnionitis, wait 6 to 12 hours for spontaneous delivery. If there is no spontaneous delivery, then induce labor.

Preterm fetuses without chorioamnionitis should be **treated with betamethasone** (to mature the lungs), tocolytics (to decrease contractions), ampicillin, and gentamicin (to decrease risk of developing chorioamnionitis while waiting for steroids to begin working). Erythromycin may be used if the patient is penicillin allergic.

Handwritten margin notes:
PROM → IF NO CHORIO, WAIT 6-12 HRS FOR DELIVERY TO START THEN INDUCE AMP/GENT ???

PPROM → STEROIDS TOCOLYTICS AMP/GENT

"PROLONGED ROM" >18 HRS FROM ROM TO DELIVERY GIVE AMOX FOR GBS

IF CHORIO → ZOSYN

Third-Trimester Bleeding

Placenta Previa

Placenta previa is an **abnormal implantation** of the placenta **over the internal cervical os**. Placenta previa is the cause of about 20% of all prenatal hemorrhages. There is an increased risk of placenta previa with:

- Previous cesarean deliveries
- Previous uterine surgery
- Multiple gestations
- Previous placenta previa

A 24-year-old woman in her 32nd week of pregnancy presents to the emergency department. She states that she woke up in her bed in a pool of blood. She has had no contractions or pain. Her heart rate is 105 bpm and blood pressure is 110/70 mm Hg.

Which of the following is the best next step in the management of this patient?

a. Digital vaginal exam
b. Transabdominal ultrasound
c. Immediate vaginal delivery
d. Immediate cesarean delivery
e. Transvaginal ultrasound

Answer: The correct answer is (B). Transabdominal ultrasound is done before a digital vaginal exam in all third-trimester bleeding. This patient has painless vaginal bleeding, which may be indicative of placenta previa. If a digital vaginal exam is done, it can result in increased separation of the placenta and the uterus, leading to an increase in bleeding. Delivery is premature at this point. Do an ultrasound to distinguish between cesarean and vaginal delivery modes should it become necessary.

Digital vaginal exam is contraindicated in third-trimester vaginal bleeding. It may lead to increased separation between placenta and uterus, resulting in a severe hemorrhage.

PRESENTATION   *PAINLESS*

- Painless vaginal bleeding
- Usually presents after 28 weeks

DIAGNOSTIC TESTS

A transabdominal ultrasound is done to see where the placenta is lying in the uterus. A **transvaginal** ultrasound is **not** done for the same reason that a **digital vaginal exam is not done:** it is dangerous and can separate the placenta further from the uterus.

Types

Ultrasound identifies the different types of placenta previa.

Types of Placenta Previa	
Type	**Description**
Complete	Complete covering of the internal cervical os
Partial	Partial covering of the internal cervical os, but covers more than the marginal
Marginal	Marginal covering of the internal cervical os
Vasa previa	Fetal vessel is present over the cervical os
Low-lying placenta	Placenta that is implanted in the lower segments of the uterus but **not** covering the internal cervical os

Complete   Partial   Marginal   Low lying

Figure 16.6: Types of placenta previa. *Source: Elizabeth August, MD.*

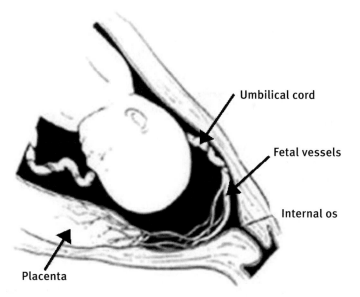

Figure 16.7: Vasa previa. *Source: Elizabeth August, MD.*

TREATMENT

Treatment of placenta previa is done when there is large-volume bleeding or a drop in hematocrit. Treatment consists of **strict pelvic rest**, with nothing put into the vagina (intercourse). There are several indications for immediate cesarean delivery including:

- Unstoppable labor (cervix dilated more than 4 cm)
- Severe hemorrhage
- Fetal distress

Prepare for life-threatening bleeding by type and screen of blood, CBC, and prothrombin time.

Preterm fetuses should also be prepared for delivery with betamethasone to mature the fetus' lungs. Should delivery occur, cesarean birth is the mode of choice.

Placental Invasion (Accreta, Increta, Percreta)

The placenta may also invade into different areas of the uterus (**placenta accreta**), which is associated with placenta previa. This becomes a problem when the placenta must detach from the uterus after the fetus is born. Often placental invasion cannot be seen on prenatal ultrasound, but does result in a significant amount of postpartum hemorrhage. Patients are usually asymptomatic, unless invasion into the bladder or rectum results in hematuria or rectal bleeding.

Placenta accreta: invades into the superficial uterine wall

Placenta increta: invades into the uterine myometrium

Placenta percreta: invades into the uterine serosa, bladder wall, or rectum wall

> Complete: full moon
> Partial: half moon
> Marginal: crescent moon

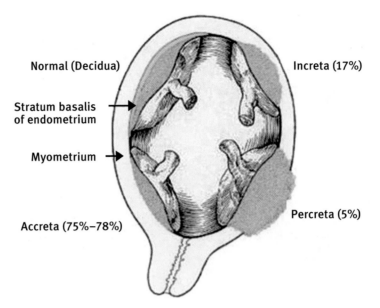

Normal (Decidua)

Stratum basalis
of endometrium

Myometrium

Increta (17%)

Percreta (5%)

Accreta (75%–78%)

Figure 16.8: Types of placental invasion. *Source: Elizabeth August, MD.*

If the placenta cannot detach from the uterine wall after delivery of the fetus, the result is catastrophic hemorrhage and shock. Patients often require hysterectomy.

Placental Abruption

Placental abruption is **premature separation of the placenta** from the uterus. This results in tearing of the placental blood vessels and hemorrhaging into the separated space. This can occur before, during, or after labor. If the separation is large enough and **life-threatening bleeding** occurs, premature delivery, uterine **tetany**, **disseminated intravascular coagulation**, and hypovolemic shock can occur. However, if the degree of separation is small with minor hemorrhage, then there may be no clinical signs or symptoms.

ETIOLOGY

The primary etiology is unknown. However, there are several precipitating factors including:

- Maternal **hypertension** (chronic, preeclampsia, eclampsia)
- Prior placental **abruption**
- Maternal **cocaine use**
- Maternal **external trauma**

PRESENTATION   PAINFUL

- Third-trimester vaginal bleeding
- Severe abdominal pain
- Contractions
- Possible fetal distress

DIAGNOSTIC TEST

Placental abruption can present in a similar fashion to placenta previa. In order to distinguish between the two, a transabdominal ultrasound is done. However, placental abruption still may not be seen on ultrasound.

▶ **TIP**

Placenta previa presents with **painless** vaginal bleeding, while placental abruption presents with **painful** vaginal bleeding.

Types of Placental Abruption		
Type	**Description**	**Complications**
Concealed	• Blood is within uterine cavity • Placenta more likely to be completely detached	Serious complications: • Disseminated intravascular coagulation • Uterine tetany • Fetal hypoxia • Fetal death • Sheehan syndrome (postpartum hypopituitarism)
External	• Blood drains through cervix • Placenta more likely to be partially detached	Usually smaller with minimal complications

TREATMENT

Indications for cesarean delivery are:

• Uncontrollable maternal hemorrhage
• Rapidly expanding concealed hemorrhage
• Fetal distress
• Rapid placental separation

Vaginal deliveries are indicated if:

• Placental separation is limited
• Fetal heart tracing is assuring
• Separation is extensive and fetus is dead

Uterine Rupture

Uterine rupture is life-threatening to both the mother and the fetus and usually occurs during labor.

Life-threatening to mother or baby = immediate delivery

Risk Factors

- Increased risk with previous cesarean deliveries (both types)
  - Classical (longitudinal along uterus): higher risk of uterine rupture
  - Low transverse (more recent use)

> Uterine rupture means there is a hole in the uterus.

Low transverse incision   Classical incision

Low vertical incision

Figure 16.9: Types of cesarean scars. *Source: Elizabeth August, MD.*

- Trauma (most commonly motor vehicle accidents)
- Uterine myomectomy
- Uterine overdistention
  - Polyhydramnios
  - Multiple gestations
- Placenta percreta

PRESENTATION

- Sudden onset of extreme abdominal pain
- Abnormal bump in abdomen
- No uterine contractions
- Regression of fetus: fetus was moving toward delivery, but is no longer in the canal because it withdrew into the abdomen

TREATMENT

Treatment is an **immediate laparotomy** with delivery of the fetus. A cesarean delivery is **not** done, because the **baby may not be in the uterus**, but floating in the abdomen. Repair of the uterus or hysterectomy will follow. If the patient undergoes a repair of the uterus, all subsequent pregnancies will be delivered via cesarean birth at 36 weeks.

> Uterine rupture requires immediate laparotomy and delivery of the fetus.

Rh Incompatibility

Rh incompatibility occurs when the **mother is Rh negative and the baby is Rh positive**. This is generally **not a problem in the first pregnancy**, as the mother has not developed antibodies to the "foreign" Rh positive blood yet. When the first baby is delivered, **fetal red blood cells cross the placenta into the mother's bloodstream**. She makes antibodies against the Rh positive blood. When the mother gets pregnant for the second time, her antibodies attack the second Rh positive baby. This leads to hemolysis of the fetus' red blood cells or hemolytic disease of the newborn.

Hemolytic Disease of Newborn

Hemolytic disease of the newborn results in **fetal anemia** and **extramedullary production of RBCs** because the baby's bone marrow is not able to make enough RBCs, so the liver and spleen help. Hemolysis results in increased heme and bilirubin levels in plasma. **Bilirubin can be neurotoxic**. These effects can lead to erythroblastosis fetalis, characterized by high fetal cardiac output (CHF).

▶ **TIP**

Extramedullary means "outside the bone marrow."

Initial Prenatal Visit

During the initial prenatal visit, an Rh antibody screening test is done. Patients who are Rh negative have an Rh antibody titer done. Patients who are Rh negative but have no antibodies to Rh are "unsensitized." Patients who are Rh negative but have antibodies to Rh are "sensitized."

▶ **TIP**

Antibody screen: done to see if mother is Rh– or Rh+

Antibody titer: done to see how many antibodies to Rh+ blood the mother has

Unsensitized Patients

Unsensitized patients do not yet have antibodies to Rh positive blood. The goal is to keep it that way, so any time that fetal blood cells may cross the placenta, anti-D Rh immunoglobulins (RhoGAM) are given. The following are some scenarios where fetal blood cells may cross into the mother's blood:

- Amniocentesis
- Abortion
- Vaginal bleeding
- Placental abruption
- Delivery

RhoGAM IF:
- 28 weeks & Rh ⊖
- DELIVERY & Rh ⊖
- D & C
- POST PARTUM HEMORRHAGE
- THIRD TRIMESTER BLEED

Prenatal Antibody Screening

Prenatal antibody screening is done at 28 and 35 weeks. Patients who continue to be **unsensitized** at 28 weeks should **receive anti-D Rh immunoglobulin** prophylaxis. At delivery, if the baby is Rh positive, the mother should be given anti-D Rh immunoglobulin again.

> Unsensitized = no anti-Rh antibodies present

Sensitized Patients

Patients who are sensitized already have antibodies to Rh positive blood. On the initial visit, if the patient is Rh negative and has antibodies, an antibody titer needs to be done via the indirect antiglobulin test. The patient is considered sensitized if she has a titer level more than 1:4. If the titer is less than 1:16, no further treatment is necessary. However, if it reaches 1:16 at any point during the pregnancy, serial amniocentesis should be done. Serial amniocentesis allows for evaluation of the fetal bilirubin level.

TRANSCRANIAL DOPPLER TO LOOK AT MCA FLOW IS TEST OF CHOICE TO CHECK FOR ANEMIA

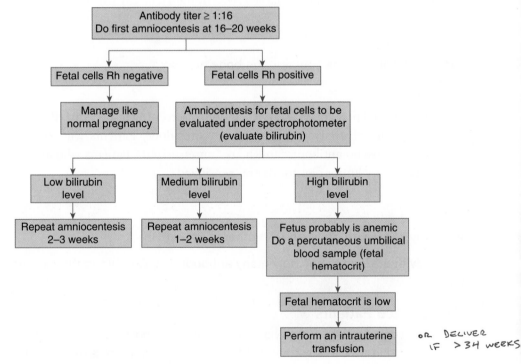

OR DELIVER IF >34 WEEKS

Figure 16.10: Incompatibility Algorithm

A 29-year-old woman G$_2$P$_1$ in her 30th week of pregnancy presents for a routine prenatal visit. She says she has no real complaints except that her wedding ring is getting too tight. On physical exam, her blood pressure is 150/100 mm Hg, heart rate is 92 bpm, respiratory rate is 12, and temperature is 99°F. Urine dipstick done in the office reveals 1+ protein.

Which of the following is the most likely diagnosis?

a. Chronic hypertension
b. Gestational hypertension
c. HELLP syndrome
d. Preeclampsia
e. Eclampsia

Answer: The correct answer is (D). Preeclampsia is characterized by hypertension, edema, and proteinuria. Eclampsia is preeclampsia with seizures. HELLP syndrome is a complication of preeclampsia with elevated liver enzymes and low platelets. Chronic hypertension is increased blood pressure that was present before the patient became pregnant. Gestational hypertension begins during pregnancy but has no edema or proteinuria.

Hypertension

Chronic Hypertension

Chronic hypertension is hypertension defined as a BP above 140/90 **before** the patient became pregnant. It may lead to preeclampsia. Treat the patient with **methyldopa**, **labetalol**, **or nifedipine**.

Gestational Hypertension

Gestational hypertension is defined as a BP above 140/90 mm Hg that **starts after 20 weeks gestation**. There is **no proteinuria and no edema**.

The patient is treated only during pregnancy with methyldopa, labetalol, or nifedipine.

> ACE inhibitors and ARBs cause fetal malformations. Do not use them in pregnancy.

Preeclampsia Risk Factors

- Chronic hypertension
- Renal disease
- Hx of Pre Eclampsia
- 1st Pregnancy
- Fam Hx
- Very Young / very old
- Multiples

> The only definitive treatment in preeclampsia is delivery.

Presentation of Types of Preeclampsia		
	Mild preeclampsia	**Severe preeclampsia**
Hypertension	>140/90	>160/110
Proteinuria	Dipstick 1+ to 2+; 24-hour urine >300 mg	Dipstick 3+; 24-hour urine >5 grams
Edema	Hands, feet, face	Generalized
Mental status changes	No	Yes
Vision changes	No	Yes
Impaired liver function	No	Yes

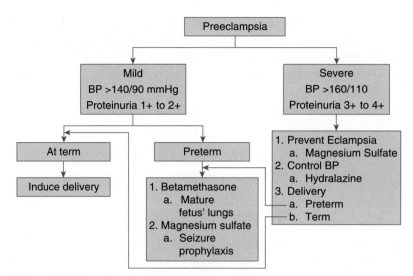

Figure 16.11: Preeclampsia Algorithm

Eclampsia

Eclampsia is defined as a **tonic-clonic seizure** occurring in a patient with a history of preeclampsia.

TREATMENT

First stabilize the mother, then **deliver the baby**. Seizure control should be done with magnesium sulfate and blood pressure control with hydralazine.

HELLP Syndrome

Patients have:

HELLP = **h**emolysis; **e**levated **l**iver enzymes; **l**ow **p**latelets

Treatment is the same as for eclampsia.

Diabetes

A 28-year-old woman in her 27th week of gestation presents for a routine pre-natal visit. She doesn't have any complaints. On physical examination her temperature is 99°F, blood pressure is 120/80 mm Hg, and heart rate is 87 bpm. The patient is asked to ingest 50 mg of glucose and have her blood glucose checked in one hour; it returns as 145 mg/dL.

Which of the following is the best next step in the management of this patient?

a. Treat with insulin

b. Treat with sulfonylurea

c. Do a fasting blood glucose level

d. Perform oral glucose tolerance test

Answer: The correct answer is (D). An oral glucose tolerance test should be done after a positive glucose load test (described in the question). Two fasting blood glucose levels above 126 mg/dL is the diagnostic test for overt diabetes. Treatment with insulin is premature without a diagnosis of gestational diabetes. Sulfonylurea use is contraindicated in pregnant patients.

Pregestational Diabetes

Pregestational diabetes means that a woman had diabetes before she became pregnant. She can be a Type 1 or a Type 2 diabetic.

Complications of Pregestational Diabetes

- Maternal
  - Four times more likely to have preeclampsia
  - Two times more likely to have a spontaneous abortion
  - Increased rate of infection
  - Increased postpartum hemorrhage

- Fetal
  - Increase in congenital anomalies (heart and neural tube defects)
  - Macrosomia
    ○ Shoulder dystocia (fetus' shoulder gets stuck under the symphysis pubis during delivery) is one complication associated with macrosomia.

- Preterm labor

Evaluation

These tests should be done in addition to the usual prenatal tests:

- EKG
- 24-hour urine for baseline renal function
  - Creatinine clearance
  - Protein
- HbA_1C
- Ophthalmological exam for baseline eye function and assessing the condition of the retina

Treatment of Diabetes		
Type of diabetes	**Route of administration**	**Type of insulin**
Type 1	Insulin pump	NPH
Type 2	Subcutaneous insulin	NPH, lispro

> **Do not use** sulfonylureas during pregnancy.

Fetal Testing		
Age	**Test needed**	**Reason**
32–36 weeks	Weekly nonstress test (NST) and ultrasound	NST: fetal well-being Ultrasound: fetal size
>36 weeks	Twice-weekly testing; one NST and one biophysical profile (BPP)	NST: fetal well-being BPP: amount of amniotic fluid and fetal well-being
37 weeks	Lecithin/sphingomyelin ratio (L/S ratio)	L/S ratio: assess fetal lung maturity test (if mature → delivery)
38–39 weeks (if patient refuses L/S ratio)	No test, just induction of labor	N/A

Gestational Diabetes

Complications

- Preterm birth
- **Fetal macrosomia**
- Birth injuries from fetal macrosomia
- Neonatal hypoglycemia: There is an increase in fetal insulin, secondary to living in a hyperglycemic environment. When the fetus leaves the hyperglycemic environment, the excess insulin causes the glucose to drop.
- Mothers with gestational diabetes are 4 to 10 times more likely to develop Type 2 diabetes after the delivery.

Evaluation

Gestational diabetes is routinely screened for between 24 and 28 weeks of gestational age. A glucose **load** test is done first. It consists of nonfasting ingestion of **50 g** of glucose, with a measurement of serum glucose **one hour later**. If the serum glucose is above 140 mg/dL, then a glucose **tolerance** test is done. The glucose tolerance test consists of the ingestion of **100 mg** of glucose after fasting, with **3 measurements** of serum glucose at 1, 2, and 3 hours. If any of the serum glucose measurements are elevated, gestational diabetes is confirmed.

GLUCOSE LOAD TEST

50g GLUCOSE ≥ 140mg/dL
↓
OGTT

100g GLUCOSE @ 1 Hour > 180
2 Hour > 155
3 Hour > 140

FASTING ≥ 125

Figure 16.12: Gestational Diabetes Testing Algorithm

TREATMENT

Diabetic **diet** and **exercise** (walking) are first-line treatments for gestational diabetes. However, if this fails to control blood sugars adequately (fasting greater than 95 mg/dL and one hour postprandial greater than 140 mg/dL), medication is indicated. Treatment with **insulin** should be given with NPH before bed and aspart before meals. Do not give sulfonylureas.

> **▶ TIP**
>
> Do **not** tell pregnant patients to lose weight. It is the most common **wrong** answer. Once patients are put on insulin, they should follow the fetal testing schedule starting at 32 weeks.

FETAL GROWTH ABNORMALITIES

Intrauterine Growth Restriction

Fetuses with intrauterine growth restriction (IUGR) weigh in the bottom 10% for their gestational age.

Types of IUGR	
Type	**Characteristic**
Symmetric	• Brain in proportion with the rest of the body • Occurs before 20 weeks gestation
Asymmetric	• Brain weight is **not** decreased • Abdomen is smaller than the head • Occurs after 20 weeks

ETIOLOGY

- Chromosomal abnormalities
- Neural tube defects
- Infections
- Multiple gestations
- Maternal hypertension or renal disease
  - Maternal malnutrition and maternal substance abuse (smoking is the number-one preventable cause in the United States)

COCAINE
SMOKING
ALCOHOL

DIAGNOSTIC TESTS

Ultrasound is done to confirm the gestational age and fetal weight.

Complications

- Premature labor
- Stillbirth
- Fetal hypoxia
- Lower IQ
- Seizures
- Mental retardation

TREATMENT

There is no conclusive treatment for IUGR other than to try to prevent it:

- Quit smoking.
- Prevent maternal infection with immunizations.

Macrosomia

Fetuses with an estimated birth weight over 4500 g are considered macrosomic babies.

Risk factors

- Maternal diabetes or obesity
- Advanced maternal age
- Postterm pregnancy

DIAGNOSTIC TESTS

On physical exam, normally the fundal height should equal the gestational age in weeks (ie, if the patient is 28 weeks, the fundal height should be 28 cm). In macrosomia, the fundal height will be at least 3 cm greater than the gestational age (ie, the patient is 28 weeks and the fundal height is 31 cm).

If the fundal height is more than 3 cm greater than the gestational age, an ultrasound should be done.

Fundal Height > 3cm GA
↓
U/S

Ultrasound confirms the estimated gestational weight by:

- Femur length
- Abdominal circumference
- Head diameter

Complications
- Shoulder dystocia
- Birth injuries
- Low Apgar scores
- Hypoglycemia

TREATMENT
- Induction of labor should be considered if the lungs are mature **before** the fetus is above 4500 g in weight.
- Cesarean delivery is indicated if fetus is above 4500 g in weight.

FETAL TESTING

Nonstress Test

The NST allows the physician to check for fetal well-being while still in the uterus. NST measures fetal movements and assesses the fetal heart rate. A reactive NST is defined as:

- Detection of two fetal movements
- Acceleration of fetal heart rate greater than 15 bpm lasting 15 to 20 seconds over a 20-minute period

A reactive NST shows the fetus is doing well, and no further testing is indicated. If the nonstress test is **non**reassuring, the fetus could be sleeping. Vibroacoustic stimulation is done to wake up the baby.

Biophysical Profile

Biophysical profile (BPP) consists of:

- NST
- Fetal chest expansions (count episodes of fetal chest expansions; normal is 1 or more episodes in 30 minutes)
- Fetal movement (count fetal movements; normal is more than 3 in 30 minutes)
- Fetal muscle tone (fetus flexes an extremity)
- Amniotic fluid index (volume of amniotic fluid based on sonogram)

Each category is worth 2 points; a BPP of 8 to 10 is normal, 4 to 8 is inconclusive, and below 4 is abnormal.

NORMAL LABOR

Electronic Fetal Monitoring

When a patient presents in labor, an external tocometer is placed on the gravid abdomen to measure the fetal heart rate and uterine contractions.

Fetal Heart Rate

Normal: 110 to 160 beats per minute

Bradycardia: below 110 beats per minute

Tachycardia: above 160 beats per minute

Accelerations

Normal accelerations are an **increase in heart rate of 15 or more** beats per minute above the heart rate baseline for longer than 15 to 20 seconds. If this happens twice in 20 minutes, it is reassuring or normal.

	Decelerations		
	Type	**Description**	**Cause**
	Early decelerations	Decrease in heart rate that occurs with contractions	Head compression
	Variable decelerations	Decrease in heart rate and return to baseline with no relationship to contractions	Umbilical cord compression
	Late decelerations (most serious and dangerous)	Decrease in heart rate after contraction started. No return to baseline until contraction ends	Fetal hypoxia

(handwritten margin notes: PRETERM, TOCOLYTICS, TERBUTALINE – β-AGONIST, NIFEDIPINE, MAG SULFATE, INDOMETHICIN; OK, OK, BAD)

Figure 16.13: Early decelerations. *Source: Elizabeth August, MD.*

Physiological Changes Before Labor

- **Lightening:** fetal descent into the pelvic brim
- **Braxton-Hicks contractions:** benign contractions that do not result in cervical dilation; they routinely start to increase in frequency towards the end of the pregnancy
- **Bloody show:** blood-tinged mucus from vagina that is released with cervical effacement

Stages of Labor		
Stages	**Beginning to end**	**Duration**
Stage 1	Onset of labor → full dilation of cervix	Primipara: ~~6–18 hours~~ ≤ 20 Hrs Multipara: ~~2–10 hours~~ ≤ 14 Hrs
Latent phase	Onset of labor → 4 cm dilation	Primipara: 6–7 hours Multipara: 4–5 hours
Active phase	4 cm dilation → full dilation	Primipara: ~~1~~ 1.2 cm per hour (minimum) Multipara: ~~1.2~~ 1.5 cm per hour (minimum)
Stage 2	Full dilation of cervix → delivery of neonate	Primipara: 30 minutes–3 hours Multipara: 5–30 minutes
Stage 3	Delivery of neonate → delivery of placenta	30 minutes

[handwritten notes: ASSESS Power / PASSAGE / PASSENGER]

[handwritten: STAGE 4 — 2 Hours Post Placenta → STABILITY]

Stage 1

Monitor the following:

- Maternal blood pressure and pulse
- Electronic fetal monitor: fetal heart rate and uterine contractions *[handwritten: → 3/30 min & > 40 mmHg]*
- Examine cervix every 2 hours to monitor the progression of labor for:
  - Cervical dilation
  - Cervical effacement

- Station
  - ◦ Where the fetus' head is located in relationship to the pelvis
  - ◦ Measured –3 through +3

Figure 16.14: Stages of fetal head descent. *Source: Elizabeth August, MD.*

Stage 2

Stage 2 begins when the cervix is fully dilated and the mother wants to push. The rate of fetal head descent determines the progression of this stage. The fetus goes through several steps in this stage:

1. Engagement
   - Fetal head enters the pelvis occiput first.

2. Descent
   - Progresses as uterine contractions and maternal pushing occur.
   - Descent continues until the fetus is delivered.

3. Flexion
   - Fetal head flexion

4. Internal Rotation
   - When fetus' head reaches the ischial spines, the fetus starts to rotate.
   - Rotation moves the sagittal sutures into the forward position.

5. Extension
   - Occurs so that the head can pass through vagina (oriented forward and upward).

6. External Rotation
   - During fetal head delivery, external rotation occurs, giving the shoulders room to descend.
   - Anterior shoulder goes under the pubic symphysis first.

7. Delivery of Anterior Shoulder
   - Gentle downward pressure on the fetal head will aid in delivery of anterior shoulder.

8. Delivery of Posterior Shoulder
   - Gentle upward pressure on the fetal head will aid in delivery of posterior shoulder.
   - The rest of the fetus will follow.

Stage 3

Immediately after delivery, inspect and repair lacerations of the vagina while waiting for placental separation.

Signs of placental separation include:

- Fresh bleeding from vagina
- Umbilical cord lengthening
- Uterine fundus rising
- Uterus becoming firm

Induction of Labor

Induction of labor means to start labor via medical means.

Medications

- **Prostaglandin E$_2$** is used for cervical ripening
- **Oxytocin**
  - Exaggerates uterine contractions
  - Normally found in the posterior pituitary (drug is a version of the naturally occurring substance)
- **Amniotomy**
  - Puncture of the amniotic sac via an amnio hook
    - Inspect for a prolapsed umbilical cord before puncturing the amniotic sac.

METHERGEN = ERGOTAMINE
⤷ DON'T GIVE TO HTN

HEMABATE = PROSTAGLANDIN
⤷ DON'T GIVE TO ASTHMATICS

Do not give prostaglandin to asthmatic patients; it may provoke bronchospasm.

BE SURE HEAD IS ENGAGED, OR CORD CAN COME OUT

COMPLICATIONS OF LABOR AND DELIVERY

A 22-year-old primipara in her 39th week of pregnancy presents with intense abdominal pain that is intermittent. She claims that she felt a gush of fluid from her vagina almost 3 hours ago. On physical exam her cervix is 3 cm dilated and 50% effaced, and the fetus' head is felt at the −2 station. For the next 3 hours she continues to progress so that her cervix is 5 cm dilated, 60% effaced, and fetal head is felt at −1 station. Six hours after presentation, her cervix is 5 cm dilated and 60% effaced, and fetal head is felt at 0 station.

Which of the following is the most likely diagnosis?

a. Prolonged latent stage
b. Protracted cervical dilation
c. Arrest of descent
d. Arrest of cervical dilation

Answer: The correct answer is (D). Arrest of cervical dilation is when there is no dilation of the cervix for more than 2 hours. Patients who are more than 4 cm dilated are considered to be in active stage 1 labor. Patients with prolonged latent stage take more than 20 hours (in primipara) to reach 4 cm of dilation. Protracted cervical dilation occurs when the primipara's cervix does not dilate more than 1.2 cm in one hour. It is dilating slowly, but still dilating. Arrest of descent is when the fetal head does not move down into the canal.

Prolonged Latent Stage

Prolonged latent stage occurs when the latent phase lasts longer than 20 hours for primipara and longer than 14 hours for multipara.

ETIOLOGY

- Sedation
- Unfavorable cervix
- Uterine dysfunction with irregular or weak contractions

TREATMENT

The treatment is rest and hydration. Most will convert to spontaneous delivery in 6 to 12 hours.

Protracted Cervical Dilation

SLOW DILATION DURING ACTIVE PHASE

Protraction occurs when there is slow dilation during the active phase of stage 1 labor, less than 1.2 cm per hour in primipara women, and less than 1.5 cm per hour in multipara.

ETIOLOGY

The 3 P's are:

- **Power:** strength and frequency of uterine contractions → oxy
- **Passenger:** size and position of fetus
- **Passage:** if passenger is larger than pelvis = cephalopelvic disproportion > c/s

TREATMENT

Treatment of cephalopelvic disproportion is **cesarean delivery**. If the uterine contractions are weak, **oxytocin** may be given.

Arrest Disorders

Types

- Cervical dilation: no cervical dilation for 2 hours
- Fetal descent: no fetal descent for 1 hour

ETIOLOGY

- Cephalopelvic disproportion
  - Accounts for half of all arrest disorders
  - Treat via cesarean delivery
- Malpresentation
  - Fetus is older than 36 weeks with the presenting part something other than the head, meaning the head is not downward.
- Excessive sedation/anesthesia

Malpresentation

A 25-year-old woman in her 35th week of gestation presents for a routine prenatal check up. She has no complaints. On physical examination her temperature is 98°F, blood pressure 130/90 mm Hg, heart rate 87 bpm, and respiratory rate 12 per minute. Her abdomen is gravid. On palpation of the abdomen, a hard circular surface is felt in the proximal part of the uterus.

Which of the following is the next step in the management of this patient?

a. External cephalic version
b. Ultrasound
c. CT scan
d. X-ray

Answer: The correct answer is (B). This patient is showing signs of a possible breech presentation on physical exam (the hard circular surface is the fetal head). Breech presentation should be confirmed via ultrasound before therapeutic measures such as external cephalic version are implemented. X-ray and CT scan are avoided during pregnancy secondary to the radiation exposure.

PRESENTATION

- Lower half of fetus (pelvis and legs) is the presenting part.
  - The presenting part is the part of the fetal body that is closest to the vaginal canal and will be engaged when labor starts. Normally it is the head (cephalic presentation); however, in malpresentation, it can be a foot or a buttock.
- Can be felt on physical exam
  - Leopold maneuvers are a set of 4 maneuvers that estimate the fetal weight and the presenting part of the fetus.
  - Vaginal exam: With malpresentation, you feel a soft mass instead of the normal hard surface of skull.

Diagnostic Evaluation

The fetus needs to be visualized with ultrasound to confirm the diagnosis.

Types of Breech Presentation	
Type	**Description**
Frank breech	Fetus' hips are flexed with extended knees bilaterally
Complete breech	Fetus' hips and knees are flexed bilaterally
Footling breech	Fetus' feet are first: one leg (single footling) or both legs (double footling)

Frank breech

Figure 16.15: Frank breech. *Source: Elizabeth August, MD.*

Complete breech

Figure 16.16: Complete breech. *Source: Elizabeth August, MD.*

Footling breech
(incomplete breech)

Figure 16.17: Footling breech. *Source: Elizabeth August, MD.*

TREATMENT

With external cephalic version, the caregiver maneuvers the fetus into a cephalic presentation (head down) through the abdominal wall. You should not perform this maneuver until after 36 weeks gestation. The fetus **can maneuver itself** into a cephalic presentation (head first) before 36 weeks.

Shoulder Dystocia

Shoulder dystocia occurs when the fetus' head has been delivered but the anterior shoulder is stuck behind the pubic symphysis.

Figure 16.18: Shoulder dystocia. *Source: Elizabeth August, MD.*

> Any factor that indicates that a fetus is too big or the pelvis is too small is a risk factor for shoulder dystocia.

Risk Factors

- Maternal diabetes and obesity causes fetal macrosomia.
- Postterm pregnancy allows the baby more time to grow.
- History of prior shoulder dystocia

TREATMENT

Treatment should follow these sequential steps:

1. McRoberts maneuver

Figure 16.19: McRobert's maneuver. *Source: Elizabeth August, MD.*

- First-line treatment
- Maternal flexion of knees into abdomen with suprapubic pressure

2. Rubin maneuver
   - Rotation of the fetus' shoulders by pushing the posterior shoulder towards the fetal head

3. Woods maneuver
   - Rotation of the fetus' shoulders by pushing the posterior shoulder toward the fetal back

4. Delivery of posterior arm
5. Deliberate fracture of fetal clavicle
6. Zavanelli maneuver
   - Push fetal head back into the uterus and perform cesarean delivery.
   - High rate of both maternal and fetal mortality
   - Last maneuver to try

POSTPARTUM HEMORRHAGE

DEFINITION

Postpartum hemorrhage is defined as bleeding more than 500 mL after delivery. **Early** postpartum bleeding occurs within 24 hours of delivery, while **late** postpartum bleeding occurs 24 hours to 6 weeks later.

> 500 mL w/ VD
> 1000 mL w/ c/s

ETIOLOGY

Normally, postpartum, the uterine contractions compress the blood vessels to stop blood loss. In uterine atony, this does not occur.

↳ M.C.C.

a = without
tony = contractions

Risk Factors

- Anesthesia
- Uterine overdistention (such as in twins and polyhydramnios)
- Prolonged labor
- Laceration
- Retained placenta (can occur with placenta accreta)
- Coagulopathy | DIC

UTERINE INVERSION = PPH ╎ ABSENT
UTERUS
↳ TRANS VAG SURGERY

↳ D&C
↳ TAH
↳ FOLLOW QUANT

IF PRECIPITOUS BIRTH | MACROSOMIA)
EPISIOTOMY
↳ MORE CHANCE ↑ FOR
VAG LAC

TREATMENT

Examine the uterus by bimanual examination. **Assure that there is no rupture of the uterus** and that there is no retained placenta. If the examination is unremarkable, bimanual **compression and massage** should be done. This will control most cases of postpartum bleeding. If the bimanual massage does not control the postpartum bleeding, administer **oxytocin** to make the uterus contract, constricting the blood vessels and decreasing the blood flow.

PUBERTY

GROWTH SPURT   GRAB PAM   13 YEARS OLD AVG FOR MENARCHE
BREASTS
2-3 YRS. PUBIC HAIR
ADRENARCHE
MENARCHE

PRECOCIOUS PUBERTY = DEVELOPMENT BEFORE 8 YEARS OLD

FAMILIAL
CENTRAL - ALL HORMONES FOLLOWED NML. → ↑ GH/GnRH →↑ LH/FSH
                                                   →CT/MRI
PSEUDO - EXOGENOUS HORMONES → CT ABDOMEN   → GnRH CONTINUOUSLY
                             → EXCISION

MENOPAUSE

51 YEAR OLD AVG | PREMATURE IS BEFORE 40 45 | 1 YEAR OF AMENORRHEA IN
                                              WOMAN OVER 40 = MENOPAUSE
OSTEOPOROSIS | CAD

ESTROGEN REPLACEMENT HELPS SYMPTOMS & REDUCES OSTEOPOROSIS
   ↳ CAUSES BREAST & ENDOMETRIAL CANCER & STROKE
   ↳ MUST GIVE PROGESTERONE IF STILL HAVE UTERUS

GYNECOLOGY

By Elizabeth V. August, MD

PREMENSTRUAL SYNDROME AND PREMENSTRUAL DYSPHORIC DISORDER

Premenstrual syndrome (PMS) and premenstrual dysphoric disorder (PMDD) begin when women are in their 20s to 30s. PMDD is a more severe version of PMS that will disrupt the patient's daily activities.

Symptoms

- Headache
- Breast tenderness
- Pelvic pain and bloating
- Irritability and lack of energy

DIAGNOSTIC TESTS

There are no tests for the diagnosis of PMS or PMDD. The patient should chart her symptoms. The following must be present to meet the diagnostic criteria:

- Symptoms should be present for 2 consecutive cycles
- Symptom-free period of 1 week in the first part of the cycle (follicular phase)
- Symptoms must be present in the second half of the cycle (luteal phase)

[handwritten margin note: ≥ 2 consecutive cycles / 1 week Sx free / LUTEAL PHASE Sxs]

TREATMENT

Patient should decrease consumption of caffeine, alcohol, cigarettes, and chocolate. If symptoms are severe, give SSRIs.

AVG AGE IS 51
45-55 IS "NML"

↑ FSH | ↑ LH
↓ ESTROGEN | ↓ PROGESTERONE

MENOPAUSE

Menopause occurs in patients aged 48 to 52. It starts with irregular menstrual bleeding. The oocytes produce less estrogen and progesterone, and both the LH and FSH start to rise. Women are symptomatic for an average of 12 months, but some women can experience symptoms for years.

Symptoms

- Menstrual irregularity
- Sweats and hot flashes★
- Mood changes
- Dyspareunia (pain during sexual intercourse)

Physical Exam Findings

- Decrease in breast size
- Vaginal and cervical atrophy

↓ CV EVENTS ???
↓ OSTEOPOROSIS
HRT → ↑ ENDO CANCER
       ↑ BREAST CANCER

DIAGNOSTIC TESTS/TREATMENT

If the diagnosis is unclear, an increased FSH level is diagnostic. Hormone replacement therapy (HRT) is indicated for short-term symptomatic relief as well as the prevention of osteoporosis.

> HRT is associated with endometrial hyperplasia and can lead to endometrial carcinoma.

Contraindications

- Estrogen-dependent carcinoma (breast or endometrial cancer)
- History of pulmonary embolism or DVT

ABNORMAL UTERINE BLEEDING

★
> Postcoital bleeding is cervical cancer until proven otherwise.

Types of Abnormal Uterine Bleeding		
Type	**Description**	**Etiology**
Menorrhagia ↑ BLEEDING AMOUNT	• Heavy and prolonged menstrual bleeding • "Gushing" of blood • Clots may be seen	• Endometrial hyperplasia • Uterine fibroids • Dysfunctional uterine bleeding • Intrauterine device
Hypomenorrhea ↓ BLEEDING AMOUNT	• Light menstrual flow • May only have spotting	• Obstruction (hymen, cervical stenosis) • Oral contraceptive pills

NON PREGNANT REPRODUCTIVE AGE BLEEDING
    M.C. FIBROIDS → U/S → MRI TO R/O LEIOMYOSARCOMA
              WANTS KIDS → MYOMECTOMY
              Ø WANT KIDS → TAH
              LEUPROLIDE TO SHRINK → SURGERY

Type	Description	Etiology
Metrorrhagia	Intermenstrual bleeding	• Endometrial polyps • Endometrial/cervical cancer • Exogenous estrogen administration
Menometror-rhagia	Irregular bleeding • Time intervals • Duration • Amount of bleeding	• Endometrial polyps • Endometrial/cervical cancer • Exogenous estrogen administration • Malignant tumors
Oligomenorrhea	Menstrual cycles >35 days long	• Pregnancy • Menopause • Significant weight loss (anorexia) • Tumor secreting estrogen
Postcoital bleeding	Bleeding after intercourse	• Cervical cancer • Cervical polyps • Atrophic vaginitis

(handwritten) Metrorrhagia — TIMING
(handwritten) Menometror-rhagia — TIMING & AMOUNT

(handwritten margin note) "THE METRO STOPS & STARTS"

DIAGNOSTIC TESTS

- CBC to see if hemoglobin and hematocrit have dropped
- PT/PTT to evaluate for coagulation disorder
- Pelvic ultrasound to visualize any anatomical abnormality *(handwritten) I.E. FIBROIDS/POLYPS*

(handwritten right margin)
AXIS
HYPOTHALAMUS
↓ GnRH
ANT PITUITARY
↓ FSH/LH
OVARIES
↓ ESTROGEN/PROGESTERONE
ENDOMETRIUM

Dysfunctional Uterine Bleeding

Dysfunctional uterine bleeding (DUB) is **unexplained abnormal bleeding**. DUB also occurs when patients are anovulatory. The ovary produces estrogen, but no corpus luteum is formed. Without the corpus luteum, progesterone is not produced. This prevents the usual withdrawal bleeding. The continuously high estrogen continues to stimulate growth of the endometrium. Bleeding occurs only once the endometrium outgrows the blood supply.

DIAGNOSTIC TESTS

Rule out systemic reasons for anovulation, such as hypothyroid and hyperp-rolactinimia. **Endometrial biopsy for women over 35 to exclude carcinoma.**

▶ **TIP**

There is no specific test for DUB. Confirm by excluding other causes.

> Any patient older than 35 with abnormal bleeding should undergo endometrial biopsy to rule out endometrial carcinoma.

(handwritten bottom section)
BLEEDING
GIRLS < 11 Y.O. → M.C. FOREIGN BODY, ABUSE, PRECOCIOUS PUBERTY →
↓ SPECULUM EXAM
GnRH STIM TEST
↳ IF ↑ LH = CENTRAL I.E. TUMOR
↳ IF ∅ Δ LH = PERIPHERAL
↳ U/S ABDOMEN/ADRENALS/OVARIES
TEST/ 17-OH-PROG/ DHEA-S
↳ LOOK FOR TUMOR
TO RESECT

483

SEVERE BLEED

IV ESTROGEN
↓
ARTERY LIGATION
↓
TAH

EMERGENCY CONTRACEPTIVES

MIFEPRISTONE
COPPER IUD
PROGESTERONE

6 HOURS BY
6 HOURS AFTER

TREATMENT

Oral contraceptive pills (OCP):

D & C
↓
OCP
↓
ABLATION
↓
HYST

- Adolescents and young women who are anovulatory
- Women over 35 who have a normal endometrial biopsy

Acute hemorrhage:

- D&C is done to stop the bleeding

DUB is severe if patients are anemic, are not controlled by OCPs, or report that their lifestyle is compromised. Treat with endometrial ablation or hysterectomy.

CONTRACEPTION

Female Condoms

The female condom has 2 rings and a thin material in between. One ring is placed deep into the vagina while the other ring is left at the introitus. Female condoms offer some protection against HIV and STDs and are under female control. They are larger and bulkier than male condoms.

Vaginal Diaphragm

A vaginal diaphragm is a circular ring with contraceptive jelly that covers the cervical canal. The diaphragm without the contraceptive jelly is ineffective. The contraceptive jelly is also used as a lubricant while placing the diaphragm. The diaphragm should be placed 6 hours before intercourse and left in for at least 6 hours after intercourse. The disadvantages of a diaphragm are:

- Need to be fitted properly (can change with weight gain or pregnancies)
- Proper use of diaphragm requires advance preparation
- Improper placement or dislodging of diaphragm reduces efficacy

Oral Contraceptive Pills

OCPs are most commonly a combination pill of both estrogen and progesterone. The pill is taken for 21 days and a placebo is taken for 7 days. During the 7 days of the placebo pills, the patient will experience menstruation. Women should start using the oral contraceptive pills on the Sunday after menstruation. OCPs reduce the risk of ovarian carcinoma, endometrial carcinoma, and ectopic pregnancy. OCPs give a slight increase in the risk of thromboembolism.

CONTRA INDICATED IN SMOKERS OVER 35 / MIGRAINE WITH AURA / CC
PROGESTIN ONLY POST PARTUM BREAST FEEDING

IF BREAK THROUGH BLEEDING → ↑ ESTROGEN

IF TOO MANY S.E. → ↓ PROGESTIN

Vaginal Ring

A flexible vaginal ring that releases both estrogen and progesterone is inserted into the vagina for 3 weeks. Hormones are released on a constant basis. When the ring is removed, withdrawal bleeding will occur. The vaginal ring has similar side effects and efficacy to OCPs.

Transdermal Patch

A transdermal patch with a combination of estrogen and progesterone is placed on the skin for 7 days. Each week the previous patch is removed and a new patch is placed. Three weeks of patches are followed by a patch-free week, during which the patient will experience withdrawal bleeding. Patches should not be placed on the breast. The side effects and efficacy are the same as OCPs.

Intrauterine Device

An intrauterine device (IUD) is placed into the uterus and provides contraception for 10 years. There are 2 types, a copper device and a levonorgestrel device. These devices are associated with pelvic inflammatory disease when they are placed.

CONTRAINDICATED IF LIKELY TO GET STDs

↑ INCIDENCE OF ECTOPIC, BUT STILL ↓ B/c LESS LIKELY TO GET PREGNANT

Sterilization

Surgical sterilization can be done on both men and women. Sterilization via tubal ligation and vasectomy is permanent and irreversible.

↳ SORT OF

Tubal Ligation

Tubal ligation is a surgical procedure that women may choose to undergo for permanent contraception. The risk of pregnancy is very low, but if it occurs, there is an increased incidence of ectopic pregnancy.

Vasectomy

Vasectomy is a surgical procedure in which ligation of the vas deferens is performed.

VULVA AND VAGINA

Labial Fusion

Labial fusion occurs when **excess androgens** are present. This can occur with extraneous androgen administration or by increased androgen production. The most common cause of labial fusion is **21-B hydroxylase deficiency**. The treatment of labial fusion is **reconstructive surgery**.

Epithelial Abnormalities			
Abnormality	**Age group affected**	**Description**	**Treatment**
Lichen sclerosus	Any age can be affected; however, if postmenopausal, there is an increased risk of cancer.	White, thin skin extending from labia to perianal area	Topical steroids
Squamous cell hyperplasia	Any age; patients who have had chronic vulvar pruritus	Patients with chronic irritation develop hyperkeratosis (raised white lesion).	Sitz baths or lubricants (relieve the pruritus)
Lichen planus	30s–60s	Violet, flat papules	Topical steroids

Bartholin Gland Cyst

Bartholin glands are located on the lateral sides of the vulva. They secrete mucus and can become obstructed, leading to a cyst or abscess that causes **pain**, **tenderness**, and **dyspareunia**. Physical exam shows edema and inflammation of the area with a deep fluctuant mass.

Treatment is similar to other cysts or abscesses. It needs to be drained. A simple **incision and drainage (I&D)** should be done. If they continue to recur, then marsupialization should be done. During I&D, the fluid released should be cultured for sexually transmitted diseases (STDs) such as *Neisseria gonorrheae* and *Chlamydia trachomatis*.

Marsupialization is a form of I&D in which the open space is kept open with sutures. This allows the space to remain open, and decreases the risk of a recurrent Bartholin gland cyst.

Vaginitis

A 19-year-old woman presents for vaginal pruritus and discharge for one week. She complains that the discharge is green and profuse. She has had multiple sexual partners in the past 2 months. Her last menstrual period was 2 weeks ago. On wet mount, the vaginal discharge has motile flagellates present.

Toxic shock = Staph Aureus

Which of the following is the most likely diagnosis?

a. Chlamydia

b. Bacterial vaginosis

c. Neisseria gonorrhoeae

d. Candidiasis

e. Trichomonas vaginalis

*Answer: The correct answer is (**E**). **Trichomonas** presents with a profuse, green, frothy discharge. **Neisseria** is a bacterial infection that is identified by culture. Chlamydia is diagnosed by serology DNA probe. Candidiasis is associated with white, cheesy vaginal discharge. Bacterial vaginosis is associated with vaginal discharge and a fishy odor, which does not cause pruritus.*

Risk Factors

Risk factors include any factor that will increase the pH of the vagina, such as:

- Antibiotic use (*Lactobacillus* **normally keeps the vaginal pH below 4.5**)
- Diabetes
- Overgrowth of normal flora

Symptoms

Patients present with itching, pain, abnormal odor, and discharge.

Types of Vaginitis				
Disease	**Pathogen**	**Symptom**	**Diagnostic Test**	**Treatment**
Bacterial vaginosis	*Gardnerella*	Vaginal discharge with fishy odor; gray white	Potassium hydroxide (KOH) shows **clue cells**.	Metronidazole or clindamycin
Candidiasis	*Candida albicans*	White, cheesy vaginal discharge	KOH shows **pseudohyphae**; vaginal culture is most specific.	Miconazole or clotrimazole, econazole, or nystatin
Trichomonas (the most common nonviral STD)	*Trichomonas vaginalis*	Profuse, green, frothy vaginal discharge	KOH shows **motile flagellates**.	Treat both patient and partner with metronidazole.

▶ TIP

If trichomonas is diagnosed, both partners need to be treated.

Malignant Disorders

Paget Disease

Paget disease is an intraepithelial neoplasia that most commonly occurs in postmenopausal Caucasian women. Paget presents with vulvar soreness and pruritus appearing as a **red lesion with a superficial white coating**. A **biopsy** is needed for a definitive diagnosis. Treatment for a bilateral lesion is a **radical vulvectomy**. If there is a **unilateral lesion, a modified vulvectomy** can be done.

Squamous Cell Carcinoma

Squamous cell carcinoma is the most common type of vulvar cancer. It presents with **pruritis**, bloody vaginal discharge, and postmenopausal bleeding. The physical exam can range from a small ulcerated lesion to a large cauliflowerlike lesion. A **biopsy is essential for diagnosis**. Staging is done while the patient is in surgery and is determined as follows.

Staging of Squamous Cell Carcinoma	
Stage	**Findings**
0	Carcinoma in situ
I	Limited to vaginal wall <2 cm
II	Limited to vulva or perineum >2 cm
III	Tumor spreading to lower urethra or anus, unilateral lymph nodes present
IV	Tumor invasion into bladder, rectum, or bilateral lymph nodes
IVa	Distant metastasis

Treatment of unilateral lesions without lymph node involvement is a modified radical vulvectomy. Treatment for bilateral involvement is radical vulvectomy. Lymph nodes that are involved must undergo lymphadenectomy.

UTERINE ABNORMALITIES

Adenomyosis

Adenomyosis is the invasion of endometrial glands into the myometrium. This usually occurs in women between the ages of 35 and 50. **Risk factors** for adenomyosis are **endometriosis** and **uterine fibroids**. It presents with **dysmenorrhea** and **menorrhagia**.

Adenomyosis is a clinical diagnosis. On physical examination the uterus is large, globular, and boggy. MRI is the most accurate test. **Hysterectomy** is the only definitive treatment. It is also the only way to diagnose adenomyosis definitively.

Endometriosis

Endometriosis is the **implantation** of endometrial tissue **outside of the endometrial** cavity. Although the endometrial tissue can implant anywhere, the most common sites are the ovary and pelvic peritoneum. Endometriosis occurs in women of reproductive age and is **more common** if a **first-degree relative** (mother or sister) has endometriosis.

Endometriosis presents with **cyclical pelvic pain** that starts **1 to 2 weeks before menstruation** and peaks 1 to 2 days before menstruation. The pain ends with menstruation. **Abnormal bleeding is common**. The **physical exam** reveals a **nodular uterus** and **adenexal mass**.

DIAGNOSTIC TESTS

Diagnosis can be made only by direct visualization via laparoscopy. Direct visualization of the endometrial implants looks like rusty or dark brown lesions. On the ovary, a cluster of lesions called an endometrioma looks like a "chocolate cyst."

TREATMENT

Analgesia can be done with NSAIDs. Patients with mild symptoms may be placed on **OCPs** to interrupt the menstrual cycle and stop ovulation.

Patients with moderate to severe symptoms should be placed on either danazole or leuprolide acetate (leupron). Both of these drugs are used to decrease FSH and LH.

Danazol is an androgen derivative that is associated with acne, oily skin, weight gain, and hirsutism.

Leuprolide acetate (leupron) is a GnRH agonist and when given continuously **suppresses estrogen**. Leuprolide is associated with hot flashes and decreased bone density.

Surgical treatment is considered for patients who have severe symptoms or are infertile. Surgery attempts to remove all of the endometrial implants and adhesions, and to restore pelvic anatomy. Patients who have completed their childbearing may undergo total abdominal hysterectomy and bilateral salpingo-oophorectomy.

OVARIAN ABNORMALITIES

Polycystic Ovarian Syndrome

Symptoms

These symptoms occur in women of reproductive age:

- **Amenorrhea** or **irregular menses**
- **Hirsutism and obesity**
- Acne
- Diabetes mellitus Type 2 (increased insulin resistance)

DIAGNOSTIC TESTS

Pelvic ultrasound will show **bilaterally enlarged ovaries** with **multiple cysts** present. Free testosterone will be elevated secondary to the high androgens. The high androgen level and obesity lead to an increase in estrogen formation

> Dysmenorrhea and dyspareunia are common in endometriosis.

outside the ovary. This stimulates LH secretion while inhibiting FSH secretion, leading to an **LH to FSH ratio of more than 3:1**.

TREATMENT

- **Weight loss:** Patients who are obese should be counseled to lose weight, which will decrease the insulin resistance.
- **OCPs** control the amounts of estrogen and progestin that are in the body. This both controls the androgen levels and prevents endometrial hyperplasia. This should be used only if the patient does not wish to have children.
- **Clomiphene and metformin** should be used in patients who wish to conceive.

SECTION 7
RADIOLOGY

PLAIN X-RAYS

Chest X-rays

A **chest x-ray** is the best initial radiologic test for all forms of **pulmonary complaints** such as:

- Cough
- Shortness of breath (dyspnea)
- Chest pain, particularly when pleuritic or changing with respirations
- Sputum and hemoptysis

The chest x-ray is also the best initial radiologic test for all forms of abnormalities on the physical examination of the lungs, including:

- Rales and rhonchi
- Wheezing
- Dullness to percussion
- Chest wall tenderness
- Tracheal deviation
- Possible superior vena cava syndrome (jugulovenous distention, plethora of the face, venous distention of the chest wall)

Posterior/anterior (PA) films: The PA film is the standard of care when a chest x-ray is done. To get films, the patient must be able to stand up.

Anterior/posterior (AP) films: AP films are the answer for an **unstable patient** who is **too sick to stand up for a PA film.** They are often done with portable chest x-ray equipment. Chest x-rays in the **intensive care unit** are **AP films.**

Decubitus films: These x-rays are done to evaluate a **pleural effusion** found on a PA film. The patient lies down on each side and an effusion is confirmed if the fluid in the chest is **freely mobile and forms a layer** on the side of the x-ray.

> Widening of the mediastinum on a PA film is the best initial test of a dissection of the thoracic aorta.

491

► **TIP**

Decubitus x-rays are the answer when the diagnosis of an infiltrate from pneumonia cannot be distinguished from an effusion.

Apical lordotic films: Lordotic films are almost never the right answer. Lordotic x-ray of the chest is done with the patient leaning backward to take ribs out of the way in order to examine the upper lobes. Lordotic films were originally the best initial test for **tuberculosis**, which has an increased predilection for the apices of the lung. However, **whenever apical lordotic films might be done, a CT scan of the chest is generally the best initial study.**

Lateral chest X-ray: A lateral x-ray is done to help identify the **precise location of an infiltrate** found on a PA film. Lateral x-rays are the best initial test for an **effusion** since they detect as little as 50 to 75 mL of effusion. The PA chest x-ray becomes abnormal with an effusion only when 200 to 300 mL of fluid have accumulated.

Abdominal X-ray

Abdominal x-ray has very few indications. **The best indication for an abdominal film is ileus or small bowel obstruction.** Abdominal x-ray of ileus will show multiple air-fluid levels in the small bowel. However, abdominal x-ray is **not accurate for stones of the kidney** and will miss at least 20% of cases. Abdominal x-ray does **not reliably find air under the diaphragm** because it does not always visualize the top of the diaphragm, especially in a tall person.

> Abdominal x-ray is good only for an ileus.

► **TIP**

For perforation of the bowel, get an upright chest x-ray, not an abdominal x-ray.

Bone X-ray

X-ray of the bone is the **best initial test for osteomyelitis**. You will see **elevation of the periosteum**. Long-standing bone infection gives destroyed bond with periosteal new bone formation. Although it will take at least two weeks for the bone x-ray to become abnormal with osteomyelitis, you should still do this study first. You will only obtain an MRI of the bone or a nuclear bone scan if the x-ray does not show osteomyelitis.

Skull X-rays

There is no first-class indication for skull x-ray. **Skull x-ray is not the best initial or most accurate test for anything.** A normal skull x-ray does not exclude intracranial hemorrhage, and an abnormal x-ray does not mean there is a hemorrhage.

▶ **TIP**

Skull x-rays are rarely correct for any question.

COMPUTERIZED TOMOGRAPHY (CT SCAN)

Head CT

Non-contrast head CT is the best initial test for:

- Severe **head trauma**, especially with loss of consciousness or altered mental status
- **Stroke**
- Any form of intracranial **bleeding** including subarachnoid hemorrhage

CT scan with **contrast**:

- **Cancer and infection** will enhance with contrast. You cannot distinguish between neoplastic disease and an abscess by CT scan or MRI, but the head CT with contrast is the best initial test for any form of intracranial mass lesion.

- Do not order contrast with severe renal failure.
- Hydrate with saline and possibly use bicarbonate or N-acetylcysteine with mild renal insufficiency.
- Stop metformin prior to using contrast.

Abdominal CT

This study should be performed with both **intravenous and oral contrast**. Oral contrast is indispensible in outlining abdominal structures that are pressed against each other and would otherwise be difficult to visualize.

Abdominal CT is also good for:

- **Retroperitoneal structures:** Organs such as the **pancreas** are difficult to visualize with sonography. In sonography, the transducer is placed against the anterior abdominal wall. This makes it difficult to visualize structures that are further away from the anterior abdominal wall.
- **Appendicitis and other intra**abdominal infections
- Most accurate test for **nephrolithiasis**; this is a case in which contrast is not needed
- **Masses within abdominal organs** such as the liver and spleen

CT is the "most accurate test" for **diverticulitis**.

Choose abdominal CT to visualize the pancreas.

> **TIP**
CT is the "most accurate test" for kidney stones.

Chest CT

When is chest CT the answer on the test?

- Hilar **nodes** such as sarcoidosis
- **Mass lesions** such as cancer
- **Cavities**
- **Interstitial lung disease:** Chest CT adds considerable definition to the chest x-ray. The chest x-ray shows only interstitial infiltrates. CT shows much more detail in evaluating **parenchymal lung disease**.
- **Pulmonary emboli:** The spiral CT or CT angiogram has supplanted the V/Q scan in confirming pulmonary emboli.

CT is neither the "best initial" nor "most accurate" test of bone.

MRI

MRI is the most accurate test of all **central nervous system diseases** with the exception of looking for hemorrhage. The indication for the use of contrast with MRI is the same as with CT scans. Contrast detects cancer and infectious mass lesions.

When is MRI the answer on the test?

- **Demyelinating** diseases such as **multiple sclerosis**
- **Posterior fossa** lesion in the cerebellum
- **Brainstem**
- **Pituitary** lesions
- Facial structures such as the orbits and sinuses
- Bone lesions, particularly **osteomyelitis**. MRI is the best visualization of bone, although it cannot determine a precise microbiologic etiology.
- **Spinal cord and vertebral lesions**

> **TIP**
With cancer and infection, the radiologic test is never the most accurate test; biopsy is.

ULTRASOUND (SONOGRAPHY)

When is ultrasound the answer?

- **Gallbladder disease**, including the ducts for **stones** and obstruction
- **Renal disease**, although CT is more sensitive for nephrolithiasis

- **Gynecologic organs:** uterus, ovaries, adnexa
- Prostate evaluation (transrectal approach)

Endoscopic Ultrasound

Endoscopic ultrasound (EUS) is the most accurate method of assessing:

- **Pancreatic lesions**, particularly in the head
- Pancreatic and biliary ductal disease
- **Gastrinoma localization** (Zollinger-Ellison syndrome)

With EUS a sonographic device is placed at the end of the scope and placed into the duodenum to allow outstanding visualization of hard-to-reach intra-abdominal structures.

NUCLEAR SCANS

- **HIDA (hepatobiliary) scan** is the only functional test of the biliary system that allows detection of **cholecystitis**.
- **Bone scan:** Although equal in sensitivity to the MRI in detecting osteomyelitis, bone scan is **not nearly as specific as an MRI**. Bone scan is good as a sensitive test to detect occult metastases from cancer.
- **Gallium scan: fever of unknown origin.** Gallium follows iron metabolism and is transported on transferrin. Gallium increases in uptake with infection and in some cancers because of increased iron deposition.
- **Indium scan:** Another test for **fever of unknown origin**; superior in assessing the abdomen, which can be obscured in gallium scanning. Indium is a tagged white blood cell scan: The patient's white cells are tagged with indium, then reinjected to see where they localize to **detect infection**.
- **Ventilation/perfusion (V/Q) scanning:** A normal V/Q scan essentially excludes a pulmonary embolus. **Low-probability** scans **still have a clot in 15%** of cases and **high-probability** scans do **not** have a clot **in 15%** of cases. V/Q is no longer the standard of care in detecting pulmonary emboli. It has been replaced by the spiral CT (CT angiogram) in the confirmation of pulmonary emboli.
- **Multiple-gated acquisition scan (MUGA)** or nuclear ventriculography is the most accurate method to measure **ejection fraction**.

SECTION 8
OPHTHALMOLOGY

CONJUNCTIVITIS

Comparison of Viral and Bacterial Conjunctivitis	
Viral conjunctivitis MOST COMMON	**Bacterial conjunctivitis**
Bilateral	Unilateral
Watery discharge	Purulent, thick discharge
Easily transmissible	Poorly transmissible
Normal vision	Normal vision
Itchy	Not itchy
Preauricular adenopathy	No adenopathy
No specific therapy	Topical antibiotics

ADENOVIRUS   GONORRHEA or CHLAMYDIA

Handwritten margin note:
ALLERGES
BILATERAL
WATERY
NO
NORMAL
ITCHY
NO

▶ **TIP**

The "must know" subjects in ophthalmology are:

- The red eye (emergencies)
- Diabetic retinopathy
- Artery and vein occlusion
- Retinal detachment

Handwritten note:
UVEITIS
INFLAMMATION BY A.I. OR INFLAMMATORY DISEASE OR INFECTION
→ PAIR → PSORIATIC | A.S. | I.B.D. | REITER'S
PAIN | PHOTOPHOBIA | INFLAMMATION
ANTIBIOTICS OR STEROIDS

THE RED EYE (OPHTHALMOLOGIC EMERGENCIES)

Etiologies of The Red Eye				
	Conjunctivitis	**Uveitis**	**Glaucoma**	**Abrasion**
Presentation	Itchy eyes, discharge	Autoimmune diseases	Pain	Trauma
Eye findings	Normal pupils	Photophobia	Fixed midpoint pupil	Feels like sand in eyes
Most accurate test	Clinical diagnosis	Slit lamp examination	Tonometry	Fluorescein stain
Best initial therapy	Topical antibiotics *IF BACTERIAL*	Topical steroids	Acetazolamide, mannitol, pilocarpine, laser trabeculoplasty	No specific therapy; patch not clearly beneficial

Glaucoma

Chronic Glaucoma

FREQUENTLY CHANGING PRESCRIPTIONS

CUP : DISK RATIO >50%

Chronic glaucoma is most **often asymptomatic** on presentation and is diagnosed by routine screening. Confirmation is with **tonometry** indicating extremely elevated intraocular pressure. Treat with medications to decrease the production of aqueous humor or to increase its drainage.

- **Prostaglandin analogues:** latanoprost, travoprost, bimatoprost
- **Topical beta blockers:** timolol, carteolol, metipranolol, betaxolol, or levobunolol
- **Topical carbonic anhydrase inhibitors:** dorzolamide, brinzolamide *(ACETAZOLAMIDE)*
- **Alpha-2 agonists:** apraclonidine
- **Pilocarpine**
- Laser **trabeculoplasty:** performed if medical therapy is inadequate

Acute Angle-Closure Glaucoma

Look for the **sudden onset of an extremely painful, red eye** that is **hard to palpation**. Walking into a dark room can precipitate pain because of pupilary dilation. The cornea is described as "steamy" and the **pupil does not react to light** because it is stuck. The cup-to-disc ratio is greater than the normal 0.3. The diagnosis is confirmed with tonometry. Treat with:

- Intravenous **acetazolamide**
- Intravenous **mannitol** to act as an osmotic draw of fluid out of the eye
- **Pilocarpine** and beta blockers to constrict the pupil and enhance drainage
- Laser **iridotomy**

Herpes Keratitis

Keratitis is an infection of the cornea. The eye may be very red, swollen, and painful, but do not use steroids. **Fluorescein staining** of the eye helps confirm the dendritic pattern seen on examination. Steroids markedly increase the production of the virus.

Treat with **oral acyclovir, famciclovir, or valacyclovir.** Topical antiherpetic treatment is trifluridine and idoxuridine.

> Beware of steroid use for herpes keratitis. Steroids make the condition worse.

CATARACTS

There is no medical therapy for cataracts. **Surgically remove the lens** and replace with a new intraocular lens. The new lens may automatically have a bifocal capability. Early cataracts are diagnosed with an ophthalmoscope or slit lamp exam. Advanced cataracts are visible on examination.

DIABETIC RETINOPATHY

Annual screening exams should detect retinopathy before serious visual loss has occurred. Nonproliferative or "background" retinopathy is managed by controlling glucose level. The most accurate test is fluorescein angiography. **Proliferative retinopathy is treated with laser photocoagulation.** Vascular endothelial growth factor inhibitors (VEGF) are injected in some patients to control neovascularization.

Vitrectomy may be necessary to remove a vitreal hemorrhage obstructing vision.

Neovascularization

Figure 19.1: New blood vessel formation obscures vision.
Source: Conrad Fischer, MD.

RETINAL ARTERY AND VEIN OCCLUSION

Both conditions present with the sudden onset of monocular visual loss. You cannot make the diagnosis without retinal examination. There is no conclusive therapy for either condition.

Figure 19.2: Retinal artery occlusion presents with sudden loss of vision and a pale retina and dark macula. *Source: Conrad Fischer, MD.*

Figure 19.3: Retinal vein occlusion leads to extravasation of blood into the retina. *Source: Conrad Fischer, MD.*

The macula is described as "cherry red" in artery occlusion because the rest of the retina is pale.

Treatment of artery occlusion is attempted with 100% oxygen, acetazolamide to decrease intraocular pressure, and thrombolytics.

RETINAL DETACHMENT

Risks include trauma to the eye, extreme myopia that changes the shape of the eye, and diabetic retinopathy. Anything that pulls on the retina can detach it.

Detachment presents with the sudden onset of **painless**, unilateral loss of vision that is described as "a curtain coming down."

Reattachment is attempted with a number of **mechanical methods** such as surgery, laser, cryotherapy, and the injection of an expansile gas that pushes the retina back up against the globe of the eye.

Figure 19.4: Sudden, painless loss of vision "like a curtain coming down."
Source: Conrad Fischer, MD.

MACULAR DEGENERATION

Macular degeneration is now the **most common cause of blindness in older persons** in the United States. The cause is unknown. There is an atrophic (dry) type and a neovascular (wet) type.

Visual loss in macular degeneration:

- Far more common in older patients
- Bilateral
- Normal external appearance of the eye
- Loss of central vision

Neovascular disease is more rapid and more severe. New vessels grow between the retina and the underlying Bruch membrane. The neovascular or wet type causes 90% of permanent blindness from macular degeneration.

FLUORESCIN ANGIOGRAPHY SHOWS NEOVASCULARIZATION

VITAMINS

> Atrophic macular degeneration has no proven effective therapy.

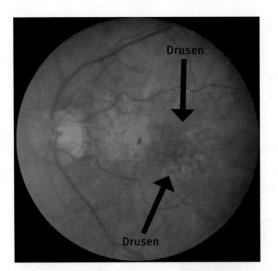

Figure 19.5: Macular degeneration can be diagnosed only by visualization of the retina. *Source: Conrad Fischer, MD.*

The **best initial therapy for neovascular disease is VEGF inhibitors** such as ranibizumab and bevacizumab. They are injected directly into the vitreous chamber every few weeks. Over 90% of patients will experience a halt of progression, and one-third of patients will have improvement in vision.

SECTION 9
PSYCHIATRY

By Alina Gonzalez-Mayo, MD

CHILDHOOD DISORDERS

Mental Retardation

DEFINITION

In order to determine the level of retardation, patients must exhibit **deficits in both intellectual functioning** (eg, cognitive abilities) as well as social adaptive functioning (eg, the ability to do daily activities). Mental retardation is **more frequent in boys** with the highest incidence being in school-age children.

Types of Mental Retardation		
Degree of mental retardation	**IQ range**	**Level of functioning**
Mild	50–55 to 70	Reaches sixth grade level of education, can work and live independently, needs help in difficult or stressful situations
Moderate	30–40 to 50–55	Reaches second grade level of education, may work with supervision and support, needs help in mildly stressful situations
Severe	20–25 to 35–40	Little or no speech, very limited abilities to manage self care
Profound	Below 20	Needs continuous care and supervision

TREATMENT

- **Genetic counseling**, prenatal care, and safe environments for expectant mothers
- If due to medical conditions, effective treatment for disorder

- Special education to improve level of functioning
- Behavioral therapy to help reduce negative behaviors

Pervasive Developmental Disorders

DEFINITION

This is a group of disorders characterized by problems in social interactions, behavior, and language that tend to occur in children before the age of 3.

Childhood Developmental Disorders			
Disorder	**Epidemiology**	**Characteristics**	**Treatment**
Autistic disorder	Greater incidence in boys than girls	Lacks peer relationships, poor eye contact and social smile. Absent or bizarre speech. Repetitive behaviors such as spinning or banging head as well as self-injurious behavior.	Improve ability to develop relationships, attend school, and achieve independent living. May benefit from behavioral modification programs. If aggressive, use antipsychotic medications.
Rett disorder	Greater incidence in girls	Progressive encephalopathy, microcephaly, hand-wringing, loss of speech, ataxia, and psychomotor retardation	Treatment is symptomatic. Behavior therapy for self-injurious behavior. Physiotherapy for muscular dysfunction.
Childhood disintegrative disorder	Greater incidence in boys	Normal development for 2 years, then marked regression in functioning. This includes loss of language, social interaction, motor function, and bladder function. Also have repetitive and stereotyped behaviors.	Improve ability to develop relationships, go to school, and achieve independent living. May benefit from behavioral modification programs. If aggressive, use antipsychotic medications.
Asperger disorder	Greater incidence in boys	Problems in social interaction and behaviors, but with no language or intellectual deficits. Preoccupied with rules.	Improve relationships with others

Gabriel is a healthy 2-year-old boy whose parents have taken him to the pediatrician. His problems started at 18 months of age, when he did not speak much. He does not have much attachment to his parents and seems aggressive toward other children.

What is the most likely diagnosis?

a. Deafness

b. Schizophrenia, childhood onset

c. Rett disorder

d. Autism

e. Learning deficit

Answer: The correct answer is (D). Autism is seen more frequently in boys and usually starts by the age of 3. Children with autism tend to have problems with language and aggression, lack separation anxiety, and are withdrawn. Deafness should be ruled out if parents report that a child does not respond when his or her name is called.

Attention Deficit Hyperactivity Disorder

DEFINITION

Attention deficit hyperactivity disorder (ADHD) is a disorder characterized by **inattention**, **short attention span**, **or hyperactivity** that is severe enough to **interfere with daily functioning** in school, home, or work. The symptoms must be present for **more than 6 months** and usually appear **before the age of 7.** The symptoms may persist into adulthood.

Diagnosis

Symptoms must be present in at least 2 areas, such as **home and school**. At home, children interrupt others, fidget in chairs, and run or climb excessively; are unable to engage in leisure activities; and talk excessively. At school, they are unable to pay attention, make careless mistakes in schoolwork, do not follow through with instructions, have difficulties organizing tasks, and are easily distracted.

TREATMENT

1. First line in the treatment of ADHD includes methylphenidate and dextroamphetamine. **Side effects include insomnia, decreased appetite, and headache**.
2. Second-line treatment includes atomoxetine, a norepinephrine reuptake inhibitor.

▶ **TIP**

On the USMLE Step 2 CK, atomoxetine is usually chosen over the first-line treatment, given the side-effect profiles of those treatments.

Disruptive Behavioral Disorders			
Disorder	**Epidemiology**	**Features**	**Treatment**
Oppositional defiant disorder	Usually noted by age 8; seen more in boys than girls before puberty, but equal incidence after puberty	Often argue with others, lose temper, easily annoyed by others, and blame others for their mistakes. Tend to have problems with authority figures and justify their behavior as response to others' actions.	Teach parents appropriate child management skills and how to lessen the oppositional behavior.
Conduct disorder	Seen more frequently in boys and in children whose parents have antisocial personality disorder and alcohol dependence	Persistent behavior where rules are broken. These include aggression to others such as bullying, cruelty to animals, fighting, or using weapons. Destroy property such as vandalism or setting fires. Steal items from others or lie to obtain goods from others. Violate rules (eg, truancy, running away from home, breaking curfew).	Behavioral intervention using rewards for prosocial and nonaggressive behavior. If aggressive, antipsychotic medications have been used.

A 10-year-old boy was seen by a school counselor after the teachers complained of his behavior in school. He frequently becomes angry towards others and loses his temper in class. His parents report that at home, he refuses to comply with house rules, often stays up later than he is supposed to, and frequently talks back to them.

What is the most likely diagnosis?

a. Conduct disorder
b. Tourette disorder
c. Adjustment disorder
d. Oppositional defiant disorder
e. Learning disorder, not otherwise specified

Answer: The correct answer is (D). Children with oppositional defiant disorder usually have problems with authority figures such as parents and teachers. Unlike children with conduct disorder, they do not break rules of society and do not commit crimes.

Tourette Disorder

Tourette disorder is characterized by the onset of multiple **tics**, lasting more than one year, and is seen before the age of 18. The motor tics most commonly involve the muscles of the face and neck, such as **head shaking and blinking**. The vocal tics include **grunting, coughing, and throat clearing**. The disorder is seen more frequently in boys than in girls and will begin by the age of 7. Treatment includes dopamine antagonists, such as antipsychotic medications like risperidone, COUNSELLING

DEEP BRAIN STIM

MOOD DISORDERS

Major Depression ↓NE ↓DOPA ↓SEROTONIN

DEFINITION

Mood disorders present with at least a 2-week course of symptoms that is a change from the previous level of functioning. The symptoms include depressed mood or **anhedonia** (absence of pleasure) and 4 others including depressed mood most of the day, **weight changes**, **sleep changes**, psychomotor disturbances, fatigue, **poor concentration**, and thoughts of death and worthlessness.

Diagnosis

Rule out any medical causes, the most common of which is hypothyroidism. The most common neurological associations are Parkinson disease and dementia. HYPERPARATHYROIDISM | STROKE | CNS NEOPLASM | PANC CANCER
DRUGS - ANTIHISTAMINES/SEDATIVES | STIMULANT WITHDRAWL | METHYLDOPA | GLUCOCORTICOIDS

TREATMENT

First-line treatment is often a selective serotonin reuptake inhibitor (SSRI) such as fluoxetine, paroxetine, sertraline, citalopram, or escitalopram. SSRIs are chosen due to their effectiveness and relatively mild side effects, and because they are less toxic in overdose than other antidepressants.

- If some improvement is noted, but it is not a full response, increase the dose of the SSRI.

- Psychotherapy such as cognitive therapy has been proven to be effective. The goal of cognitive therapy is to reduce depression by teaching patients to identify negative cognitions and develop positive ways of thinking.

> SSRIs should not be taken with MAO inhibitors as they will cause a dramatic increase in serotonin.

Exceptions to SSRI Use	
Variety of depression	**Specific alternative to SSRIs**
Patient with depression and neuropathic pain	Use desvenlafaxine since it is approved for both depression and neuropathy.
Patient with depression who is fearful of weight gain or sexual side effects	Use bupropion since it has fewer sexual side effects and less weight gain than SSRIs. May also be used as adjunct treatment for SSRI-induced sexual side effects.

DEPRESSION WITH PSYCHOTIC FEATURES → PSYCH FEATURES NOT PRESENT W/O DEPRESSION

SCHIZOAFFECTIVE → PSYCHOTIC THEN MOOD DISORDER

▶ **TIP**

The USMLE Step 2 CK will not give you 2 SSRIs from which to choose.

A 45-year-old woman was recently seen by her primary care physician due to complaints of depressed mood, lack of pleasure, sleep problems, decreased appetite and weight, decreased energy, and problems with concentration. She states that these symptoms started when she was fired from her job about 4 weeks ago, and that since then, she has been unable to function.

What is the most indicated treatment at this time?

a. Alprazolam
b. Paroxetine
c. Bupropion
d. Venlafaxine
e. Trazodone
f. Electroconvulsive therapy

Answer: The correct answer is (B). She has a diagnosis of major depression and the first-line treatment is the use of an SSRI medication because of a better side-effect profile compared to the other therapies. All others, except alprazolam and electroconvulsive therapy, would be useful but not the first choice. Alprazolam is simply a benzodiazepine and acts as an anxiolytic, not an antidepressant. Electroconvulsive therapy might be useful if initial therapy did not work or the depression was far more severe and was associated with psychotic features.

> The choices on the USMLE Step 2 CK may include an SSRI and another antidepressant medication. Pick the cleanest, which is the SSRI.

Bipolar Disorder   MANIA ↑ NE ↑ SEROTONIN

DEFINITION

Bipolar disorder is a mood disorder where the patient experiences manic symptoms that last at least one week and cause significant distress in the level of functioning. **Manic** symptoms include **elevated mood, increased self-esteem, distractibility, pressured speech, decreased need for sleep, an increase in goal-directed activity, racing thoughts, and excessive involvement in pleasurable activities**. This disorder typically starts with depression.

Diagnosis

Make sure the condition is not secondary to drug use, such as **cocaine** or **amphetamine use**. Obtain a good history and urine drug screen.

Classification

The difference between **mania** and **hypomania** has to do with the **severity of symptoms**, level of functioning, and duration. Manic symptoms last more than one week, affect functioning, and are severe enough to warrant hospitalization. Hypomanic symptoms last less than one week, do not severely affect functioning, and are not severe enough to warrant hospitalization.

Types of Bipolar Disorders	
Bipolar disorder type I	Mania and depression
Bipolar disorder type II	Hypomania and depression

A 21-year-old college student was taken to the university clinic after she was noted to be acting bizarrely in class. She is talking fast and reported that she has not slept for over 4 days. She appears to be giggling and not paying attention in class. Her roommate reported that she has been drinking alcohol excessively over the last few days and has had many sexual contacts with unknown men.

What is the most likely diagnosis?

a. Alcohol-induced mood disorder
b. Bipolar disorder type I
c. Bipolar disorder type II
d. Major depression with psychosis
e. Cyclothymia

*Answer: The correct answer is **(B)**. The patient is exhibiting mania, as shown by her pressured speech, decreased sleep, increased libido, and inappropriate behavior. The symptoms are severe enough that her level of functioning is affected. Bipolar disorder occurs more frequently in young individuals.*

TREATMENT

- You must distinguish whether you are treating acute mania or bipolar depression.
- If **acute mania**, **use lithium**, valproic acid, and atypical antipsychotics as first-line treatments.
- If bipolar depression, lithium or lamotrigine is indicated.
- If acute mania with severe symptoms, consider the use of atypical antipsychotics due to shorter onset of action. If kidneys are compromised, do not use lithium.

▶ **TIP**

Lithium is the **correct** answer to most **bipolar questions.**

A 33-year-old man was taken to the emergency room by the police after neighbors complained about his behavior. His family informed the doctor that he has been diagnosed with bipolar disorder and was recently started on lithium. While in the emergency room, he became combative and punched a nurse on the mouth.

What is the next step in the management of this patient?

a. Obtain lithium level
b. Admit to psychiatric unit
c. Refer to psychiatry
d. Add valproic acid
e. Olanzapine

*Answer: The correct answer is (E). The patient is exhibiting mania and **you do not need to verify the lithium level given that his symptoms are acute.** He apparently has been noncompliant with medications and obtaining a level is not the correct answer. He needs to be medicated, and antipsychotics are considered first-line treatment for bipolar patients, especially if acutely and severely manic. Admitting an agitated patient to the psychiatric unit is not as important as administering adequate treatment. "Refer to psychiatry" is never the correct answer on Step 2 CK.*

Dysthymia

Dysthymia is characterized by the presence of **depressed mood** that lasts most of the day and is present almost continuously. Symptoms must be present for **more than 2 years**. Treatment is with **antidepressant medications and psychotherapy.** No hx of MOD or suicidal ideation

Cyclothymia

Cyclothymia is characterized by the presence of **hypomanic episodes** and mild **depression**. Symptoms must be present for more than 2 years. Treatment is with lithium, valproic acid or carbamazepine, and psychotherapy.

Atypical Depression

Atypical depression is characterized by **reverse vegetative changes** such as **increased sleep**, **increased weight**, and **increased appetite**. Mood tends to be worse in the evening and patients may complain of extremities feeling "heavy." Treatment is with **SSRIs** or **MAOIs**. SSRIs have a better side-effect profile. If MAOIs and SSRIs are in the same question, choose SSRIs because of the side-effect profile.

▶ **TIP**

Usually **MAOIs** are the correct answer on USMLE Step 2 CK for the treatment of **atypical depression**.

Seasonal Affective Disorder

Seasonal affective disorder (SAD) is characterized by seasonal changes in mood during fall and winter. Symptoms include weight gain, increased sleep, and lethargy. Treat with **phototherapy** and bupropion.

Postpartum Disorders				
Disorder	**Onset**	**Symptoms**	**Mother's feelings toward baby**	**Treatment**
Postpartum blues or "baby blues"	Immediately after birth up to 2 weeks	Sadness, mood lability, tearfulness	No negative feelings	Supportive, usually self-limited
Postpartum depression	Within 1–3 months after birth	Depressed mood, weight changes, sleep disturbances, and excessive anxiety	May have negative feelings toward baby	Antidepressant medications
Postpartum psychosis	Within 2–3 weeks after birth	Depression, delusions, and thoughts of harm	May have thoughts of harming baby	Antipsychotic medication, lithium, and possibly antidepressants

Bereavement (Grief)

Normal bereavement typically begins after the **death of a loved one** and includes feelings of **sadness**, **worrying about the deceased**, irritability, sleep difficulties, poor concentration, and tearfulness. It **typically lasts less than 6 months**, but can go on longer. Treatment is generally limited to supportive **psychotherapy. Medical therapy is a wrong answer.**

Diagnosis of major depression (greater severity than bereavement):

- Thoughts of death
- Morbid preoccupation with **worthlessness**
- Marked psychomotor retardation
- Psychosis
- Prolonged functional impairment
- **Symptoms last longer than 2 months** and adversely affect functioning

---

A 65-year-old man was brought to the office by his daughter after she became concerned about him. He has been hopeless and helpless since his wife died 3 months ago. His daughter is worried about his isolative behavior and lack of appetite. He has lost over 30 pounds. He does not seem interested in getting better and believes he should have died with his wife.

What is the most likely diagnosis?

a. Bereavement
b. Dysthymia
c. Major depression
d. Adjustment disorder
e. Bipolar disorder

Answer: The correct answer is (C). Although it has been less than 6 months since his wife died, his symptoms are severe enough to warrant a diagnosis of major depression. He has no interest in things, has lost weight, feels hopeless and helpless, and believes he should have died as well. He needs to be treated with antidepressants, and you must ensure that he is not suicidal since he is at high risk.

TREATMENT

Antidepressants, Mood Stabilizers, Electroconvulsive Therapy	
Type of medication	**Adverse effects**
Tricyclic antidepressants (amitriptyline, nortriptyline, imipramine)	Hypotension, dry mouth, constipation, confusion, arrhythmias, sexual side effects, weight gain, GI disturbances
Monoamine oxidase inhibitors (phenelzine, isocarboxazid, tranylcypromine)	Monitor diet, given that food rich in tyramine will produce hypertension. Safe foods include white wine and processed cheese. Unsafe foods include red wine, aged cheese, and chocolate.
Serotonin selective reuptake inhibitors (fluoxetine, paroxetine, sertraline, citalopram, escitalopram, fluvoxamine)	Headaches, weight changes, sexual side effects, GI disturbances
Serotonin norepinephrine reuptake inhibitors (venlafaxine, duloxetine, desvenlafaxine)	Hypertension, blurry vision, weight changes, sexual side effects, GI disturbances
Others (bupropion, mirtazapine, trazodone)	Bupropion has increased risk for seizures, trazodone has increased risk for priapism, and mirtazapine has increased risk for weight gain and sedation.
Lithium	Tremors, weight gain, GI disturbance, nephrotoxic, teratogenic, leukocytosis, diabetes insipidus. Severe toxicity gives confusion, ataxia, lethargy, and abnormal reflexes.
Valproic acid	Tremors, weight gain, GI disturbances, alopecia, teratogenic, hepatotoxic. Must monitor levels; toxicity causes hyponatremia, coma, or death.
Lamotrigine	Stevens-Johnson syndrome
Electroconvulsive therapy	Headaches, transient memory loss

What is the single most effective treatment for depression?

a. Electroconvulsive therapy

b. Fluoxetine

c. Venlafaxine

d. Imipramine

e. Phenelzine

Answer: The correct answer is (A). Although electroconvulsive therapy (ECT) is usually used for suicidal patients or those who do not respond to treatment, it is considered the best treatment for depression. All others are equally efficacious, but the SSRIs are used more frequently due to side-effect profiles.

Serotonin Syndrome

Serotonin syndrome is a potentially life-threatening disorder occurring as a result of therapeutic drug use of SSRIs, often with inadvertent interactions between drugs, overdose, or recreational use of drugs that are serotonergic in origin.

Common symptoms include:

- **Cognitive effects:** agitation, confusion, hallucinations, hypomania
- **Autonomic effects:** sweating, hyperthermia, tachycardia, nausea, diarrhea, shivering
- **Somatic effects:** tremors, myoclonus

TREATMENT

- Stop SSRI medication.
- Symptomatic treatment of fever, diarrhea, hypertension
- Cyproheptadine (serotonin antagonist)

BENZO's

PSYCHOTIC DISORDERS

Classification of Psychotic Disorders			
Disorder	**Duration of symptoms**	**Symptoms**	**Treatment**
Brief psychotic disorder	More than 1 day but less than 1 month	Delusions, hallucinations, disorganized speech, grossly disorganized or catatonic behavior	Antipsychotic medication
Schizophreniform disorders	More than 1 month but less than 6 months	Delusions, hallucinations, disorganized speech, grossly disorganized or catatonic behavior, and negative symptoms (flat affect, poor grooming, social withdrawal)	Antipsychotic medication
Schizophrenia	More than 6 months	Delusions, hallucinations, disorganized speech, grossly disorganized or catatonic behavior, and negative symptoms. Severely affects level of functioning.	Antipsychotic medication

DISORGANIZED SPEECH
DISORGANIZED DRESS
+ Sx → DELUSIONS | HALLUCINATIONS
— Sx → FLAT AFFECT | POVERTY OF SPEECH

513

▶ **TIP**

Be careful with **duration of symptoms**; it is the only thing that **distinguishes brief psychosis, schizophreniform, and schizophrenia.** If no time is mentioned, always choose schizophrenia as the correct answer to the "What is the most likely diagnosis?" question.

Schizophrenia   ↑ DOPAMINE

DEFINITION

Schizophrenia is a thought disorder that impairs **judgment, behavior,** and the **ability to interpret reality.** The symptoms must be present for at least 6 months and it must affect functioning. There is an equal incidence in men and women but it **affects men earlier** due to earlier age of onset. Urine drug screen is important in order to **rule out cocaine or amphetamine use.**

BRIEF PSYCHOSIS < 1 month
SCHIZOPHRENIFORM >1 month < 6 months
SCHIZOPHRENIA >6 months

MIGHT SEE ENLARGED VENTRICLES ON IMAGING

Types of Schizophrenia	
Type of schizophrenia	**Specific features/diagnostic criteria**
Paranoid	Characterized by **delusions** or **hallucinations,** mostly of the persecutory or grandiose type. Most common type of schizophrenia and has a later age of onset.
Catatonic	Characterized by **psychomotor disturbances,** ranging from retardation to excitation. These include stupor, rigidity, excitement, or posturing. Mutism is common.
Disorganized	Characterized by marked regression to **disinhibited behavior** with little contact with reality. Patients typically **appear disheveled** and have **bizarre emotional responses.** These patients have the worst prognosis and **earliest age of onset.**
Residual	Characterized by **lack of positive symptoms** (hallucinations, delusion) but presence of **negative symptoms** (flat affect, poor grooming, social withdrawal).
Undifferentiated	Characterized by **not meeting criteria for other types.**

TREATMENT

- **Hospitalize** patients who are acutely psychotic.
- Ensure patient safety and use an atypical antipsychotic, such as risperidone, olanzapine, quetiapine, ziprasidone, aripiprazole, or paliperidone.

- In emergency situation where intramuscular medication is needed, consider olanzapine or ziprazidone; haloperidol may be used, but has more side effects.
- If noncompliant with medication, consider a long-acting antipsychotic medication such as risperidone as first-line treatment. Haloperidol may be used but it has more side effects.
- **Clozapine is used when patients do not respond to an adequate trial of typical** or atypical antipsychotics; **never used as a first-line treatment.**

▶ **TIP**

You need to know the differences in the side-effect profiles of the atypical antipsychotics. It is common to have 2 appear on the test and you need to pick the best one based on side effects for that patient.

TYPICALS — CHLORPROMAZINE (LP)
  THIORIDIZINE (LP)

HALOPERIDOL (HP)
DROPERIDOL (HP)

Adverse Effects of Atypical Antipsychotic Medications	
Antipsychotic medication	**Specific adverse effects**
Olanzapine	Greater incidence of **diabetes** and **weight gain**; avoid in diabetic and obese patients
Risperidone	Greater incidence of **movement disorders**
Quetiapine	**Less incidence of movement disorders**
Ziprasidone	Increased risk of **prolongation of QT interval**; **avoid in patients with conduction defects**
Clozapine	High risk of agranulocytosis need to **monitor CBC** on regular basis; never used as first-line treatment given side-effect profile

ARIPIPRAZOLE

A 22-year-old woman was recently diagnosed with schizophrenia. She is 30 pounds overweight and suffers from diabetes Type 2. She is concerned about her medications and asks for your advice.

Which of the following would be most indicated in this patient?

a. Aripiprazole
b. Olanzapine
c. Quetiapine
d. Clozapine
e. Risperidone

*Answer: The correct answer is (A). Aripiprazole and ziprasidone are the **least likely to cause weight gain, diabetes**, and metabolic syndrome. Clozapine and olanzapine have the highest risk of metabolic abnormalities. Risperidone and quetiapine have medium risk.*

Management of Adverse Effects of Antipsychotic Medications			
Disorder	**Onset of symptoms**	**Symptoms**	**Treatment**
Acute dystonia	Hours to days	Muscle spasms, such as torticollis, laryngeal spasms, occulogyric crisis	Benztropine, trihexyphenidyl, diphenhydramine *(ANTI CHOLINERGIC)*
Akathisia	Weeks	Generalized restlessness, pacing, rocking, inability to relax	Reduce dose, beta blockers, switch to atypical medication
Tardive dyskinesia	Rare before 6 months *>6 months*	Abnormal involuntary movements of head, limb, and trunk. Perioral movements are the most common.	Switch to atypical antipsychotic. Clozapine has least risk.
Neuroleptic malignant syndrome	Not time limited	Muscular rigidity, fever, autonomic changes, agitation, and obtundation	Dantrolene or bromocriptine

You have recently diagnosed a 23-year-old man with schizophrenia and started him on haloperidol. Within a few hours he develops muscle stiffness, and his eyes roll upward and he cannot move them down.

What is the most likely diagnosis?

a. Tardive dyskinesia
b. Neuroleptic malignant syndrome
c. Akathisia
d. Serotonin syndrome
e. Acute dystonic reaction

*Answer: The correct answer is (E). Acute dystonic reactions develop within hours of the use of medications. This side effect is typical for haloperidol. The treatment of choice is **benztropine** or **diphenhydramine**, which can be given with the haloperidol or after should side effects occur.*

Delusional Disorder

Delusional disorder is characterized by the prominence of **non-bizarre delusions** for more than one month and **no impairment in level of functioning**. In other words, the patient may believe the country is about to be invaded, but he or she **still obeys the law, goes to work, and pays bills**. Hallucinations are not present. Treatment is with atypical antipsychotic agents as first-line therapy. You may also consider psychotherapy to help promote reality testing.

ANXIETY DISORDERS ↑ NE ↓ SEROTONIN ↓ GABA

Panic Disorder

DEFINITION

Panic disorder is the experience of **intense anxiety** along with feelings of **dread** and doom. This is accompanied by at least 4 symptoms of autonomic hyperactivity, such as **diaphoresis**, **trembling**, **chest pain**, **fear of dying**, **chills**, **palpitations**, **shortness of breath**, nausea, dizziness, dissociative symptoms, and paresthesias. These sensations typically **last less than 30 minutes** and may be accompanied by **agoraphobia**, defined as the fear of places where escape is felt to be difficult.

Panic disorder is typically seen in women, can occur at any time, and usually has no specific stressor. It is important to ensure that thyroid disease, hypoglycemia, and cardiac disease have been ruled out.

TREATMENT

- **SSRIs**, typically fluoxetine, paroxetine, and sertraline, are indicated for this disorder.
- Along with SSRIs, patients may benefit from benzodiazepines such as alprazolam. Begin with both and then taper the benzodiazepine given the potential for abuse.
- Behavioral and individual therapy are also helpful, but are not sufficient as the only treatment without medication.

*Which is considered to be first-line treatment for panic **disorder**?*

a. Alprazolam
b. Buspirone
c. Sertraline
d. Imipramine
e. Fluvoxamine

*Answer: The correct answer is (**C**). SSRIs are considered to be first-line treatment. If the question is panic **attack**, then alprazolam is the correct answer; if a single panic attack is the diagnosis, a benzodiazepine is the treatment. If panic **disorder** is the diagnosis, then pick the SSRI.*

Phobias

A phobia is the **fear of an object or situation** and the need to avoid it. Phobias may be learned and involve 2 main types.

Two Types of Phobias	
Type of phobia	**Characteristic of the phobia**
Specific phobia	Fear of an object, such as animals, heights, or cars
Social phobia	Fear of a situation, such as public restrooms, eating in public, or public speaking. These involve situations where something potentially embarrassing may happen.

Diagnosis

The diagnosis usually can be made by obtaining a good history where patients indicate anxiety symptoms in specific situations or when in contact with feared objects.

TREATMENT

- **Behavioral modification** techniques such as systematic desensitization expose individuals to their feared objects, moving from the least anxiety-provoking to the most anxiety-provoking.
- Patients are also taught **relaxation techniques** such as breathing or guided imagery.

> Beta blockers such as atenolol or propanolol are only used for performance anxiety such as stage fright. They are given 30 minutes to 1 hour before the performance.

A 40-year-old man was referred to a psychiatrist by his physician because he is "too shy." He has problems going to parties, feels anxious about getting close to others, and stays at home in fear that others would laugh at him. When confronted by others, he develops severe anxiety as well as hyperventilation and increased sweating.

Which is the most likely diagnosis?

a. Panic disorder
b. Social anxiety
c. Generalized anxiety disorder
d. Specific phobia
e. Acute stress disorder

Answer: The correct answer is (B). Social anxiety is characterized by fear of embarrassment in social situations. These patients have problems going out in fear that others will laugh at them.

OBSESSIVE COMPULSIVE DISORDER

DEFINITION

Obsessive compulsive disorder (OCD) is a disorder where patients typically experience either **obsessions alone** or, most commonly, a combination of obsessions and compulsions typically **affect the individual's level of functioning**.

Difference between Obsessions and Compulsions	
Obsessions	**Thoughts** that are intrusive, senseless, and distressing to the patient, thus increasing anxiety. These include fear of contamination.
Compulsions	**Rituals**, such as counting and checking, that are done to neutralize thoughts. These are time consuming and tend to lower anxiety.

Diagnosis

OCD is seen more frequently in young patients. There is an equal incidence in men and women. OCD can coexist with Tourette disorder.

TREATMENT

- **SSRIs are the treatment of choice.** Fluoxetine, paroxetine, sertraline, citalopram, or fluvoxamine are most commonly used as first-line agents.
- The main behavioral therapy used is exposure and response prevention.

POSTTRAUMATIC STRESS DISORDER AND ACUTE STRESS DISORDER

DEFINITION

In both posttraumatic stress disorder (PTSD) and acute stress disorder, **individuals have been exposed to a stressor** to which they react with fear and helplessness. **Patients continually relive the event** and avoid anything that reminds them of the event. These stressors are usually overwhelming and involve such events as war, rape, hurricanes, or earthquakes. The **symptoms adversely affect the patient's level of functioning**. Other symptoms include increased startle response, hypervigilance, sleep disturbances, anger outbursts, and concentration difficulties.

Difference between Posttraumatic Stress Disorder and Acute Stress Disorder	
Posttraumatic stress disorder	Symptoms last for more than **1 month**
Acute stress disorder	Symptoms last for **more than 2 days** and a **maximum of 1 month**. They occur within 1 month of the traumatic event.

Diagnosis

The **main feature** in correctly identifying the diagnosis is determining the **time period** when the traumatic events occurred in relationship to the symptoms. Depression and substance abuse must be ruled out since both worsen the diagnosis.

TREATMENT

- First-line treatment includes **paroxetine and sertraline**.
- **Relaxation techniques** and hypnosis have been proven to be helpful in these patients.
- Psychotherapy after traumatic events will allow for the development of coping techniques and acceptance of the event.

A 35-year-old woman has complained of palpitations, dizziness, and increased sweating for at least 8 months. She has visited numerous physicians and none have been helpful. Her husband is concerned because she cannot relax and worries about everything. She worries about her parents' health even though they are healthy. She worries about her finances, although her husband assures her they are financially secure.

What is the most likely diagnosis?

a. Generalized anxiety disorder
b. Phobias
c. Panic disorder
d. Adjustment disorder
e. Social anxiety

Answer: The correct answer is (A). The main feature of generalized anxiety disorder is the chronic worrying about things that do not merit concern. It is also accompanied by other symptoms of anxiety, as well as sleep and concentration problems.

GENERALIZED ANXIETY DISORDER

This is a disorder in which patients experience **excessive anxiety and worry** about most things, lasting more than 6 months. Typically, the **anxiety is out of proportion to the event**. This is accompanied by **fatigue**, concentration difficulties, sleep problems, muscle tension, and restlessness. Patients are usually **women** and complain of feeling anxious as long as they can remember.

TREATMENT

- **SSRIs** such as fluoxetine, paroxetine, sertraline, or citalopram are indicated in this disorder.
- **Venlafaxine and buspirone have** also been used.
- Psychotherapy and behavioral therapy are beneficial as well but are not considered first-line agents in most patients.

Antianxiety Medications and Their Adverse Effects

Antianxiety medication	Adverse effects
Benzodiazepines (diazepam, lorazepam, clonazepam, alprazolam, oxazepam, chlordiazepoxide, temazepam, flurazepam)	Sedation, confusion, memory deficits, respiratory depression, and addiction potential
Buspirone	Headaches, nausea, dizziness

Antianxiety Medications and Their Specific Indications

Antianxiety medication	Specific indications
Lorazepam	Used frequently in emergency situations because it can be given intramuscularly
Clonazepam	May be used if addiction is a concern given it has a longer half-life
Chlordiazepoxide, oxazepam	Used frequently in treatment of alcohol withdrawal
Alprazolam	Used frequently in panic disorder
Flurazepam, temazepam, triazolam	Approved as hypnotics (rarely used)

Flumazenil is a benzodiazepine antagonist used only when:

- The overdose is acute

and

- You are certain that there is no chronic dependence

Flumazenil can cause seizures in benzodiazepine-dependent patients. It causes acute withdrawal, which can be tremor or seizures similar to delirium tremens (alcohol withdrawal).

SUBSTANCE-RELATED DISORDERS

Definition of Specific Substance Abuse Disorders

Substance abuse disorder	Definition of specific substance abuse disorder
Intoxication	Reversible experience with a substance that leads to either psychological or physiological changes
Withdrawal	**Cessation or reduction** of a substance leading to either **psychological or physiological changes**
Abuse	Maladaptive pattern of use of substances that leads to engaging in hazardous situations, legal problems, inability to fulfill obligations, and **continued use despite adverse consequences**
Dependence	Maladaptive pattern of use of substances that leads to tolerance. There is **withdrawal when trying to cut down**. Patients spend a great deal of time engaging in drug use. There is continued use despite adverse consequences.

		Presentation and Treatment of Intoxication and Withdrawal		
Substance	Signs and symptoms of intoxication	Treatment of intoxication	Signs and symptoms of withdrawal	Treatment of withdrawal
Alcohol	Talkative, sullen, gregarious, moody, disinhibited	Mechanical ventilation if severe	Tremors, hallucinations, seizures, delirium tremens	Benzodiazepines, thiamine, multivitamins, folic acid
Amphetamines and cocaine	Euphoria, hypervigilance, autonomic hyperactivity, weight loss, pupillary dilatation, perceptual disturbances	Antipsychotics and/or benzodiazepines and/or antihypertensives	Anxiety, tremulousness, headache, increased appetite, depression, risk of suicide	Bupropion and/or bromocriptine
Cannabis	Impaired motor coordination, slowed sense of time, social withdrawal, increased appetite, conjunctival injection	None	None	None
Hallucinogens	Ideas of reference, perceptual disturbances, impaired judgment, tremors, incoordination, dissociative symptoms	Antipsychotics and/or benzodiazepines and/or talking down	None	None
Inhalants	Belligerence, apathy, aggression, impaired judgment, stupor, or coma	Antipsychotics	None	None
Opiates	Apathy, dysphoria, pupillary constriction, drowsiness, slurred speech, coma, or death	Naloxone	Fever, chills, lacrimation, abdominal cramps, muscle spasms, diarrhea	Clonidine, methadone, or buprenorphine
Phencyclidine (PCP)	Belligerence, psychomotor agitation, violence, nystagmus, hypertension, seizures	Antipsychotics and/or benzodiazepines and/or talking down	None	None
Anabolic steroids	Irritability, aggression, mania, psychosis	Antipsychotics	Depression, headaches, anxiety, increased concern over body's physical state	SSRIs

If you suspect someone is an alcoholic, do the **CAGE** test. Two positive responses to the four questions are considered a positive test and indicate that further assessment is warranted.

TREATMENT

- **Detoxification:** usually 5 to 10 days, mostly in hospital settings to assure safe detoxification
- **Rehabilitation:** usually 28 days or more, with a focus on relapse prevention techniques
- Alcoholics Anonymous
- Narcotics Anonymous
- Pharmacologic treatments: often include disulfram (acetaldehyde dehydrogenase inhibitor), naltrexone (opioid receptor antagonist), and acamprosate

A 65-year-old engineer is taken to the emergency room after being involved in a motor vehicle accident. He suffered a fracture of the femur and some cuts and bruises. He is admitted to the medicine floor and started on oxycodone. The day after admission, he appears confused and has observable tremors in both extremities. He becomes concerned about "bugs on the walls" in his room and asks for your help.

What is the most likely explanation for his symptoms?

a. Brain concussion
b. Alcohol withdrawal
c. Oxycodone intoxication
d. Brief psychotic disorder
e. Schizophrenia

*Answer: The correct answer is **(B)**. Most withdrawal questions are asked in a hospital setting on the next day after admission. He presents with uncomplicated alcohol withdrawal, characterized by visual hallucinations and tremors.*

SOMATOFORM DISORDER, FACTITIOUS DISORDER, AND MALINGERING

Somatoform Disorders

DEFINITION

Somatoform disorders are a group of conditions characterized by the presentation of **physical symptoms with no medical explanation**. Typically the symptoms are severe enough to **adversely affect level of functioning**. They are seen more frequently in **young women** and usually have some **psychological component** of which the patient is unaware. **Psychotherapy is the treatment** of choice given that the source of the symptoms is psychological in nature.

Types of Somatoform Disorders	
Type of somatoform disorder	**Definition/diagnostic criteria**
Somatization disorder	Patients must have at least 4 **pain**, 2 **gastrointestinal**, **1 sexual**, and **1 pseudoneurological** symptom.
Hypochondriasis	Patients believe that they have some **specific disease despite constant reassurance.**
Conversion	Typically affects **voluntary motor or sensory functions** that are indicative of a medical condition but are usually caused by psychological factors. Can be associated with "la belle indifference," where the **patient is unconcerned about his or her impairment.**
Body dysmorphic disorder	Patients **believe** that some part of **the body is abnormal**, defective, or misshapen.
Pain disorder	The **presence of pain** is the main complaint, and must have **psychological factors** associated with the pain.

A 35-year-old married woman with 3 children is taken to the doctor's office after frequent complaints of dizziness, nausea, diarrhea, vomiting, pain during intercourse, paresthesias, leg pain, stomach pain, food intolerance, and headaches. She has these complaints frequently. She has been tried on numerous medications but none have proven to be beneficial. A neurological examination is normal.

What is the next step in the management of this patient?

a. Lorazepam
b. Sertraline
c. Individual psychotherapy
d. Lithium
e. Risperidone

Answer: The correct answer is (C). She has somatization disorder, which is treated with individual psychotherapy given that psychological issues are the cause of her symptoms. She should have one primary caretaker and not be sent to specialists. SSRIs such as sertraline treat fibromyalgia and depression. Lorazepam, a benzodiazepine, treats anxiety disorder. Lithium treats bipolar disorder. Risperidone is for psychosis.

Factitious Disorder

DEFINITION

In **factitious disorder**, an individual **fakes an illness** in order to get attention and emotional support in the patient role. This can be either a psychological or physical illness. Psychological symptoms include hallucinations, delusions, depression, and bizarre behavior. Physical symptoms include abdominal pain, fever, nausea, vomiting, or hematomas. At times, **they may inflict life-threatening injuries on themselves in order to get attention**. This behavior may be compulsive at times. Factitious disorder was formerly known as **Münchausen syndrome**. If factitious disorder is by proxy, the caretaker will fake signs and symptoms in another person, usually a child, in order to assume the sick role by proxy as the caregiver.

Diagnosis

Typically, patients with this disorder are **women** who may have a **history of being employed in healthcare**. Men more often have **physical symptoms**. The patient's ultimate goal is to gain admission to the hospital. You must always exclude any medical disorder with similar symptoms.

> Factitious disorder cannot be diagnosed without first confirming that a legitimate medical illness is not present.

TREATMENT

No specific therapy has been proven to be effective in these patients. When a child is involved in factitious disorder by proxy, child protective services should be contacted to ensure the child's safety.

Malingering

Malingering is characterized by the **conscious production of signs and symptoms for an obvious gain,** such as avoiding work, evading criminal prosecution, or achieving financial gain. **Malingering is not a mental illness**.

Diagnosis/Management

Malingering is seen more frequently in prisoners and military personnel. It is typically **diagnosed when there is a discrepancy between the patient's complaints and the actual physical or laboratory findings**. If medical evaluation reveals malingering, then confront the patient with the outcome.

> A lack of cooperation from patients is characteristic of malingering.

ADJUSTMENT DISORDER

Adjustment disorder is characterized by a **maladaptive reaction to an identifiable stressor,** such as loss of job, divorce, or failure in school. The symptoms usually occur within 3 months of the stressor and must remit within 6 months of removal of the stressor. The symptoms include **anxiety, depression, or disturbances of conduct**. They are severe enough to cause **impairment in functioning**. Psychotherapy is the treatment of choice. Both individual and group therapy have been used effectively.

PERSONALITY DISORDERS

This is a group of disorders characterized by personality patterns that are pervasive, inflexible, and maladaptive.

Types of Personality Disorders	
Type of personality disorder	**Definition/diagnostic criteria**
Paranoid	**Suspicious**, **mistrustful**, secretive, isolated, and questioning of the loyalty of family and friends
Schizoid	Choice of **solitary activities**, lack of close friends, **emotional coldness**, no desire for or enjoyment of close relationships
Schizotypal	Ideas of reference, **magical thinking**, odd thinking, eccentric behavior, increased social anxiety, **brief psychotic episodes**
Histrionic	**Must be the center of attention**, inappropriate sexual behavior, self-dramatization, use physical appearance to draw attention to self
Antisocial	**Failure to conform to social rules**, deceitful, lack of remorse, impulsive, **aggressive towards others**, irresponsible, must be over the age of 18
Borderline	Unstable relationships, impulsive, recurrent suicidal behaviors, **chronic feelings of emptiness**, **inappropriate anger**, dissociative symptoms when severely stressed, brief psychotic episodes
Narcissistic	**Grandiose sense of self**, belief that they are special, lack empathy, sense of entitlement, require excessive admiration
Avoidant	**Unwilling to get involved with people**, views self as socially inept, reluctant to take risks, **feelings of inadequacy**
Dependent	Difficulty making day-to-day decisions, **unable to assume responsibility**, unable to express disagreement, fear of being alone, seeks relationship as source of care
Obsessive compulsive	**Preoccupied with details**, rigid, orderly, perfectionistic, excessively devoted to work, inflexible

TREATMENT

- Individual **psychotherapy**
- Medications if mood or anxiety symptoms are present

Which of the following personality disorders has been associated with positive psychotic symptoms?

a. Borderline
b. Histrionic
c. Schizoid
d. Paranoid
e. Antisocial

Answer: The correct answer is (A). Borderline and schizotypal personality disorders may have short-lived psychotic episodes that are brief and usually occur after stressful situations.

EATING DISORDERS

A 15-year-old girl is brought to the clinic by her mother, who found her vomiting in the bathroom. Her mother reports that the girl vomits daily after each meal. She is sometimes observed exercising excessively. She has numerous calluses on her hands as well as cavities. She is 5'5'' and weighs 90 pounds.

What is her most likely diagnosis?

a. Bulimia nervosa
b. Anorexia nervosa
c. Eating disorder not otherwise specified
d. Obesity
e. Atypical depression

Answer: The correct answer is (B). The main focus of this question is the height and weight. She should weigh about 110 pounds but weighs only 90 pounds. This is indicative of the weight loss seen in anorexia nervosa. She obviously purges and as a result has calluses and cavities. Amenorrhea, significant weight loss, and abnormal preoccupation with body image are the key to the diagnosis of anorexia.

Anorexia Nervosa

DEFINITION

Anorexia is characterized by **failure to maintain a normal body weight**, fear and preoccupation of gaining weight, and **body image disturbance**. There is an unrealistic self-evaluation as overweight. Amenorrhea is common from low body weight. These patients tend to **deny their emaciated condition**. They show **great concern with appearance** and frequently examine and weigh themselves. They typically lose weight by maintaining strict caloric control, excessive exercise, **purging**, and **fasting**, with **laxative and diuretic abuse**.

Diagnosis

Anorexia is seen more frequently in **teenage girls** between the ages of 14 and 18. There is evidence of severe weight loss. Hypotension, bradycardia, lanugo hair, and edema may be present. EKG changes such as rhythm disorders occur as a result of potassium deficiency. Arrhythmia is the most common cause of death.

REFEEDING SYNDROME

TRANSFER FROM FAT METAB TO CARB METAB.

- ↓ PHOSPHATES
- RHABDOMYOLYSIS
- CARDIOVASCULAR COLLAPSE
- SEIZURES

TREATMENT

- **Hospitalization** to prevent **dehydration, starvation, electrolyte imbalances**, and death
- **Psychotherapy**
- Behavioral therapy
- **SSRIs** have been used to promote weight gain.

Bulimia Nervosa

DEFINITION

Bulimia is characterized by **frequent binge eating**, as evidenced by eating large amounts of food in a discrete amount of time, as well as a **lack of control of overeating episodes**. This is accompanied by a compensatory behavior to prevent weight gain in the form of **purging, misuse of laxatives and diuretics, fasting**, and **excessive exercise**. The patient's self-evaluation is unduly influenced by body shape and weight.

Diagnosis

Bulimia is seen more frequently in women and occurs **later in adolescence than anorexia nervosa**. Most of these women are of **normal weight** but do have a **history of obesity**.

TREATMENT

- **Does not require hospitalization unless severe electrolyte abnormality is present**
- Psychotherapy
- SSRIs

Eating Disorder Not Otherwise Specified

A designation of eating disorder not otherwise specified (NOS) is used when patients do not meet criteria for either anorexia nervosa or bulimia nervosa.

Examples include:

- Criteria for anorexia present in girls but menstruation is normal
- Anorexic patient with normal weight
- Use of compensatory behavior after eating normal amounts of food

SLEEP DISORDERS

Narcolepsy

Characterized by **excessive daytime sleepiness** and abnormalities of REM sleep, narcolepsy most frequently begins in young adulthood. Sleep studies are usually indicated in the diagnosis. No therapy has been found to be curative.

The patient is managed with **forced naps during the day. Modafinil** is a medication used to maintain alertness.

Psychiatric and Physical Symptoms of Narcolepsy (Sleep Disorder)	
Specific feature of narcolepsy	**Characteristics of sleep disorders**
Sleep attacks	Episodes of **irresistible sleepiness** and feeling **refreshed upon awakening**
Cataplexy	**Sudden loss of muscle tone**: considered pathognomonic and may be precipitated by loud noise or emotions
Hypnogogic and hypnopompic hallucinations	**Hallucinations** that occur as the patient is **going to sleep and waking up**
Sleep paralysis	**Patient awake but unable to move**; this typically occurs upon awakening

Insomnia

Insomnia is a disorder characterized by the **inability to initiate or maintain sleep**. Insomnia may be due to anxiety and depression. It is severe enough to adversely affect level of functioning. It is typically seen in women who complain of feeling tired or have increased appetite and yawning. Treatment consists of **sleep hygiene techniques** such as going to bed and waking up at the same time, avoiding caffeinated beverages, and avoiding daytime naps. Behavioral modification techniques include using the bed only for sleeping and not for reading, watching TV, or eating. Medical therapy consists of zolpidem, eszopiclone, or zaleplon.

LONG TERM USE OK.

HUMAN SEXUALITY

Terminology of Human Sexuality	
Sexual characteristic	**Definition**
Sexual identity	Based on a person's secondary sexual characteristics
Gender identity	Based on a person's sense of maleness or femaleness, established by the age of 3
Gender role	Based on external patterns of behavior that reflect inner sense of gender identity
Sexual orientation	Based on person's choice of love object; may be heterosexual, homosexual, bisexual, or asexual

Masturbation

- Normal precursor of object-related sexual behavior
- All men and women masturbate.
- Problematic only if it adversely interferes with daily functioning

Homosexuality

- Not considered a mental illness unless it is ego-dystonic (person not happy with sexual orientation)
- May be considered normal experimentation in teenagers

Sexual Dysfunction

Types of Sexual Dysfunction		
Disorder	**Definition**	**Treatment**
Impotence	Persistent or recurrent inability to attain or maintain an erection until completion of the sexual act	Rule out medical causes or medication, psychotherapy, couples sexual therapy
Premature ejaculation	Ejaculation before penetration or just after penetration, usually due to anxiety	Psychotherapy, behavioral modification techniques (stop and go, squeeze), SSRI medication
Dyspareunia	Pain associated with sexual intercourse, not diagnosed if due to medical condition	Psychotherapy
Vaginismus	Involuntary constriction of the outer third of the vagina preventing penile insertion	Psychotherapy, dilator therapy

Paraphilias

Paraphilias are a group of disorders that are **recurrent**, **sexually arousing**, and seen more frequently in men. They usually focus on humiliation, nonconsenting partners, or use of nonliving objects. Must occur for more than 6 months and cause distress as well as adversely affect level of functioning. Do not diagnose if done in experimentation.

Types of Paraphilias	
Type of paraphilia	**Definition**
Exhibitionism	Recurrent urge to expose oneself to strangers
Fetishism	Recurrent use of nonliving objects to achieve sexual pleasure
Pedophilia	Recurrent urges or arousal toward prepubescent children
Masochism	Recurrent urge or behavior involving the act of humiliation
Sadism	Recurrent urge or behavior involving acts in which physical or psychological suffering of victim is exciting
Transvestic fetishism	Recurrent urge or behavior involving cross dressing for sexual gratification; usually found in heterosexual males
Frotteurism	Rubbing, usually one's pelvis or erect penis, against a nonconsenting person for sexual gratification

TREATMENT

- Individual psychotherapy
- Behavioral modification techniques such as aversive conditioning
- Antiandrogens or SSRIs to reduce sexual drive

Gender Identity Disorder

This is a disorder characterized by the persistent discomfort and sense of inappropriateness regarding the patient's assigned sex.

Diagnosis

Gender identity disorder will manifest by wearing the opposite gender's clothes, using toys assigned to the opposite sex, play with opposite-sex children when young, and feeling unhappy about the person's own sexual assignment. Patients will take hormones when older to deepen voice, if female, or soften voice, if male. Women may bind their breasts and men may hide their penis and testicles. It is seen more frequently in young men.

TREATMENT

- Sexual reassignment surgery if approved
- Individual psychotherapy

SUICIDE

PRESENTATION

- Recent suicide attempt
- Complaints of suicidal thoughts
- Admission of suicidal thoughts
- Demonstration of suicidal behaviors (eg, buying weapons, giving away possessions, or writing a will)

Risk Factors

- Men
- Older adults
- Social isolation
- Presence of psychiatric illness/drug abuse
- Perceived hopelessness
- Previous attempts

TREATMENT

- Hospitalize patient
- Take all threats seriously

Section 10
Emergency Medicine

Toxicology/Poisoning/Overdose
Initial Management of Poisoning

A 32-year-old woman with a history of depression comes to the emergency department 30 minutes after taking a bottle of pills in an attempt to commit suicide. Blood pressure is 118/70, pulse is 90 per minute, and respirations are normal at 14 per minute. She refuses to tell you what she took.

What is the most appropriate next step in the management of this patient?

a. Induce emesis with ipecac
b. Gastric lavage
c. Psychiatric consultation
d. Serum chemistry
e. Urine toxicology screen
f. Cathartics/laxatives
g. Whole bowel irrigation
h. Naloxone
i. Flumazenil

Answer: The correct answer is (B). When ingestion is extremely recent, it is possible to try to remove the substance from the body prior to its absorption. Gastric emptying has very limited value because there is not much time between the ingestion and passage of the pills beyond the pyloric sphincter from where they cannot be removed. Pills, on an empty stomach, can leave in as little as 30 to 60 minutes. Gastric lavage can be attempted up to 2 hours after ingestion, but it will remove only 50% of pills at one hour and 15% at 2 hours. After 2 hours, it is useless. Although serum chemistry and urine toxicology screen should be done, they are not helpful this soon after ingestion. Ipecac and the induction of vomiting is wrong when a patient is already in the emergency department. Inducing vomiting needs 15 to 20 minutes to work, and only delays the administration of antidotes such as N-acetylcysteine which can be given orally.

Gastrointestinal Emptying

Gastric lavage may be useful in the first hour of ingestion. It is **dangerous** in:

- **Altered mental status:** may cause aspiration
- **Caustic ingestion:** causes burning of the esophagus and oropharynx

---

Gastric lavage is rarely done.

- Removes 50% of pills at 1 hour
- Removes 15% of pills at 2 hours

▶ **TIP**

Ipecac is always a **wrong answer** in the emergency department.

Ipecac

Although ipecac has been used as a home remedy in those with accidental overdose or pill ingestion **prior to coming to the hospital,** there is no benefit in using ipecac in the hospital. Ipecac needs 15 to 20 minutes to work and delays the administration of antidotes.

Cathartics

Cathartic agents such as sorbitol are **always a wrong answer.** Speeding up gastrointestinal transit time **does not eliminate the ingestion** without absorption.

Forced Diuresis

Giving **fluids and diuretics** to accelerate urinary excretion is **always a wrong answer.** More patients are **harmed** with **pulmonary edema** with this method than are helped.

Whole Bowel Irrigation

Placing a gastric tube and flushing out the GI tract with polyethylene glycol-electrolyte solution (GoLYTELY; Braintree Laboratories, Braintree, Massachusetts) is **almost always wrong.** Indications for this method are very narrow and limited to massive iron ingestion, lithium, and swallowing drug-filled packets (eg, smuggling).

Gastric emptying of any kind is always wrong with:

- Caustics (acids and alkali)
- Altered mental status

▶ TIP

When the answer is not clear and the **cause of overdose** is asked, say:

- Acetaminophen
- Aspirin

They are, by far, the most common cause of death by overdose.

▶ TIP

What to do is often unclear. **What is useless or dangerous** (ipecac, forced diuresis, cathartics) **is very clear.**

A woman comes to the emergency department one hour after taking a bottle of pills. Blood pressure is 118/70, pulse is 90/min, and respirations are 14/min. She is confused, disoriented, and lethargic.

What is the most appropriate next step in the management of this patient?

a. Flumazenil
b. Gastric lavage
c. Psychiatric consultation
d. Naloxone and dextrose
e. Intubation

Answer: The correct answer is (D). The best initial management of altered mental status of unclear etiology is an opiate antagonist and glucose. Opiate ingestion and diabetes are extremely common. Naloxone and glucose work instantaneously and have no adverse effects. If they do not work, perform intubation to protect the airway, possibly followed by gastric lavage. Intubation should not be done first. Naloxone is faster and emergency intubation is associated with aspiration, trauma to teeth, and the possibility of intubating the esophagus. Flumazenil reverses benzodiazepines, but can cause seizures from instant withdrawal.

▶ TIP

Psychiatric consultation is indicated when the overdose is from a suicide attempt, but is a wrong answer on USMLE Step 2 CK when specific antidotes and diagnostic tests are needed. You do not need a consultant to tell you to give naloxone and dextrose.

- **Opiate** overdose is **fatal: Give naloxone** immediately.
- **Benzodiazepine** overdose by itself is **not fatal** and acute withdrawal causes seizures. **Do not give flumazenil.**

Charcoal

Charcoal is benign and should be **given to anyone with a pill overdose.** Charcoal may not be effective for every overdose, but it is **not dangerous** in anyone. Charcoal can also remove toxic substances even after they have been absorbed. Blood levels of toxins drop faster in those given repeated doses of charcoal. **Charcoal is superior to lavage and ipecac.**

▶ **TIP**

When you don't know what to do in toxicology, give charcoal.

Acetaminophen

> Alcoholism decreases the amount of acetaminophen needed to cause toxicity.

Legal drugs kill more people in the United States than illegal drugs because they are less expensive and more available. Toxicity of acetaminophen may occur with ingestions greater than 8 to 10 grams. Fatality may occur with ingestions above 12 to 15 grams.

Four Most Common Acetaminophen Overdose Questions

1. If a clearly **toxic amount of acetaminophen has been ingested (more than 8–10 grams)**, the answer is **N-acetylcysteine.**
2. If the overdose was **more than 24 hours ago**, there is **no therapy.**
3. If the amount of **ingestion is unclear**, get a **drug level.**
4. **Charcoal** does **not make N-acetylcysteine ineffective.** Charcoal is not contraindicated with N-acetylcysteine.

Aspirin Overdose

The most common question is "What is the most likely diagnosis?" Look for:

- **Tinnitus** and **hyperventilation**
- **Respiratory alkalosis progressing to metabolic acidosis**
- Renal toxicity and altered mental status
- Increased anion gap

> Tinnitus, respiratory alkalosis, and metabolic acidosis are the key to diagnosing aspirin overdose.

Aspirin causes diffuse, multisystem toxicity. It causes ARDS. It interferes with prothrombin production and raises the prothrombin time (PT). The **metabolic acidosis is from lactate.** Aspirin interferes with oxidative phosphorylation and results in anaerobic glucose metabolism, which produces lactate.

Treatment is **alkalinizing the urine, which increases the rate of aspirin excretion.**

▶ **TIP**

Know the blood gas in aspirin overdose.

Which of the following is most likely to be found in aspirin overdose?
(Normal values: pH 7.40 pCO$_2$ 40 HCO$_3^-$ 24)

a. pH 7.55 pCO$_2$ 50 HCO$_3^-$ 24
b. pH 7.25 pCO$_2$ 62 HCO$_3$ 38
c. pH 7.46 pCO$_2$ 22 HCO$_3$ 16
d. pH 7.35 pCO$_2$ 32 HCO$_3$ 20

Answer: The correct answer is *(C)*. The blood gas shows a respiratory alkalosis with a low pCO_2 and a metabolic acidosis with decreased bicarbonate. Because the pH is alkalotic, we know that the respiratory alkalosis is not simply compensation for a metabolic acidosis. If it were respiratory compensation, the pH would be below 7.4 as in choice *(D)*. Choice *(D)* is a primary metabolic acidosis with respiratory alkalosis as compensation as would occur in sepsis, DKA, or uremia. Choice *(B)* shows an increased pCO_2 and an elevated bicarbonate. This represents a primary respiratory acidosis with bicarbonate retention at the kidney as compensation. This is characteristic of COPD.

*A patient with depression presents with altered mental status from ingesting multiple toxic substances. You know for certain that he took some lorazepam **only today, for the first time**. There is no response to naloxone or dextrose. The patient is given flumazenil and immediately seizes.*

What is the most likely cause of the seizure?

a. Cocaine withdrawal
b. Opiate withdrawal
c. Tricyclic antidepressants
d. SSRIs
e. Aspirin

Answer: The correct answer is *(C)*. Although flumazenil can cause seizures from reversing chronic benzodiazepine dependence, this case quite specifically states the benzodiazepine ingestion was today only. Benzodiazepines, however, can prevent seizures from tricyclic toxicity. When you reverse the benzodiazepines, you remove the suppression of the tricyclic toxicity. Opiate withdrawal does not cause seizures. Cocaine toxicity causes seizures, not withdrawal. Coingestion of tricyclics and benzodiazepines is very common.

What is the best initial test for the patient previously described?

a. Urine toxicology
b. Electroencephalogram
c. EKG
d. Head CT
e. Potassium level

Answer: The correct answer is *(C)*. Tricyclic antidepressant toxicity is rapidly detectable on EKG. The EKG will show widening of the QRS complex.

Undulating amplitude like it is 'twisting around a point'

Figure 21.1: Tricyclic antidepressant toxicity prolongs the QT until torsade develops. *Source: Pablo Lam, MD and Eduardo Andre, MD.*

Tricyclic Antidepressants

Tricyclic antidepressant (TCA) toxicity can cause seizures and arrhythmia leading to death. A wide QRS will tell who is about to have an arrhythmia. TCAs cause signs of anticholinergic effects such as:

- Dry mouth
- Constipation
- Urinary retention

None of these effects causes death.

Treatment of TCA overdose is with **sodium bicarbonate. Bicarbonate will protect the heart** against arrhythmia. The **bicarbonate** does **not increase urinary excretion** of TCAs as it does for aspirin.

Caustics

Caustic ingestion of acids and alkalis (eg, drain cleaner) causes **mechanical damage** to the oropharynx, esophagus, and stomach including **perforation. Do not give alkali to reverse acids**, or give acids to reverse alkali. This would cause the release of heat from an exothermic reaction and would only make it worse. **Flush out the caustics.** Use water in high volumes. Endoscopy is performed to assess the degree of damage.

> Steroids do not prevent injury from caustics.

Carbon Monoxide Poisoning

Carbon monoxide (CO) poisoning is the **most common cause of death in fires**. 60% of deaths on the first day after a fire are from CO poisoning. Also look for a history of:

- Gas heaters or **wood-burning stoves**
- **Automobile exhaust**, particularly in an enclosed environment

CO binds oxygen to hemoglobin so tightly that carboxyhemoglobin **will not release oxygen to tissues**. Carboxyhemoglobin **acts functionally like anemia**. There is no functional difference between the absence of blood and carboxyhemoglobin; 60% carboxyhemoglobin acts like the loss of 60% of blood. CO poisoning presents with **dyspnea**, lightheadedness, **confusion**, seizures, and ultimately death from a **myocardial infarction**.

> The left ventricle cannot distinguish between anemia, carboxyhemoglobin, and a stenosis of the coronary arteries.

> Carbon monoxide poisoning gives a normal pO_2 because oxygen does not detach from hemoglobin.

Which of the following blood gas results would you find in carbon monoxide poisoning?

a. pH 7.55 pCO_2 50 HCO_3^- 24
b. pH 7.25 pCO_2 62 HCO_3 38
c. pH 7.46 pCO_2 22 HCO_3 16
d. pH 7.35 pCO_2 26 HCO_3 18

Answer: The correct answer is (D). Carbon monoxide poisoning prevents oxygen release to tissues, so lactic acidosis develops.

DIAGNOSTIC TESTS/TREATMENT

Since **routine oximetry will be falsely normal**, the most accurate test is a level of carboxyhemoglobin. You should expect to find a **low bicarbonate** and **low pH** (metabolic acidosis) when carbon monoxide levels are very high.

The best initial therapy is to remove the patient from exposure and **give 100% oxygen**, which detaches carbon monoxide from hemoglobin and shortens the half-life of carboxyhemoglobin. **Severe disease is treated with hyperbaric oxygen**. Hyperbaric oxygen shortens the half-life of carboxyhemoglobin even more than 100% oxygen. "Severe" symptoms are defined as:

- **CNS** symptoms
- **Cardiac** symptoms
- Metabolic **acidosis**

Whenever any of these are in the question, the answer is hyperbaric oxygen.

Methemoglobinemia

Methemoglobin is oxidized hemoglobin that is locked into the ferric state. **Oxidized hemoglobin is brown and will not carry oxygen**. Methemoglobinemia occurs from an idiosyncratic reaction of hemoglobin to certain drugs such as:

- Benzocaine and other **anesthetics**
- **Nitrites** and nitroglycerin
- Dapsone

PRESENTATION

The effects of methemoglobinemia are similar to carboxyhemoglobin. Oxygen is not delivered to tissues. In methemoglobinemia, hemoglobin will never pick up the oxygen. With carboxyhemoglobin, the oxygen is picked up, but will not release it to tissues. Severe symptoms appear when blood levels rise above 40% to 50%. There is no functional difference for end organs such as the brain and heart. The symptoms are the same and include:

- **Dyspnea** and cyanosis
- Headache, **confusion, and seizures**
- **Metabolic acidosis**

> Carbon monoxide: blood is abnormally **red**.
> Methemoglobinemia: blood is abnormally **brown**.

DIAGNOSTIC TESTS/TREATMENT

Both methemoglobinemia and carboxyhemoglobin can give a **normal pO2 on blood gas**. At the same time, there is no delivery of oxygen to tissues. The most accurate test is a methemoglobin level. The best initial therapy is 100% oxygen. The most effective **therapy is methylene blue**, which decreases the half-life of methemoglobin.

▶ **TIP**

Cyanosis + normal pO_2 = methemoglobinemia

Organophosphate (Insecticide) Poisoning and Nerve Gas

Organosphosphates and nerve gas are identical in their effects. **Nerve gas is faster and more severe**. It causes a massive increase in the level of acetylcholine by inhibiting its metabolism. Patients present with:

- Salivation
- Lacrimation
- Polyuria
- **Diarrhea**
- Bronchospasm, bronchorrhea, and **respiratory arrest** if severe

> Acetylcholine causes constriction of bronchi and an increase in bronchial secretions.

A 56-year-old military commander has been attacked with nerve gas. He presents with salivation, lacrimation, urination, defecation, and shortness of breath. His pupils are constricted.

What is the first step in the management of this patient?

a. Atropine
b. Decontaminate (wash) the patient
c. Remove his clothing
d. Pralidoxime
e. No therapy is effective

*Answer: The correct answer is (**A**). Atropine blocks the effects of acetylcholine that is already increased in the body. Atropine dries up respiratory secretion. Although removing clothes and washing the patient to prevent further absorption is good, this will do nothing for symptoms that are already occurring. Pralidoxime is the specific antidote for organophosphates. **Pralidoxime reactivates acetylcholinesterase**. It does not work as instantaneously as atropine.*

> Nerve gas and organophosphates are absorbed through the skin.

Digoxin Toxicity

ETIOLOGY

Hypokalemia predisposes to digoxin toxicity because potassium and digoxin compete for binding at the same site on the sodium/potassium ATPase. **When less potassium is bound, more digoxin is bound.**

PRESENTATION

The most common presentation of digoxin toxicity is **gastrointestinal problems** such as **nausea**, **vomiting**, and abdominal pain. Other symptoms are:

- **Hyperkalemia** from the inhibition of the sodium/potassium ATPase
- Confusion

- **Visual disturbance** such as **yellow halos around objects**
- **Rhythm disturbance** (bradycardia, atrial tachycardia, AV block, ventricular ectopy, and arrhythmias such as atrial fibrillation with a slow rate)

DIAGNOSTIC TESTS

The most accurate test is a digoxin level. The best initial tests are a potassium level and an EKG. The EKG will show a **downsloping of the ST segment** in all leads. Atrial tachycardia with variable AV block is the most common digoxin toxic arrhythmia.

TREATMENT

Control potassium and give **digoxin-specific antibodies**. Digoxin-binding antibodies will rapidly remove digoxin from circulation.

Lead Poisoning

Lead is diffusely toxic throughout many organs in the body. Patients present with:

- **Abdominal pain (lead colic)**
- Renal tubule toxicity (**ATN**)
- **Anemia** (sideroblastic)
- Peripheral neuropathies such as **wrist drop**
- CNS abnormalities such as **memory loss** and confusion

The **most accurate test is a lead level**. Lead interferes with hemoglobin production. This gives anemia. The best initial diagnostic test is an **increased level of free erythrocyte protoporphyrin**.

▶ **TIP**

The most accurate test for sideroblastic anemia is a **Prussian blue stain.** This detects increased iron built up in red cell mitochondria.

TREATMENT

Chelating agents remove lead from the body. **Succimer** is the only oral form of lead chelator. **Ethylenediaminetetraacetic acid (EDTA) and dimercaprol (BAL)** are parenteral agents that bind and remove lead from the body.

Mercury Poisoning

Orally ingested mercury causes **neurological problems**. Inhaled mercury vapor produces **lung toxicity** that presents as **interstitial fibrosis**. Neurological problems present with patients who are **nervous, jittery, twitchy, and sometimes hallucinatory**.

Hypokalemia → digoxin toxicity
Digoxin toxicity → hyperkalemia

Digoxin can produce **any** arrhythmia.

The strongest indication for digoxin-binding antibodies are CNS and cardiac involvement.

There is **no therapy to reverse the pulmonary toxicity**. Chelating agents can remove mercury from the body. Chelating agents such as **dimercaprol and succimer are effective** in removing lead from the body and decreasing neurological toxicity. The can prevent progression of pulmonary disease, but cannot reverse fibrosis.

Toxic Alcohols: Methanol and Ethylene Glycol

Both methanol and ethylene glycol produce **intoxication** and **metabolic acidosis** with **an increased anion gap**. Both give an **osmolar gap** and are **treated with fomepizole and dialysis**.

Differences between Methanol and Ethylene Glycol		
	Methanol	**Ethylene glycol**
Source	Wood alcohol, cleaning solutions, paint thinner	Antifreeze
Toxic metabolite	Formic acid/formaldehyde	Oxalic acid/oxalate
Presentation	Ocular toxicity	Renal toxicity
Initial diagnostic abnormality	Retinal inflammation	Hypocalcemia, envelope-shaped oxalate crystals in urine

Osmolar Gap

The osmolar gap is the difference between the **measured** serum osmolality and the **calculated** osmolality.

Serum osmolality = 2 times the sodium + BUN/2.8 + glucose/18

If you **calculate** the serum osmolality to be 300, but on **measurement** you find the osmolality to be 350, it is possible that a toxic alcohol such as methanol or ethylene glycol is accounting for the extra osmoles. Ordinary alcohol **(ethanol) also increases the osmolar gap**.

TREATMENT

The **best initial therapy is fomepizole**, which inhibits alcohol dehydrogenase and prevents the production of the toxic metabolite. Fomepizole does not remove the substance from the body. Only **dialysis will effectively remove methanol and ethylene glycol** from the body.

Snake Bites

The **most common injury** from snake bites is the **local wound**. 25% to 35% of bites are not deep enough to deliver venom to the bloodstream, but they do deposit venom into the tissues. Proteases and lipases in the venom **damage tissue locally**.

Death from snake bites is from:

- **Hemolytic toxin: hemolysis** and **DIC** and damage to the endothelial lining of tissues
- **Neurotoxin:** can result in **respiratory paralysis**, ptosis, dysphagia, and diplopia

Treatment of Snake Bites	
Ineffective or dangerous treatment	**Beneficial therapy**
Tourniquets blocking arterial flow	Pressure
Ice	Immobilization decreases movement of venom
Incision and suction, especially by mouth	Antivenin

CLEAN WOUND

Spider Bites

All spider bites present with a sudden, sharp pain that the patient may describe as "I stepped on a nail" or "A piece of glass was in my shoe."

Differences between Types of Spider Bites		
	Black widow	**Brown recluse**
Presentation	Abdominal pain, muscle pain	Local skin necrosis, bullae, and blebs
Lab test abnormalities	Hypocalcemia	None
Treatment	Calcium, antivenin	Debridement, steroids, dapsone

TETANUS TOXOID
ANALGESIA   *ERYTHROMYCIN*

Dog, Cat, and Human Bites

Management of dog, cat, and human bites is essentially identical. They are managed with:

- Amoxicillin/clavulanate
- Tetanus vaccination booster if more than 5 years since last injection

Dog and Cats: *Pasteurella multocida*

Humans: *Eikenella corrodens*

> Human bites are **more damaging** than dog and cat bites.

> **Rabies vaccine only if:**
>
> - Animal has **altered mental status/bizarre behavior.**
> - Attack was unprovoked, by a **stray dog** that cannot be observed or diagnosed.

HEAD TRAUMA

Any head trauma resulting in sufficient injury to cause altered mental status or loss of consciousness (**LOC**) is **managed first with a head CT**. It does not matter how minor the trauma is if it results in LOC. Head CT without contrast is the best initial test to detect blood. Contrast detects mass lesions such as cancer and abscess, not blood.

▶ **TIP**

LOC = CT

- **Concussion:** no focal neurological abnormalities. **Normal CT** scan.
- **Contusion:** occasionally (rarely) has focal findings. **Ecchymoses** found on CT (blood mixed in with brain parenchyma).

Figure 21.2: Blood mixed in with brain but not collected in a way that allows drainage. *Source: Saba Ansari, MD.*

- **Subdural and epidural hematomas:** usually associated with more severe trauma than a concussion. **Impossible to distinguish without a head CT,** even though epidural hematoma is more frequently associated with skull fracture.

Figure 21.3: Lenticular hemorrhage from higher pressure artery. *Source: Saba Ansari, MD.*

Lucid Interval

A **lucid interval is a second loss of consciousness** occurring several minutes to several hours after the initial loss of consciousness. The patient wakes up after the initial LOC, but loses consciousness a second time due to the accumulation of blood. **The time between the first and second episodes of LOC is the lucid interval.**

> **Both** epidural and subdural hematomas are associated with a **lucid interval.**

TREATMENT

Concussion: no specific therapy. Wait at least 24 hours before returning to sports.

Contusion: vast majority need no specific treatment. Rarely need surgical debridement.

> Those with concussion are safe to go home. Hospitalization is not necessary. Observe at home for altered mental status.

Subdural and epidural hematoma: Treatment is **based on size** and signs of compression of the brain. Small ones are left alone. Large hematomas are managed with:

1. Intubation and hyperventilation
2. Mannitol
3. Drainage

Hyperventilation works by decreasing pCO$_2$. Normally, cerebral circulation constricts when the pCO$_2$ is low. A small decrease in volume results in a large decrease in pressure.

> Hyperventilation briefly slows herniation and is a bridge to surgery.

Mannitol is an osmotic diuretic that is used to **decrease intravascular volume**. This decreases intracranial pressure but has only a limited benefit.

545

Definition of a Large Intracranial Hemorrhage

- Compression of ventricles or sulci
- Herniation with abnormal breathing and unilateral dilation of the pupil
- Worsening mental status or focal findings

Differences between Types of Cerebral Injury

Summary of Severe Head Trauma			
Concussion	**Contusion**	**Subdural**	**Epidural**
No focal finding	Rarely focal	+/– focal findings	+/– focal findings
No lucid interval	No lucid interval	+/– lucid interval	+/– lucid interval
Normal CT	Ecchymoses	Venous, crescent	Arterial, biconvex or lens-shaped hematoma
No specific treatment; observe at home for lucid interval or new focal findings	No specific treatment; observe in hospital	Drain large ones	Drain large ones

A 25-year-old man sustains head trauma in a motor vehicle accident. A large epidural hematoma is found. Immediately after intubation and mannitol, surgical evacuation is successfully performed.

Which of the following will most likely benefit the patient?

a. Repeated doses of mannitol
b. Continued hyperventilation
c. Proton pump inhibitor (PPI)
d. Nimodipine
e. Dexamethasone

Answer: The correct answer is (C). A PPI is given to prevent stress ulcers. The only clear indications for stress ulcer prophylaxis are:

- ***Head trauma***
- *Burns*
- *Endotracheal intubation*
- *Coagulopathy (platelets below 50,000 or INR over 1.5) with respiratory failure*

*Hyperventilation has very short-term efficacy and is probably ineffective after 24 hours. Nimodipine prevents stroke after subarachnoid hemorrhage. Dexamethasone, a potent **glucocorticoid**, is **ineffective** for intracranial hemorrhage.*

> Steroids do not benefit intracranial bleeding. They decrease edema around mass lesions.

BURNS

The **best initial therapy** for those caught in a fire is **100% oxygen** to **treat smoke inhalation** and **carbon monoxide poisoning**. Airway burn is the second most common cause of death from burns **only if there has been airway injury**. Intubate the patient if there is:

- Stridor
- Hoarseness
- Wheezing
- Burns **inside** the nasopharynx or mouth

If airway burn is not present, the **second most common cause of death is volume loss**. Fluid replacement is based on the percentage of body surface area (BSA) burned.

Volume of Fluid Replacement

Replace with **Ringer lactate**. If Ringer lactate is not one of the choices, the answer is normal saline. Give one-half in the first 8 hours, a quarter in the second 8 hours, and a quarter in the third 8 hours. Give 4 mL for each percentage of BSA burned (including 2nd and 3rd degree burns) for each kilogram of body weight.

Head: 9% BSA

Arms: 9% BSA each

Legs: 18% BSA each

Chest or back: 18% BSA each

Patchy burns that are not continuous make the percentage of BSA burned hard to assess. Use the width of the patient's hand to make an estimate. **Each hand width is one percent of BSA.**

> Fluid replacement
> (4 mL) × (%BSA burned) × weight in kg

The short answer is: Give the largest amount of Ringer lactate or normal saline listed as a choice. It is probably the right answer.

What is the most common cause of death several days to weeks after a burn?

a. Infection
b. Renal failure
c. Cardiomyopathy
d. Lung injury
e. Malnutrition

Answer: The correct answer is (A). Because of loss of skin, there is a massive loss of body fluids and albumin. Fluid loss, if fatal, will occur immediately. After several days, the loss of the protective barrier of the skin leads to infection with Staphylococcus. Rhabdomyolysis causes renal failure, especially combined with volume depletion decreasing renal perfusion. This is not the most common cause of death. Lung injury is an immediate cause of death.

> **Prophylactic topical antibiotics (eg, silver sulfadiazine) are routinely used, not intravenous antibiotics.**

Heat Disorders				
	Heat cramps/ exhaustion	**Heatstroke**	**Neuroleptic malignant syndrome**	**Malignant hyperthermia**
Risk	Exertion; high outside temperatures	Exertion; high outside temperatures	Antipsychotic medications	Anesthetics administered systemically
Body temp	Normal	Elevated	Elevated	Elevated
CPK and potassium level	Normal	Elevated	Elevated	Elevated
Treatment	Oral fluids and electrolytes	IV fluids; evaporation	Dantrolene or dopamine agonists: bromocriptine, cabergoline	Dantrolene

↑ BUN/CR.

HYPOTHERMIA

Look for an **intoxicated person** with a low body temperature. Unintoxicated people do not fall asleep outside in cold temperatures. The most common cause of **death** from hypothermia is **cardiac arrhythmia**. The best initial step is **EKG**.

Figure 21.4: Hypothermia results in marked elevation of the J point. This is not ST elevation or right bundle branch block. All of these abnormalities normalized with rewarming. *Source: Juan Hernandez, MD and Eduardo Andre, MD.*

— HEATED BLANKETS
— WARMED SALINE
— WARM LAVAGE

DROWNING

Manage with airway and administer positive pressure ventilation.

- **Steroids and antibiotics are not beneficial.**
- **Salt** water drowning: acts like **CHF** with wet, heavy lungs
- **Fresh** water drowning: causes **hemolysis** from absorption of hypotonic fluid into the vasculature

▶ **TIP**

Wrong answers for drowning include:

- Steroids
- Antibiotics

CARDIAC RHYTHM DISORDERS

Initial Management of Cardiac Arrest

The first step in any potential cardiac arrest patient is to:

- Make sure the patient is truly unresponsive.
- Call for help: Call 911/activate Emergency Medical Services (EMS).

It is critical to make sure that the patient is truly unresponsive and not just sleeping or having a syncopal episode. Rescue breaths on a person who is breathing are counterproductive. Performing chest compressions on a person with a pulse is dangerous.

After the patient has been shown to be unresponsive, and EMS activated, the next step is:

1. Open the airway: head tilt, chin lift, jaw thrust.
2. Give rescue breaths if not breathing.
3. Check pulse and start chest compressions if pulseless.

> CPR does not restart the heart; CPR keeps the patient alive until cardioversion can be performed.

▶ **TIP**

When is a "precordial thump" the answer?

- Very recent onset of arrest (less than 10 minutes) with no defibrillator available
- You know it is recent because you saw it happen ("witnessed").

Pulselessness

The sudden loss of a pulse can be caused by:

- Asystole
- Ventricular fibrillation (VF)

- Ventricular tachycardia (VT)
- Pulseless electrical activity (PEA)

The best initial management of all forms of pulselessness is CPR.

Asystole

Besides CPR, **therapy for asystole** is with **epinephrine and atropine.**
Vasopressin is an alternative to epinephrine. They both constrict blood vessels in tissues such as the skin. This shunts blood into critical central areas like the heart and brain.

Ventricular Fibrillation

The best initial therapy for ventricular fibrillation (VF) is an immediate, **unsynchronized cardioversion** followed by the resumption of CPR if this was not effective. **Unsynchronized cardioversion is synonymous with defibrillation.** Generally, all electrical cardioversions should be synchronized to the cardiac cycle except VF and pulseless VT. In VF, there is no organized electrical activity to synchronize with.

> Only VF and ventricular tachycardia (VT) without a pulse get unsynchronized cardioversion.

Figure 21.5: Ventricular fibrillation with no organized electrical activity.
Source: Abhay Vakil, MD.

After another attempt at defibrillation, the most appropriate next step in management is **epinephrine or vasopressin** followed by another electrical shock. Medications do not restart the heart. They make the next attempt at defibrillation more likely to succeed.

Amiodarone or lidocaine is given next to try to get subsequent shocks to be more successful. Magnesium is given with ventricular arrhythmia without waiting for a level.

IN ACUTE CORONARY SYNDROMES
LIDOCAINE ↓ RISK OF V-FIB
↑ RISK OF ASYSTOLE

► **TIP**

Bretyllium is always a wrong answer.

Ventricular Tachycardia

VT is a wide complex tachycardia with a regular rate. **Management is entirely based on the hemodynamic status**.

- **Pulseless VT:** Manage in exactly the same way as VF.
- **Hemodynamically stable VT:** Treat with medications such as amiodarone, then lidocaine, then procainamide. If all medical therapy fails, then cardiovert the patient.
- **Hemodynamically unstable VT:** Perform electrical cardioversion several times, followed by medications such as amiodarone or lidocaine.

> VF is managed with shock, drug, shock, drug, shock, drug, and CPR at all times in between the shocks.

Figure 21.6: Short run of nonsustained ventricular tachycardia. *Source: Abhay Vakil, MD.*

Hemodynamic instability is defined as:

- Chest pain
- Dyspnea/CHF
- Hypotension
- Confusion

These qualities of instability are the same for all rhythm disturbances.

► **TIP**

Direct **intracardiac medication** administration is **always a wrong answer.**

Pulseless Electrical Activity

Pulseless electrical activity (PEA), formerly called electrical-mechanical dissociation (EMD), means that the heart is **electrically normal**, but there **is no motor contraction**. In other causes of PEA, the heart may still be contracting but without blood inside there will be no meaningful cardiac output.

> We synchronize the delivery of electricity in the cardioversion of VT to prevent worsening of the arrhythmia into ventricular fibrillation or asystole.

▶ **TIP**

To diagnose PEA, look for a patient with a normal EKG and no pulse.

TREATMENT

Since the treatment of PEA is to correct the underlying cause, knowing the etiology is identical to knowing the treatment. PEA is caused by:

- **Tamponade**
- **Tension pneumothorax**
- Hypovolemia and hypoglycemia
- Massive **pulmonary embolus (PE)**
- Hypoxia, hypothermia, metabolic acidosis
- **Potassium** disorders, either high or low

Atrial Arrhythmias

Atrial rhythm disturbances are rarely associated with hemodynamic compromise because cardiac output is largely dependent upon ventricular output, not atrial output. Look for the following findings in the history to suggest an atrial arrhythmia:

- Palpitations, dizziness, or lightheadedness
- Exercise intolerance or dyspnea
- Embolic stroke

▶ **TIP**

An irregularly irregular rhythm suggests atrial fibrillation as "the most likely diagnosis" even before an EKG is done. Atrial fibrillation is the most common arrhythmia in the United States.

Atrial Fibrillation and Atrial Flutter

These 2 disorders have nearly identical management. The major points of difference are:

- **Flutter is a regular rhythm** whereas **fibrillation is irregular**.
- **Flutter usually goes back into sinus rhythm or deteriorates into fibrillation.**

Figure 21.7: Atrial fibrillation with an irregularly irregular rhythm.
Source: Abhay Vakil, MD.

Figure 21.8: Sawtooth pattern of atrial flutter. *Source: Abhay Vakil, MD.*

TREATMENT

Hemodynamically **unstable** atrial arrhythmias are managed with **synchronized cardioversion**. Synchronization prevents electricity from being delivered during the refractory period (ST-T wave). **Synchronization helps prevent deterioration** into VT or VF. Hemodynamic instability is defined as it is for VT: hypotension, confusion, CHF, and chest pain.

Chronic Atrial Fibrillation

By definition, chronic atrial fibrillation is defined as lasting for more than 2 days. It takes several days for there to be a risk of clot formation. **Routine cardioversion is not indicated**. The majority of those who are converted into sinus rhythm will not stay in sinus. Atrial fibrillation and flutter are caused

> Chronic atrial fibrillation should be anticoagulated before cardioversion. Unstable, acute disease does not need anticoagulation.

by anatomic abnormalities of the atria from hypertension or valvular heart disease. Shocking the patient into sinus rhythm does not correct a dilated left atrium. **Over 90% will revert to fibrillation** even with the use of antiarrhythmic medications.

▶ **TIP**

Rate control and warfarin is the standard of care for atrial fibrillation.

The **best initial therapy** for fibrillation and flutter is to **control the rate** with **beta blockers**, **calcium channel blockers**, or **digoxin**. Once the rate is under 100 per minute, the most appropriate next step is **to give warfarin until the INR is between 2 and 3**. Continue rate controlling medication and warfarin indefinitely.

1. Slow the **rate**.
2. **Anticoagulate**.

The calcium blockers used to control heart rate with atrial arrhythmias are diltiazem and verapamil. These reliably block the AV node. The other calcium channel blockers control BP.

Warfarin

Without anticoagulation, there will be about **6 embolic strokes per year for every 100 patients** with atrial fibrillation (6% a year). When the INR is maintained between 2 and 3, the rate is 2% to 3%. You need to use heparin before warfarin only if there is a current clot in the atrium.

Atrial fibrillation is caused by anatomic cardiac defects dilating the atrium. These **defects do not go away with cardioversion**. That is why the **vast majority revert**. Many patients with acute atrial fibrillation from alcohol, caffeine, cocaine, or transient ischemia will simply convert back to sinus rhythm on their own. Hence, **acute disease normalizes spontaneously**; don't force it. Chronic disease reverts into the arrhythmia. Don't force it either.

Dabigatran is an alternative oral anticoagulant for a trail fibrillation. It prevents stroke and does not need to be monitored with INR.

Lone Atrial Fibrillation

Patients with a low risk of stroke can have their strokes safely prevented with using aspirin alone without warfarin as an anticoagulant. If the annual risk of stroke is only 2% to 3% per year, there is no point in subjecting these patients to the 1% a year risk of major bleeding.

Rate control drugs do not convert the patient into sinus rhythm.

No matter how much you might think it better to shock every patient into sinus, it just does not work in the long run.

Heparin is not necessary before starting a patient on warfarin.

Atrial rhythm problems can cause acute pulmonary edema from loss of atrial contribution in those with a cardiomyopathy.

Normally the atrium contributes 10% to 15% to cardiac output. In a diseased heart, this rises to 30% to 50%.

"Major" bleeding from warfarin is defined as:

- Intracranial hemorrhage
- Requiring a transfusion

Definition/Criteria for Low Risk of Stroke from Atrial Fibrillation

CHADS 2

- **No** cardiomyopathy/CHF/atherosclerosis   = 1
- **No** hypertension   = 1
- Age 75 or younger   = 1
- **No** diabetes   = 1
- **No** stroke in the past   = 2

When all of the risk factors for stroke are absent, this is called "lone" atrial fibrillation. The answer for management of lone atrial fibrillation is:

IF SCORE > 2
- WARFARIN or DABIGATRAN

- **Rate control**
- **Aspirin**

Supraventricular Tachycardia

Supraventricular tachycardia (SVT) presents with palpitations in a patient who is usually hemodynamically stable. The best initial step is:

1. **Vagal maneuvers** (eg, carotid massage, Valsalva, dive reflex, ice immersion)
2. **Adenosine** if vagal maneuvers don't work   → *BLOCKS CONDUCTION THROUGH AV NODE*
3. Beta blockers (metoprolol), calcium channel blockers (diltiazem), or digoxin if adenosine is not effective

▶ **TIP**

Adenosine is used only therapeutically for SVT.

Figure 21.9: Supraventricular tachycardia (SVT) is a narrow complex tachycardia without P See waves, fibrillatory waves, or flutter waves. Based on reentry around the AV node, patients present with palpitations. SVT is frequently curable with radiofrequency catheter ablation.
Source: Abhay Vakil, MD.

> Vagal maneuvers both slow and convert SVT. They do not convert atrial fibrillation.

Wolff-Parkinson-White Syndrome

Wolff-Parkinson-White syndrome (WPW) is an anatomic abnormality in the cardiac conduction pathway. You answer the "most likely diagnosis" question by looking for:

- **SVT alternating with ventricular tachycardia**
- SVT that gets **worse after diltiazem or digoxin**
- Observing the **delta wave** on the EKG

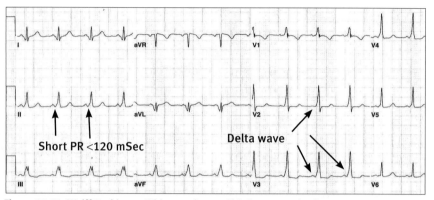

Figure 21.10: Wolff-Parkinson-White syndrome. This is a preexcitation syndrome with early depolarization of the ventricle. This gives a short PR interval. *Source: Juan Marcos Velasquez, MD.*

▶ TIP

The most accurate test for WPW is cardiac electrophysiology (EP) studies.

TREATMENT

Acute therapy: Procainamide or **amiodarone** are useful for both atrial and ventricular rhythm disturbances. Use them only if WPW is **currently** presenting with an arrhythmia.

Chronic therapy: Radiofrequency catheter ablation is curative for WPW. The tip of the catheter is heated up and simply **ablates** or eliminates the abnormal conduction tract around the AV node. **EP studies tell you where the anatomic defect is**.

Digoxin and calcium channel blockers are **dangerous in WPW**. They **block the normal AV** node and force conduction into the abnormal pathway.

Multifocal Atrial Tachycardia

Multifocal atrial tachycardia (**MAT**) is associated with **chronic lung disease** such as **COPD**. Treat the underlying lung disease. Treat MAT as you would atrial fibrillation, but **avoid beta blockers** because of the lung disease.

Figure 21.11: MAT has at least 3 different P-wave morphologies and is associated with COPD. *Source: Abhay Vakil, MD.*

Bradycardia and AV block

A woman comes to the office for routine evaluation. She is found to have a pulse of 40 and an otherwise completely normal history and physical examination.

What is the most appropriate next step in the management of this patient?

a. Atropine
b. Pacemaker
c. EKG
d. Electrophysiology studies
e. Epinephrine
f. Isoproterenol
g. Nothing; reassurance

*Answer: The correct answer is **(C)**. Bradycardia is common. The normal heart rate is between 60 and 100, but some people just normally have a heart rate that is below 60. Bradycardia can also be the initial presentation of third-degree or "complete" heart block. An EKG is mandatory to distinguish the cause of bradycardia. The most common wrong answer is "do nothing." If you confirm that this is an asymptomatic sinus bradycardia, **then** the answer is "reassurance" or "do nothing." **Atropine** is the answer for an **acutely symptomatic patient** with signs of **hypoperfusion. Pacemaker** is used for all patients with **third degree AV block. Epinephrine is dangerous,** especially since ischemia is such a common cause of bradycardia. Isoproterenol is an old, rarely used nonspecific beta agonist that speeds up the heart rate but increases ischemia.*

▶ TIP
Isoproterenol is never the right answer to anything.

Atropine and pacemaker are used for sinus bradycardia only if symptomatic.

Sinus Bradycardia

No treatment is indicated if sinus bradycardia is **asymptomatic**, no matter how low the heart rate is. **If symptomatic, use atropine as the "best initial therapy" and a pacemaker as "the most effective therapy."**

First-Degree AV block

Use the same management as sinus bradycardia.

Second-Degree AV block

Mobitz I or Wenckebach block: This is a **progressively lengthening PR interval** that results in a "dropped" beat. Mobitz I is most often a sign of **normal aging** of the conduction system. If there are no symptoms, it is managed in the same way as sinus bradycardia. **Do not treat if asymptomatic.**

Figure 21.12: Mobitz I or Wenckebach block is a benign sign of the aging of the conduction system. The PR interval gradually progresses until a beat is dropped. No treatment needed. *Source: Abhay Vakil, MD.*

Mobitz II block: Mobitz II second-degree AV block is far more pathologic than Mobitz I. **Mobitz II just drops a beat without the progressive lengthening of the PR interval.** Mobitz II progresses, or deteriorates into third-degree AV block. Treat it like third-degree AV block. **Everyone with Mobitz II block gets a pacemaker** even if they are asymptomatic.

Figure 21.13: Mobitz II block. *Source: Abhay Vakil, MD.*

Figure 21.14: Third-degree or complete heart block. The P-waves and T-waves have no fixed relationship to each other. *Source: Nishith Patel.*

ARRHYTHMIA BONUS QUESTIONS

A 58-year-old woman is admitted to the hospital with an acute myocardial infarction. On the second hospital day she develops sustained ventricular tachycardia even though she is on aspirin, heparin, lisinopril, and metoprolol.

What is the most appropriate next step in management?

a. Increase the dose of metoprolol
b. Add diltiazem
c. Angiography for angioplasty or bypass
d. Implantable defibrillator
e. EP studies

*Answer: The correct answer is **(C)**. The most common cause of death in the 72 hours surrounding an acute myocardial infarction is a ventricular arrhythmia. Manage arrhythmias from ischemia by correcting the ischemia. Don't put in an implantable defibrillator for an arrhythmia you can prevent or fix by eliminating the cause.*

Which of the following tests would you do for this patient to determine a risk of recurrence?

a. EP studies
b. Echocardiography
c. MUGA scan (nuclear ventriculography)
d. Ventilation/perfusion scan
e. Tilt-table testing

*Answer: The correct answer is **(B)**. Left ventricular function is the most important correlate of the risk of recurrence. Although nuclear ventriculography is more accurate, you would never do this test first or before you had done an echocardiogram. Tilt-table testing assesses orthostasis and autonomic instability. Tilt-table testing is done to evaluate syncope of unclear etiology particularly when there are signs of postural instability. EP studies are used when you are not certain of the diagnosis. EP studies are done if there are short runs or ventricular tachycardia or unexplained syncope and you want to see if you can induce sustained ventricular tachycardia. If the echo shows a normal ejection fraction her risk of recurrence of ventricular arrhythmia is small.*

A 73-year-old man has his third syncopal episode in the last 6 months. An EKG done in the field shows ventricular tachycardia. His stress test is normal.

What is the most appropriate next step in the management of this patient?

a. Metoprolol
b. Diltiazem
c. Angiography
d. Implantable defibrillator
e. EP studies

Answer: The correct answer is (D). There is no point in doing an EP study when the EKG shows a clear etiology of the syncope. We already know he has an unprovoked ventricular rhythm disorder. Metoprolol is not sufficient when syncope or sudden death has occurred. Calcium channel blockers like diltiazem are useless in preventing or treating ventricular tachycardia. The stress test is normal and there is no chest pain, so there is no point in doing angiography. An implantable defibrillator will prevent the next episode of sudden death or syncope.

A 46-year-old man has intermittent episodes of palpitations, lightheadedness, and near-syncope. His EKG is normal. The echo shows an ejection fraction of 42%. Holter monitor shows several runs of wide complex tachycardia lasting 5 to 10 seconds.

Which of the following is most likely to benefit this patient?

a. Pacemaker placement
b. Digoxin
c. Warfarin
d. EP studies
e. Swan-Ganz catheter

Answer: The correct answer is (D). EP studies are useful in detecting a source of ventricular arrhythmia. If you can readily induce sustained ventricular tachycardia, this person would benefit from an implantable defibrillator. He may have episodes of sustained ventricular tachycardia causing his symptoms that have not been detected by the Holter monitor. Digoxin is useless for ventricular arrhythmias. Swan-Ganz is a right heart catheter that assesses intracardiac pressure and cardiac output.

SECTION 11
ETHICS

Every human being of adult years and sound mind has the right to determine what shall be done with his own body; and a surgeon who performs an operation without his patient's consent commits an assault, for which he is liable in damages...except in cases of emergency where the patient is unconscious and where it is necessary to operate before consent can be obtained.

Justice Benjamin Cardozo, *Schloendorff v. Society of New York Hospital*, 211 NY 125, 105 NE 92 (1914)

This landmark decision states in one sentence the fundamental premise which underlies half the ethics questions on Step 2 CK of USMLE:

1. Autonomy
2. Adult
3. Capacity to understand

AUTONOMY

Patients have the sole right to determine what treatments they shall and shall not accept. Autonomy, ethically, is more important than beneficence. Beneficence, trying to do good for others, is generally a good thing—but trying to help someone is not as important as following her wishes.

A man has an ugly house that you offer to paint for free in his favorite color. Everyone on the neighborhood council agrees that the house is ugly and that what you are offering is clearly superior to what he has. The man would have no financial or other obligation in exchange. He understands everything you are offering, including the clear benefit to him. The man still refuses.

What do you do?

a. Honor the man's wishes: no paint job
b. Paint his house against his will
c. Ask the neighborhood council to consent to the paint job
d. Get a psychiatric evaluation on the man
e. Get a court order to allow the paint job

> Patients have the right to refuse treatments that are good for them if they do not want them.

f. Ask his family for consent to the paint job

g. Wait until he is out of town, then paint his house

Answer: The correct answer is (A). This seemingly silly example will allow you to answer the majority of questions. Cost and benefit and the common good are not as important as the autonomy individuals have to just do what they want with their own property. A community board is like an ethics committee. You cannot wait until a person loses consciousness or is sedated to then perform the test or treatment.

*A man comes to the emergency department after a motor vehicle accident that causes a ruptured spleen. At present, he is still **fully conscious**. He understands that he will die without splenectomy, and that he will live if he has the splenectomy. He refuses the repair and refuses blood transfusion. His whole family is present, including his brother, who is the healthcare proxy. The family and the proxy—both the agent (the person) and the document completed only a few weeks ago—clearly state, "Everything possible should be done, including surgery."*

What do you do?

a. Honor his current wishes, no surgery

b. Wait until he loses consciousness, then perform the surgery

c. Psychiatric consult

d. Ethics committee

e. Emergency court order

f. Follow what is written in the documented health-care proxy

g. See if there is consensus from the family

*Answer: The correct answer is (A). **You must follow the last known wishes of the patient**, even if they are verbal, and even if they contradict the written proxy. You cannot wait until his consciousness is lost, then go against his wishes. The family cannot go against his clearly stated wishes, even if the whole family is in agreement. The proxy cannot go against his wishes. There is no need for a psychiatric consultation if it is clear that the patient has the capacity to understand the problem and the consequences of refusing treatment. A court order or ethics committee cannot contradict an adult with capacity to understand. If a patient writes one thing and 10 minutes later changes his mind, **you go with whatever the last clear wishes are**.*

Advance Directives

Advance directives tell the caregivers the parameters of care that the patient wanted. The **agent** is the person designated by the patient to carry out the patient's wishes. This term is sometimes used interchangeably with **healthcare proxy**. The healthcare proxy is the written document outlining the parameters of care. The major problem with the proxy is that the details of care are often not clear. It is not helpful to just say, "No heroic measures." In order to be useful, the document must specifically state, "No intubation, no CPR, no chemotherapy, no dialysis." The proxy can also specifically state wishes about fluid and nutrition. If the proxy says, "No nasogastric tube, no artificial feeding," then it is useful.

The healthcare **proxy takes effect only** when the patient has **lost** the **capacity** to make decisions.

Order of Decision Making

1. A **patient with capacity** supersedes all else.

2. **Healthcare proxy that includes an agent (person) to carry out wishes**

3. **Living will:** The living will is a document outlining a patient's wishes. A document clearly stating, "I never want dialysis" is more valid than a family member or friend saying, "From what I know about him, he would not want dialysis," or "He told me he never wants dialysis." **Advance directives are a matter of documentation.** A written living will that makes concrete statements such as "I never want blood transfusion or chemotherapy" is valid.

4. **Persons clearly familiar with the patient's wishes.** The problem with this is one of documentation. If the patient loses capacity, it is difficult for a friend to document that she knew the patient's wishes better than the family. If the case clearly states that a friend knows and can prove that she knew the patient's wishes, then this is the plan of care that is followed.

5. **Family.** In general, the order of decision making starts with a spouse. If there is no spouse, then it goes to adult children, then parents, then siblings. Unlike life, USMLE Step 2 CK must provide clear circumstances in order to know what to do. If the family is split, then the answer is an ethics committee or court order.

Ethics Committee

The ethics committee is important when a patient has lost capacity to make decisions and the advance directive is missing or unclear. The ethics committee is also important on issues of **medical futility**. This is when the patient or healthcare proxy is asking for tests and treatments that may have no benefit.

Court Order

The court order is important when the patient has no capacity to understand and the family is in disagreement. It is like a house being left equally to four children who cannot agree what to do with it. Examples of when court order is the right answer:

- A patient has no capacity and no proxy; his family is split about whether to continue care.

- Caregivers want to withdraw care and the ethics committee cannot reach a conclusion.

Psychiatric Evaluation of the Patient

A psychiatric consult is important when it is **not clear** if the patient has **capacity to understand**. If the question clearly states that the patient has capacity to understand, a psychiatric evaluation is not necessary. If the patient is clearly delirious or psychotic, psychiatric evaluation is not necessary.

Minors

Minors do not have decision-making capacity. They cannot consent to or refuse medical treatments. Only the parents or legal guardian can consent and refuse. Exceptions are contraception, prenatal care, substance abuse treatment, and sexually transmitted diseases (STDs) including HIV/AIDS.

Abortion

The states are split on parental notification laws. Some require it, and some don't. Your answer will be something like "Tell the minor patient to notify her parents."

Brain Death

Brain death is considered death in our legal system. If the patient is brain dead, you do not need consent to stop therapy such as mechanical ventilation or antibiotics. Court order and ethics committee are not correct answers.

▶ **TIP**

USMLE Step 2 CK will want you to **discuss, educate, explain,** and **confer** before everything else.

IRREVERSIBLE ABSENCE OF
ALL BRAIN ACTIVITY ≥ 6 HRS
Ø CN REFLEXES
APNEA
Ø HYPOTHERMIA
Ø EEG
Ø BLOOD FLOW TO BRAIN

CONSENT

Only an adult can consent to procedures, and each procedure needs individual consent. Consent is implied in an emergency. The person doing the procedure must obtain consent. Adverse effects of a procedure must be explained to make the consent valid and the consequences of refusing a procedure must be explained to make the consent valid. Pregnant women can refuse procedures and treatments for their unborn children. Telephone consent is valid.

A patient signs consent for an ovarian biopsy on the left side. At surgery you find cancer of the right side.

What do you do?

Answer: Wake the patient up and obtain consent to remove the ovary on the right side.

A patient needs colonoscopy. The gastroenterologist asks you to obtain consent for the procedure.

What do you do?

Answer: The gastroenterologist who will perform the procedure needs to obtain consent. Do you know all the complications of the procedure and the alternatives? If you do not explain the possibility of perforation because you are unfamiliar with it, the consent is not valid. Do you know that sigmoidoscopy or barium enema are alternatives? If the patient's colon perforates and you did not explain alternate procedures, the consent is not valid.

Do Not Resuscitate Orders

Do not resuscitate (DNR) orders refer only to withholding cardiopulmonary resuscitation. They do not refer to withholding any other form of therapy.

A patient with capacity consents to DNR before losing consciousness. She needs a surgical procedure, but the surgeon refuses because the patient is DNR.

What do you do?

Answer: Perform the surgery. DNR does not mean withholding antibiotics, chemotherapy, or surgery. DNR means only that, if the patient dies, you will not attempt resuscitation.

Physician-Assisted Suicide

Physician-assisted suicide is <u>always a wrong answer.</u> This includes states in which it is legal to do so. Ethical requirements for physicians supersede legality. Physician assisted suicide is administered by the patient, but this is still unethical for the physician.

> Physician ethics come before legal requirements. You cannot do something unethical even if it is legal at the moment.

Euthanasia

Euthanasia is the physician administering treatment intended to end or shorten the life of the patient. It is <u>always wrong.</u>

Terminal Sedation and Law of Double Effect

It is acceptable to administer pain medication even if there is the possibility of the treatment shortening the patient's life. For example, **it is acceptable to give pain medications to a person with COPD who has metastatic cancer even if the only way to relieve pain is to give enough opiates that breathing may be impaired**, causing the patient to die earlier.

The question is one of intent: If the medications are given with the intent to relieve pain, and as an adverse effect they shorten life, it is ethical. If the primary intent is to shorten life, it is unethical.

Futile Care

A physician is not obligated to render care that is futile even if the family or patient wants it. If a patient is brain dead and the family insists that you continue mechanical ventilation, you are under no obligation to do so. You are under no obligation to perform tests and treatments you consider worthless.

ORGAN AND TISSUE DONATION

Payment for organ donation is unacceptable; however, payment for renewable tissues such as sperm and eggs is acceptable.

Consent for Organ Donation

Only the organ donor network should ask for consent for the organs. It is an ethical conflict of interest for the physician to ask for consent for organ donation. The organ donor network also has fewer refusals than the physician. Organ donor cards give an indication of the patient's wishes, but **the family can refuse** organ donation even if the patient has an organ donor card.

CONFIDENTIALITY

The patient's right to confidentiality **can be broken** when there is danger to others. Examples of ethically acceptable circumstances in which confidentiality can be broken are STDs, HIV/AIDS, airborne communicable diseases such as tuberculosis, and court orders demanding information.

The patient's right to confidentiality **cannot be broken** for employers, coworkers, government agencies, or family and friends.

> Confidentiality is important, but not as important as protecting others from harm.

A patient with HIV/AIDS has repeatedly refused to disclose his HIV status to his sexual partner. The partner accompanies the patient to the office visits and is in the waiting room. The patient insists you not tell the partner.

What do you do?

a. Honor the patient's wishes
b. Obtain a court order
c. Consult the ethics committee
d. Either the physician or the department of health can notify the partner

*Answer: The correct answer is **(D)**. You have the right to notify the partner or to disclose the patient's HIV status to the health department so that they can notify the partner. The confidentiality of the patient is not as important as protecting the health of the partner.*

> HIV-positive healthcare workers do **not** have to disclose their status to their patients or their employers.

A woman comes to your office with valid identification from a government agency that works in law enforcement. She requests a copy of your patient's medical records.

What do you do?

Answer: You are to provide health-related protected records to government agencies, including those from law enforcement, only if they have a valid warrant or subpoena from the courts. To do otherwise would be a violation of the constitutional protection against illegal search and seizure of property. This would also constitute a violation of HIPAA, which is designed to protect health information.

DOCTOR/PATIENT RELATIONSHIP

A physician is not obligated to accept everyone coming to him or her as a patient. The physician has the right to end the doctor/patient relationship but must give the patient sufficient time to obtain another caregiver. Small gifts from patients are acceptable as long as they are not tied to a specific treatment request. Romantic or sexual contact between patients and their current physicians is never acceptable.

Gifts from Industry

Unlike a small gift from a patient, gifts from industry such as drug companies are never acceptable. Even small items from industry such as pens, penlights, pads, and cups are **unacceptable**. Meals in direct association with educational activities are not considered gifts.

DOCTOR AND SOCIETY

Elder Abuse

You can report elder abuse against the consent of the patient. This is based on the concept that abused older adults may be too weak, fragile, or vulnerable to protect themselves or remove themselves from an environment of potential harm. Elder abuse is treated ethically like child abuse.

Domestic Violence and Spousal Abuse

Unlike child abuse, domestic abuse **cannot be reported** against the patient's wishes. You can report and intervene only with the consent of the patient.

Impaired Drivers (Seizure Disorders and Driving)

This is one of the least clear areas nationally, and the states have no uniformity of laws. You must answer "suggest that the patient find another means of transportation." **Wrong** answers would be:

- Confiscating car keys and reporting to law enforcement
- Hospitalizing the patient
- Refusing to let the patient get in her car

Execution of Prisoners

It is never ethical for a physician to participate in executions at any level. You cannot ethically formulate a lethal injection or even do so much as pronounce a prisoner dead. Even if state law makes execution legal, you as a physician are not to participate at any level.

Torture

Physicians are **never to participate in the torture** of prisoners or detainees. Even if the question states that you are in the military, your ethical obligation as a physician supersedes your obligation to the military. This would include:

- Refusing orders from military superiors to participate in torture
- Keeping the torture "safe" so that it is not fatal or damaging

The ethics questions on torture are easy to answer because your answer is "no" to any level of involvement, even if you are a military physician in a legal war zone whose role is simply to protect the patient against permanent harm.

> Torture is the ethical equivalent of child abuse. Your participation is never acceptable; you are obligated only to report it.

MALPRACTICE

DUTY OF CARE – LEGAL OBLIGATION TO CONFORM TO A REASONABLE STANDARD OF CARE

BREACH OF DUTY – FAILURE TO CONFORM TO THE STANDARD OF CARE

HARM – INJURY OR HARM TO THE PLAINTIFF

CAUSATION – BREACH OF DUTY WAS LEGAL CAUSE OF HARM

To PROVE FAULT
- "RES IPSA LOQUITUR" – IT SPEAKS FOR ITSELF
- EXPERT TESTIMONY

INDEX